SUZANNE SOMERS'
SLIM and SEXY
FOREVER

SUZANNE SOMERS'
SLIM and SEXY
FOREVER

The Hormone Solution for
Permanent Weight Loss and Optimal Living

BY SUZANNE SOMERS

Illustrations by Leslie Hamel

Foreword by David R. Allen, M.D.

CROWN PUBLISHERS
NEW YORK

Copyright © 2005 by Suzanne Somers

Foreword copyright © 2005 by David R. Allen, M.D.

Insert photographs and photographs on pages viii, 63, 80, 152, 169, 204, 205, and 220 copyright © Jeff Katz.

Published in the United States by Crown Publishers, an imprint of the Crown Publishing Group, a division of Random House, Inc., New York.

www.crownpublishing.com

CROWN is a trademark and the Crown colophon is a registered trademark of Random House, Inc.

Library of Congress Cataloging-in-Publication Data
Somers, Suzanne
Suzanne Somers' slim and sexy forever : the hormone solution for permanent weight loss and optimal living / Suzanne Somers; illustrations by Leslie Hamel.—1st ed.
  1. Reducing diets.   2. Weight loss—Endocrine aspects.
  3. Insulin.   I. Title: Slim and sexy forever.   II. Title.
RM222.2.S6558   2005
613.2'5—dc22   20004029792

ISBN 1-4000-5325-0

Printed in the United States of America

Design by Lauren Dong

10   9   8   7   6   5   4   3   2   1

First Edition

To every man and woman who has thought,
"It's all downhill from here. I'm never
going to look as good as I used to;
I'm never going to feel as good as I
used to." This one's for you!

And to Alan—you're slimmer and sexier than ever!

ACKNOWLEDGMENTS

This is always my favorite page in the book to write. No one person could possibly do all that is entailed in putting out a book with this many details. I have superb assistance with my Somersize books.

First of all . . . Caroline, Caroline, Caroline! My awesome daughter-in-law who is brilliant, brainy, and beautiful. She is my right arm, my left arm, and at times my brain. She is my rock, and without her I would be lost. Thank you, Caroline, for all your input and excellence. I love you.

A big thank-you to my stepdaughter Leslie Hamel. Her abilities are astounding. These illustrations make me laugh, especially the seven dwarfs and adrenal-burnout girl. She has humor and intelligence and consistently knows exactly how to convey the message. I love your talent, Leslie; whether it be designing my costumes, the apparel line, or illustrating the books, you always get it right. I love you and thank you once again.

Next, Kristin Kiser, my fabulous editor . . . This is our eighth book together and I continue to love working with you. I also appreciate that you do that back-of-the-book stuff that I don't enjoy doing. You have a great eye, you don't bug me when I am late turning in, and you trust me to do my thing.

The Crown group, Jenny Frost, Steve Ross, Philip Patrick, Tina Constable, and Tammy Blake. It is a joy to continue these books with you. Thank you all for your support and loyalty.

My agent, Al Lowman, while fighting for every breath, and not giving up on life when many others would, you continue to work with me, guide me, fight for me. You are an angel on earth and I pray for your life every day. You are the best agent ever. No one cares like you do, no one puts as much into each deal as you do, and no one fights for every comma like you do. I love you.

My husband, Alan Hamel, my visionary, my brilliant supermanager. Your abilities are astounding. I love you so much.

Thank you, Dr. Allen, for your supportive and informative foreword. Your understanding of my program helps to validate all of us who are looking for a better quality of life. It is doctors like yourself who are impacting medicine and driving change. As the world changes, we need to adjust. Sugar and environmental assaults are serious problems relative to today's health. Thank you for bringing light to this important message.

And thank you to Sandi Mendelson and Judy Hilsinger for your great job in getting these books to the marketplace. It takes a team and you are an important part of mine.

Marsha Yanchuk, my assistant of twenty-eight years. You were invaluable on this book. You spent the entire summer typing

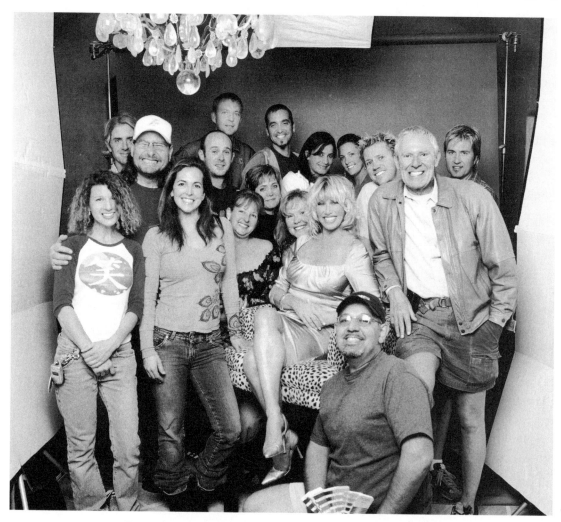

The photo team! That's Bruce and Alan to my left and Caroline to my right.

recipes, questioning amounts, reminding us of what was forgotten. You pulled together all these incredible and emotional testimonials. You are an intimate part of our company, our family, and our projects. I love you.

Marc Chamlin, my lawyer. This is the eighth book. You know I can't close the deal without you and you close so very well. Thank you.

Louise Charbonneau . . . Wow . . . is all I can say . . . the food in this book is unbelievably awesome. Uptown and understandable. Unusual and delicious. I loved working with you. Our days in the test kitchen together were memorable and amazing. You taught me many things and it excites me to pass on these new recipes and techniques to my readers. Thank you so much. I love each and every recipe. They are all part of my new repertoire and it is exciting to cook new and delicious foods.

Jeff Katz, the only photographer I work with. We have a shorthand together . . . the photos are always superb, but I think they took yet another leap forward in this book. Your excellence and caring blow me away. You are the best and I love what we did together in this book.

And Jeff's team . . . Victor Boghossian, thank you for all the photographic vignettes, you see what others do not. Jack Coyier, who also was an awesome production manager. Gabriel Hutchison, even though you are weird about "condiments," you are great to work with. Stuart Gow, thank you.

Kimberly Huson, the food styling was perfect and beautiful, and thank you, Mary Margaret Martinez, for all your wonderful, cheerful assistance. Same for Christine Langfeld and Vince Beckley. Beautiful job on all the food.

Laurie Baer did an amazing job of interpreting "my look." I know I am a stickler, but you were cheerful, accommodating, and talented. I love what you did.

And Laurie's team, Claire Harbo and Emily Golden, you are appreciated and I am thanking you for all your hard work. It's a big hill up to my house.

Petra Pfaffli on wardrobe, thank you.

And Mooney—no one does my hair like you do. I love you and I love working with you. You are talented, reliable, and artistic. You understand my "look" and always stay within those parameters. It's important to me and there is no one I would rather have around me. Thank you.

Patty Ramsey, thank you, great job. You understood my need to have makeup that suits me and you made me feel very comfortable.

And a big thanks to our production manager's assistant, Kingsley Riley. You are a doll and a real pro.

I want to thank everyone at Crown in the production and art departments who helped put this book together: Amy Boorstein, Trisha Howell, Leta Evanthes, Lauren Dong, Dan Rembert, and Kristin's assistant Lindsey Moore. I couldn't have done it without you.

And, of course, the girls in my office, Anka, Liz, and Julie. You're the best.

I am proud and privileged to work with such outstanding people. Thank you all and I'll see you on the next one (rest up, it's coming sooner than you think)!

Sincerely, Suzanne Somers

CONTENTS

FOREWORD

This book is devoted to educating people on how to achieve optimum health through proper food selection, a positive lifestyle, and responsible hormone replacement. Suzanne Somers triumphs in undertaking these complex topics and presenting them in a clear and understandable way without sacrificing the depth of each subject.

Based on my thirty years of medical experience, I eagerly endorse all that Suzanne presents here: cutting-edge information given in a way that can be absorbed and applied by anyone who is committed to good health, vitality, and longevity.

In the last quarter of a century our knowledge of nutrition and health has increased exponentially. I remember how as a senior at the UCLA School of Medicine I engaged in a debate with one of the professors. The topic was "Does Diet Affect Your Health?" The professor's position was that diet really didn't matter. If you ate from the four main food groups (meat, dairy, fruit, vegetables), that was all you needed to do to enjoy optimum health. I argued that it was much more complex than that, and, for example, there was a fifth main food group he neglected to talk about. This was a group called miscellaneous, which included soft drinks, Twinkies, Snickers, and so on. And this fifth group comprised up to 40 percent of the caloric intake of the average American. Many years later I was proved right, and now you can learn much about the devastating effects sugar and refined carbohydrates can have on your health. Suzanne explains how limiting your intake of these foods is one of the keys to health and weight loss.

A few years after graduating from medical school, my nutritional consciousness was raised in an unexpected way while I was working in an emergency room in Ojai, California. I was waiting for a patient's test results and started talking to his wife. She was a horse breeder and I casually asked her about what horses ate. She replied that it depended on the time of year, the activity level and age of the horse, and so forth. I was startled and asked, "You mean the behavior and health of a horse depends to a large degree on what the horse eats?" She said that this had been widely known for years and was surprised that I was unaware of this. She told me that people spend millions of dollars training and raising horses and diet plays an integral part in this process. I was shocked and suddenly reflected on how my medical education included *nothing* about how food and nutrients could affect human health, performance, and disease prevention.

Since I have been in practice I have tried and supervised many diets, ranging from macrobiotic, fruitarian, Pritikin, vegan, and The Zone to Atkins, raw foods, blood type, and grapefruit, just to name a few. With so much conflicting diet advice, the average person becomes confused about choosing the best way to eat.

If we look back 40,000 years, the human body then is identical to how it is today, and it's instructive to look at what millions of years of evolution designed our bodies to eat. Early humans ate a variety of foods and ate them in season. This is consistent with Suzanne's idea of proper food combining. I can imagine early humans eating some form of fruit and then walking for twenty or thirty minutes before gathering and eating something else. They ate simply and by necessity didn't combine a lot of foods. The simple

rules of proper food combining could probably eliminate up to 50 percent of all gastrointestinal problems. Imagine that!

It was only after the last Ice Age, around 8,000 years ago, that grains began to be cultivated. This means that many of us do poorly with grains, especially highly processed grain products. This does not mean that grains in their whole form should be excluded from a healthy diet. It does mean that consumption of high-glycemic carbohydrates that are derived from grains, such as white flour and sugar, should be kept to a minimum. A recent article in *The Journal of the American Medical Association* confirmed that low–glycemic index diets facilitated more weight loss than low-fat diets, reduced the incidence of diabetes, lowered cholesterol, decreased chronic inflammation, and lowered blood pressure. Appropriately enough, foods with a low glycemic index, which keep insulin levels low in the blood, form an important part of Suzanne's health program.

As a practicing physician who sees patients every day, I am aware of the problems that affect us all. Most people I see have what I call vertical illness. They are remaining vertical, not sick in bed in a horizontal position. They go to work, raise children, have relationships, and otherwise conduct their lives productively—but they don't feel good. The number one complaint of all people who come for help is fatigue. As a country we are tired. We drink coffee to charge us up in the morning and alcohol to wind us down at night. I always ask, "On a scale of one to ten, with ten being highest, what is your general energy level?" Of the people who answer between seven to nine, I find that most of them are running on wired energy, fueled by a strong will, but underneath they are exhausted more often than not. I then inquire about when they are most tired. If they are exhausted and can't get up in the morning I wonder about heavy eating at bedtime, poor sleep, or low thyroid. If they have mid- or late-afternoon fatigue, I wonder about burned-out adrenals. Late-night fatigue often relates to low growth hormone levels, and low blood sugar, estrogen, or testosterone levels can produce fatigue at any time of day.

The second most common complaint is either headache or some kind of stomach or intestinal problem. Every other commercial on TV is for headache pain or some form of stomach pain, bloating, or excess acid. Billions of dollars are spent on medications that offer only symptom relief and do nothing to address the cause of these conditions.

Another major concern among my patients is lack of sexual interest or poor performance. As baby boomers move into the summer or autumn of their lives, many are encountering this issue for the first time. How many people have just accepted this decline and resigned themselves to the loss of such an important aspect of human interaction, expression, and celebration?

The cure for the above conditions is not more Tums, Tylenol, or Viagra. As attractive as a magic bullet answer may be, it just doesn't exist! We need to be honest with ourselves and begin to take responsibility for our health. It is a big mistake to rely on medical doctors for all your information about health. Certainly working with your physician is an important part of your health program, but most doctors are disease-oriented. That is, we are taught to treat disease rather than promote health. I am, however, finding more and more patients who are well informed and eager to understand how they can participate in their own health care. The information available in *Suzanne Somers' Slim and Sexy Forever* can play a major role in informing anyone who wants to take charge of their own health care, realizing far greater energy and fewer common ailments.

In addition to serving as a wonderful guide to proper diet, *Suzanne Somers' Slim and Sexy Forever* also emphasizes the importance of bioidentical hormone replacement therapy. A few decades ago, the only hormone that was associated with aging in women was estrogen. Whether or not men experience menopause was widely debated. We now know that almost all hormones decline with age, in both men and women, and as they fall we decline in health and vitality, which can invite disease. Some important hormones include cortisone, adrenaline, insulin, testosterone, estrogen, progesterone, growth hormone, and thyroid. Hormones are important in brain and bone health. They help to keep our immune system strong, maintain our sex drive and virility, and help us to burn fat. In fact, you can't *live* without hormones. To a great extent, hormones determine who we are and how we function in all parts of our lives. And just like a finely tuned orchestra, all of our hormones need to be in balance and harmony to empower optimum function.

I am excited for those about to embark on the adventure of this new book. It's not just another volume on health and nutrition, but rather a clear and practical, medically sound program presented in an engaging way that any motivated person can use. It is through education that we can become participants in our own health care, proactive in our treatments, and, indeed, be slim and sexy forever!

DAVID R. ALLEN, M.D.

SUZANNE SOMERS'
SLIM and SEXY
FOREVER

INTRODUCTION

So here I was thinking I had it alllllllllllll figured out. With my Somersize program I had learned how to control my weight without my weight controlling me. I had tricked my forty-year-old metabolism into burning my fat as fuel by eliminating sugar and foods the body converts to sugar. I had learned to control the hormone insulin so that I could eat rich, delicious foods and watch the pounds melt away. This was a miracle! I would never have to worry about my weight again! I could eat cheese and cream sauces and steak and chocolate and all the things I loved. I could do this while improving cholesterol levels. I had found the answer! In fact, I was such a Little Miss Smarty Pants, I wrote a whole series of books to teach others how to Somersize to stay healthy and trim for all the years to come.

Surprise, surprise. I entered my fifties and my body betrayed me once again. Suddenly I was gaining weight and Somersize was not

fixing the problem. I decided I must have been cheating too much so I went back to strict Level One guidelines—I still couldn't shake the weight. I bumped up my exercise routine—I still couldn't shake the weight. My stomach was bloated. My jeans were too tight. In my bountiful closet I couldn't find an outfit that I felt good about wearing. My husband, Alan, would say things to me like, "You're not going to like the way that looks from behind." Ugh! I thought I had this thing licked. What was sabotaging my fabulous Somersize program and keeping me from losing weight?

Menopause. It ain't for sissies. In this passage women lose 90 percent of their hormones within a two-year period. You may be eating and exercising as you always have, but suddenly you find the pounds stacking up and you can't seem to stop the weight gain. Why, you ask? Loss of hormones! You try dieting, but you're not getting any results.

Loss of hormones! In fact, you're being really good on your diet, and you're adding exercise, but you're still not losing. Loss of hormones! For men hormonal loss is slower, over a ten-year period, but one day you wake up and realize that your once vital husband is a grumpy old man with too much love in those handles. Loss of hormones!

THE SEVEN DWARFS OF MENOPAUSE

Even though I was Somersizing perfectly, I was gaining weight. What was happening? No amount of eating right or exercise would help. It wasn't just the weight gain; it was as though the Seven Dwarfs of Menopause entered my life one day—Itchy, Bitchy, Sweaty, Sleepy, Bloated, Forgetful, and All Dried Up. This was no picnic, but I was not going to sit back and take it without a fight.

We begin to lose our hormones in perimenopause and then they really start dropping during menopause. The loss of hormones causes the most horrible side effects! The dwarfs are no fun. I wrote about these horrible dwarfs in *The Sexy Years,* but here's a recap for those who haven't met the dwarfs yet!

Itchy: I got an itch on my leg that just about drove me nuts. No amount of lotion would fix the problem. I wanted to scratch my leg right off.

Bitchy: I thought PMS was bad. During this phase it was like I had PMS all day—every day. The mood swings were awful. My poor husband. He hadn't done anything wrong, but I just hated him. I'd get mad at him for chewing or breathing. No wonder so many men leave their wives during this time. Bitchy is a powerful side effect and very difficult to overcome on your own.

Sweaty: Who turned on the heater? There is nothing more embarrassing than those horrid hot flashes. We pull and tug at our clothing and say things like, "Is it hot in here or is it just me?" Especially in the middle of the night; I would wake up with sweat pouring down my body like a faucet was between my breasts. Sexy, huh?

Sleepy: It's impossible to get a good night's sleep during this phase. I'd wake up at 3 A.M. and toss and turn for two hours, sweating with those awful hot flashes. I was a walking zombie during the day because I was so tired!

Bloated: Well, we've talked about this. That distended stomach with no way to suck it

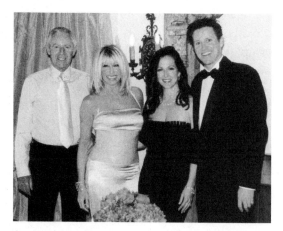

Out for a fancy night with Alan, Caroline, and Bruce.

in. In fact, my whole body started padding up. It's the body's defense mechanism to protect our bones. As we start losing estrogen, our bones become more brittle. The body naturally gives us an extra layer of padding so that when we fall we will not break our bones.

Forgetful: All of a sudden I could not keep a thought in my head. I would go to dial a number and forget whom I was calling. I remember being in an interview and I could not remember the question I wanted to ask. I thought I had Alzheimer's and it scared me.

All Dried Up: Here's the one no one likes to talk about. Did I want to be the one to discuss lack of sex drive and vaginal dryness? No, that was never my life's goal, but SOMEONE has got to talk about this passage that sucks women dry and takes the life right out of us! Intimacy had always been so important in my marriage and suddenly it was something I did because I should, not because I wanted to. And, sadly, I felt nothing.

This was no fairy tale, but fortunately it has a happily ever after. I did not want to become the poster child for menopause, but I was shocked that our mothers never talked about it! We had no preparation for this passage that would rob us of our physical and emotional well-being. There had to be a way to get through this with grace and dignity. I'm here to tell you—there is, and this book will show you step by step how to reclaim your life, your body, your relationships, and your health so you can experi-

ence optimal living. Why is this information not readily available? Why are doctors not trained to assist us during this time? I wanted answers.

Just as I had done with Somersize, I went on a hunt and did my research. I spoke with conventional doctors and got the same lame answers over and over again. I did not want to take synthetic hormones. I did not want to take a drug if I didn't have to. I heard things like, "The drug companies know best, dear." The drug companies don't know best! Not in this area. Trust me, I do not want to live in a world without pharmaceuticals, but in this case, the drugs are not best. There is a natural alternative that is better. Rather than treating the symptoms of lost hormones with synthetic hormones, we can actually replace lost hormones with an exact replica of what our bodies make.

Yes, there is an answer! It's natural, bioidentical hormones. This is the solution that will slap Bitchy across the face and bring back the pleasant woman your family loves. This is the solution that will turn off the faucet for Sweaty. This is the solution that will pop Bloated so you can return to your ideal weight. This is the solution that will give Forgetful her memory back. This is the solution that will give All Dried Up her zest for love and life. Natural, bioidentical hormones are the solution and I will explain how you can achieve these results and experience the dramatic turnaround for yourself and officially send those dwarfs packing.

If you bought this book and want the promise of the title, I will show you how to get it. *Slim and Sexy Forever*—that's exactly what you can have if you follow the advice I have collected from the cutting-edge doctors and professionals I have been working with for the past decade. When you understand the science of Somersize and the science behind our hormonal system, you will see how the combination of this weight-loss program with natural replacement of lost hormones will deliver the promise so you can live out your years looking and feeling your best.

This program is the only one that specifically addresses the needs of those wanting to lose weight in the second half of life. *If your hormones are out of balance, no weight-loss program will work for you.* You can starve yourself and exercise all day, but you still will not get results unless you first balance your hormones. This passage of life takes work, but the more you put into it, the more you'll get out of it. I have a plan of attack for you and it works. The first phase is to Balance Your Hormones. For women this begins during perimenopause, anytime from your mid-thirties to your late forties. For men it occurs in andropause, around ages forty to fifty-five. I will outline the symptoms you can expect so that they do not come as a surprise to you. As I have explained, if they catch you off guard you will experience an array of nasty symptoms that will sabotage your physical and emotional well-being, including your figure. With this information you will be ahead of the curve.

In *Slim and Sexy Forever,* you will learn all about the importance of natural, bioidentical hormone replacement—or, as I like to call it, "my happy pills." Many people are scared when they hear about hormone replacement therapy. They think of the medical studies citing increased risk of heart attack and stroke. These studies were all done with synthetic hormones. Please do not confuse these drugs prescribed by doctors around the country with the natural, bioidentical hormones I am suggesting. Again, natural, bioidentical hormones actually replace the lost hormones we lose in the aging process. Synthetic hormones only treat the symptoms. Even at that, they treat only some of the symptoms. Your hot flashes may get a little better, but good luck getting rid of that pear-shaped body with synthetic hormone replacement! You must actually replace the lost hormones and treat the root of the problem rather than addressing only the symptoms.

The second phase is to Balance Your Diet. This is the Somersize piece of the puzzle to lose the extra weight and maintain your ideal body composition for life. It has worked for countless people; in fact, an estimated ten million people are following this program with astounding results. Ten million people can't be wrong! This eating program gets back to basics. It's based on real food, the way our mothers used to prepare food before we had convenience items like TV dinners and fast-food restaurants. You simply buy fresh produce, dairy products, meat, poultry, and seafood and you are on your way. In addition, you will learn about good carbohydrates in their whole-grain form that must be included in your daily menus to experience results that will have you looking good from the inside out.

After years of research, including seven books on the subject, I can tell you that this one-two punch will eliminate the problem: *Slim, that's the Somersize piece; Sexy, that's the hormone replacement piece. Put them together and you have one happy, slim, and extremely healthy individual.* I have been talking and writing about Somersize for years, and I introduced my philosophy on hormone replacement for the first time in *The Sexy Years,* but never before have I combined these two topics to tackle weight loss and health for the second half of life. If you have been struggling with your weight and feeling run-down and don't know why, this book could change your life.

For men and women who are still making a full complement of hormones, you will not need to balance your hormones just now. Somersizing will be enough to keep you looking and feeling your best. That being said, if you think you are too young to be experiencing hormonal loss, you may be surprised to hear that many women and men as young as in their thirties experience loss of hormones that can nullify the effects of any weight-loss program. If you assume that you will start losing your hormones years, even

decades, down the road, you need to pay particular attention to the amount of stress in your life, which can lower hormone levels and thrust you into this phase much sooner than you anticipate. Stress has long been considered the culprit in several medical conditions, especially heart health. In this book you'll learn how it can affect your hormones, which affect your weight, and keep you from achieving your goals.

For those of you who are familiar with my weight-loss program, you know that I have always included whole-grain carbohydrates as a vital part of Somersize. Now I feel this information is more important than ever. The low-carb movement has exploded in this country. Much of it is good because now people understand the importance of eliminating sugar and refined carbohydrates (like white flour and white rice) from our diets. What's not good is that going too low in carbohydrates for extended periods of time creates a different type of hormonal imbalance that will also disrupt your weight loss. This is a relatively new phenomenon and in this book I will explain the importance of including whole-grain carbohydrates to achieve a balanced diet and balanced hormones.

One word that means a lot to dieters is "plateau." Unfortunately, even Somersizers can experience this stall in weight loss. You will read important information about why your body will try to keep you from shedding the pounds and how you can get over the hump and get back on your way to steady weight loss. Also, you'll learn about the important role that carbohydrates play in getting through this phase. After a decade

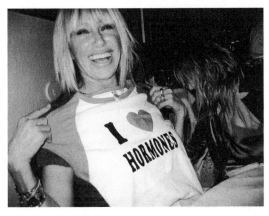

I love hormones! Leslie gave me this shirt for my birthday.

of Somersizing, we have seen a phenomenon of people who go too low in carbohydrates and end up creating hormonal imbalance by virtually eliminating this food group. This is not how Somersize was designed and not how I recommend you follow it, but sometimes people will stay away from even the whole-grain carbohydrates and end up without a balanced diet. This can lead to hormonal imbalance, and as you will learn, hormonal imbalance always leads to weight gain.

At first dieters achieve great results by cutting those carbs, but in time the weight loss stalls and they hit that dreaded plateau. In *Slim and Sexy Forever,* I'll show you how to push past those plateaus and reach your goal weight. You may be surprised to hear this, but actually *adding* a limited portion of carbohydrates to your protein meals could be the solution for you. This is new information to Somersizers and it's fascinating! It's so wonderful to add some carbs with your protein meals. The key is not overdoing it, and I will show you how to make this adjustment with the proper proportions of food.

In addition, you'll learn how important it is to include the right type of carbohydrates in your diet to correct hormonal imbalances created by stress. I'll cover the connection between adrenals and cortisol and show you the science behind this stress syndrome and how it can wreak havoc on your entire system.

We are all so overstressed, yet I don't think we realize how that stress damages our bodies. We hear about heart disease in relation to stress, yet we continue with our daily grind until the moment we drop dead of a heart attack. With heart disease as the number one killer of women, we need to listen up! When stress is abundant in our lives, we throw two major hormones out of whack—our adrenals and our cortisol. For those of us with a to-do list (most of us) that goes from here to China, we are running on overload. The constant rush from here to there maxes out our adrenals and our stress hormone cortisol. The result? The cortisol makes us gain weight—not fun. Then we reach adrenal burnout—really not fun. When it hits, it's like falling off the cliff. You just can't move anymore. Not only do you lose your energy, but you can really pack on the pounds as well.

I have burnt myself out several times in my career and it is a process to get back to that place of balance. From a diet perspective you will learn how adding the carbohydrate back to our meals is one of the ways we heal from adrenal burnout. This is just another way in which I am updating the information on the importance of carbohydrates. Oh, yeah! I even enjoy an occasional small potato with my steak! Slowly your energy comes back and the weight begins to fall off.

All of this information could not come at a better time. Obesity will soon overtake cigarette smoking as the number one preventable cause of death in this country. Think about the severity of that: Poor diet and lack of exercise is now more dangerous than smoking cigarettes! That is simply astounding. This problem is out of hand and we must get control of the situation.

After I show you how to balance your

hormones, I will show you how to lose weight in Level One by controlling your insulin levels—this means eliminating sugar and foods the body converts to sugar. Then I will teach you to enjoy protein, healthy fats, whole-grain carbs, fruits, and vegetables in a way that reprograms your metabolism to burn fat. The results are fast and astounding, as you'll see from the incredible testimonial letters of people who have lost the weight without ever going hungry.

In Level Two, I'll show you how to keep the weight off for good by sharing with you a maintenance program that works for life. In this section I'll share important scientific information about the dangers of eliminating carbohydrates for extended periods of time and how once your system is balanced you must add healthy carbs back to your protein meals to maintain that weight loss forever. The good news, once again, is that it means you even get to have some carbs with your meals again! Okay, not every meal, but this Irish girl couldn't be happier to bring back her old friend the potato.

In my favorite new section I will also share with you a Somersize Scrapbook and Photo Album. You will read just a fraction of the fabulous letters I have received from people who have balanced their hormones and lost the weight for good. These are inspiring tales that will show you how easy it is to make the changes to get in control of your life and health. And you'll love seeing the before-and-after photos as proof of their success. Amazing results are on the way for you, too.

How is it that so many have had such great success with my program? People often ask me how it differs from others on the market. I don't typically get lumped in with low-carb programs since mine includes whole grains. Here's the major difference: *This program is specifically designed for dealing with weight loss in the second half of life.* This is for the baby boomers. Our weight-loss needs are different from our younger counterparts'. I remember when I was young, I could go on any diet and lose as much as I wanted—and fast. A special party was coming up for the weekend and I would say, "I'm going to lose five pounds so that I look good in that dress on Saturday night." No problem. I could drop it in a blink. After forty, it's not so easy. This program is the only one that addresses the issue of hormonal imbalance. You will not lose weight until you fix that problem.

If you are still making a full complement of hormones or if you have your hormones balanced, Somersize is still the most delicious and wonderful way to lose weight. Here's what sets it apart from the rest—the food! I have the most delicious food.

Using everyday ingredients, I share one hundred spectacular new recipes that sound more like the menu from the town's best restaurant than from a weight-loss book. Not only will they dazzle your taste buds, they are surprisingly easy to prepare.

- Summer Tomato Soup with Basil Pistou and Parmesan Crisps
- Chopped Vegetable Salad with Roasted Chicken
- Pan-Roasted Rib-Eye Steak with Slow-Roasted Sweet Onion and Sautéed Spinach

- Grilled Halibut with Spicy Rock Shrimp Salsa
- Whole-Wheat Linguine with Candied Roma Tomatoes
- Crispy-Skinned Salmon with Roasted Garlic Aïoli and Warm Radicchio–Shiitake Mushroom Salad
- Peppered Pork Chops with Fried Sage Leaves, Smashed Tuscan Potatoes, and Braised Red Chard
- Warm Chocolate Soufflé Cakes
- Wild Berry Crostada
- Velvet Chocolate Pudding

As I have said, in order to stay young looking, slim, and sexy, we need a two-pronged attack: One, maintain hormonal balance by replacing lost hormones with natural, bioidentical hormones; two, eat right and exercise. This combination is my secret "fountain of youth" to stay young, healthy, slim, and vital for all your years to come.

"Over the hill" . . . What hill? I refuse to age gracefully if that means sweaty nights with a sexless, pear-shaped body. I will not watch my husband get plump around the middle and start dozing off in the afternoons due to lack of energy. Aging *with your health* is a wonderful phase of life. You have experience and wisdom that does not come with youth and tight skin. Rather than fight the aging process, I have found a way to embrace

aging. For these years I plan to stay as vital as I possibly can and I believe that the steps I am taking will keep me healthy and happy until the day I die. My goal is to die smiling.

In the same respect, I don't want to give in to the physical limitations many people feel as they get older. This book is a tool for you. I have done countless hours of research on weight loss and hormonal balance to figure out how to stay lean and vital. I will share the science behind it with you so that you can discover the complete health and weight-loss solution that will last your whole lifetime through.

Slim and Sexy Forever—who wouldn't want that? Especially eating food like this? Slim—that's the Somersize part to lose the weight; Sexy—that's the *Sexy Years* part to balance your hormones. Together it's a winning solution, with all the tools you need to help ensure a healthy, trim body, increased stamina, and a balanced life. Following the Somersize program and replacing lost hormones with bioidentical hormones is the answer to midlife complaints. Imagine that you could maintain your youthful figure, eat delicious foods while doing it, and have hormonal balance so that every day was a good one. Don't you want to have that? This is optimum living and I plan to have it for the rest of my life. You can have it, too; and this book will tell you how.

Part One

BALANCE YOUR HORMONES

CHAPTER 1

Hormonal Balance

If you have picked up this book, you want real answers to the questions that are affecting your life the most at this phase. You want to feel good. You want to look good. You want to be happy and you want to be in control of your body physically and emotionally. The only way to achieve these goals is through hormonal balance. Hormonal balance is something we generally take for granted. For most of our early lives it is not an issue, until we hit puberty. Remember? Suddenly things started happening to our bodies and we felt out of control. For girls the breasts swelled and the hips became rounder. For boys the voice became deeper and they began to grow facial hair. For both, pimples arrived without an invitation and hair grew on your private parts (*gasp!*). For many it was also the first time that we struggled with our weight. And quite commonly, we felt weird! We had angst and we were angry but didn't know why. Or we

were confused or depressed. Or we had strong sexual urges. This was our first experience with hormonal imbalance.

For women, we also feel hormonal imbalance at certain times of the month. PMS can be worse for some than others. I know when it hits me because I look at my darling husband, Alan, whom I adore, and think, "Why the hell did I ever marry you?" These irrational feelings are from your whacked-out hormones. (And God help Alan if he EVER insinuates that I am having PMS. He might as well put a gun to his own head.) We've all said things like, "I don't know why I'm so weepy." And, "I am just craving chocolate." That's the hormones talking!

If you've ever been pregnant, you know that your body is completely altered by hormones. Cravings, breast tenderness, weight gain, feeling tired, heightened sexual feelings, depression, an acute sense of smell,

THE SEVEN DWARFS OF MENOPAUSE

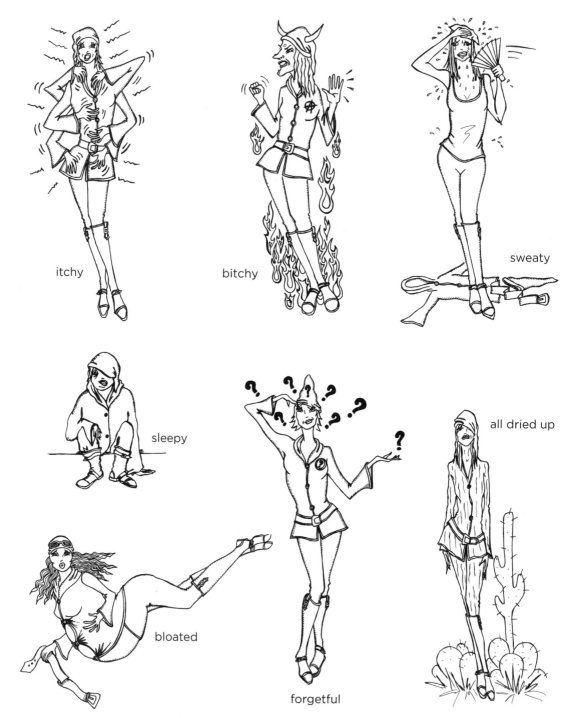

itchy

bitchy

sweaty

sleepy

bloated

forgetful

all dried up

nausea, gray hair, straight hair gone curly or curly hair gone straight. Your body is no longer your own. These are all results of hormonal changes. Our bodies are ruled by hormones!

In this book I want to talk with you again about hormones, and how they affect your weight and overall health. The second half of life gets a little tricky, but you can manage your hormones once you are armed with the proper information. You'll want to devour this material because, first of all, you are probably interested in losing weight. Am I right? You've come to the right place.

No weight-loss program will work for you until you balance your hormones.

The weight-loss piece always gets everyone's attention, because who wants to give up her favorite foods and work out and still not be able to be at her ideal weight? It's one thing if you are eating poorly and neglecting to exercise, but if you are really trying to take care of yourself and you are hitting the wall, you may very well be experiencing hormonal imbalance. In the next section of this book I will share with you my Somersize program so you can learn how to eat in a way that controls the hormone insulin. This weight-loss plan is nothing short of miraculous, as you will see from the astounding testimonials. HOWEVER, even Somersize will not work as well as you would like if you are experiencing a decline in hormone production (which occurs naturally as we age).

We will discuss weight at length, but hormonal imbalance affects much more than the size of your derriere. It affects everything!

Hormones regulate the biochemical reactions in the body. I know you're thinking, "What the hell does that mean?" Think about it this way: To keep your body alive and functioning well, you need to have chemicals that are used for structure, function, and energy. According to Dr. Diana Schwarzbein, a leading endocrinologist and my personal doctor, these chemicals are known as biochemicals. Cells, cell membranes, organs, glands, teeth, hair, skin, nails, muscles, bones, and connective tissue are all *structural* biochemicals. Hormones, neurotransmitters, enzymes, cell mediators, and antibodies are examples of *functional* biochemicals. Some of the *energy* biochemicals are sugar, ketones, triglycerides, and glycogen. They are burned for fuel to keep biochemical reactions occurring.

The hormones in your body regulate all these biochemical reactions. Everything your body does and makes is regulated by the hormones in your body. The point is, hormones are really important to our existence. If hormones regulate all of the above, then no wonder we all feel so lousy as we start to lose our hormones. Without hormones, what do you think will happen to you? Everything starts going wacky. Hormones are a language and all hormones communicate with the other hormones, so when there is a deficiency how can we expect our bodies to work properly anymore?

That is why I want you to understand the importance of *replacing* hormones lost in the aging process. When you understand the key functions hormones play in our bodies you will understand that without balanced hormones you will not be able to control your weight. You will do better at it than others if you are eating correctly, but to really be in charge and control of your weight, you need to eat properly and balance your hormones with bioidentical hormones.

I have good news for you: You can remain healthy, vital, and happy—in other words, you can age successfully—if you understand the important role that hormones play in your life. Not only will balanced hormones help you to avoid the diseases of aging, you will have restored energy, vitality, a youthful glow, sexuality, a slim figure, a good attitude, healthier bones, a healthier heart, and most important, in my opinion, a healthier brain.

Ever notice that since your estrogen levels have started to diminish you are having trouble finishing a thought? Have you secretly harbored fears that you have Alzheimer's disease because you are becoming so forgetful? I know I had these worries, but no more. Now that my hormones have returned to balance, my brain is working better than ever. My energy is fantastic, I have no plaque in my heart or arteries, I have no menopausal symptoms, my skin has become more youthful, even my breasts have a certain perkiness to them. Instead of going south they are definitely looking to the north. (Just a little side benefit.)

Mainly, I am impressed with bioidentical hormone replacement because I feel good. Isn't that what we all want . . . not to have aches and pains and stiffness, inertia, moodiness, depression, or unexplained weight gain? Don't we want to feel happy and upbeat? Well, it's available to you. The combination of eating properly (Somersize) and replacing hormones lost in the aging process, coupled with your new wisdom and life perspective, can make this passage the best ever.

The maximum life span of the human race is 120 years old, yet few of us ever live that long. Our daily habits, not genetics, determine our life span. Sometimes I wonder why we take our bodies for granted. We never appreciate them when our bodies are working perfectly. It's only when our bodies start malfunctioning that we begin to panic and change our lifestyles. Most of us take better care of our cars than we do our bodies.

Aging is loss of hormones. The less stress we have, the longer we keep our hormones in balance. That is why in some cultures people actually live to be 120 years old, because their lives are devoid of stress. Now it's not reasonable to expect all of us to suddenly throw away our cell phones and move beside a remote river, but it is definitely time to start paying attention to how our bodies are working.

MENOPAUSE: NOT FOR SISSIES

This is one heck of a passage. We women lose 90 percent of our hormones over a two-year period. Imagine! The very chemicals (hormones) that keep us alive are running out of us like water down a drain. When I discovered that I could PUT BACK what I had lost so far in the aging process, and that I could PUT BACK an exact, NONDRUG replica of the hormones my body makes (bioidentical hormones), I was pretty excited; so excited that I had to write a whole book on the subject: *The Sexy Years.* The changes in my body were profound and what I learned in researching menopause and its symptoms was so life altering that I had to share with the world what I had found out about bioidentical hormone replacement therapy (HRT).

Like you, all I had ever heard about HRT was that you got fat and that hormones were dangerous. I was going to be one of the women to "tough it out." I could get through this. No big deal! That all changed when I reached my sixth month of not sleeping for longer than fifteen-minute intervals, only to be awakened soaking wet, as if someone had thrown a bucket of water on me. I "toughed it out" until I was so exhausted that I was weepy and depressed. I remember feeling that this was all terribly unfair. Sound familiar?

I am going to explain to you the difference between HRT using bioidentical hormones—exact, non drug replicas of what your own body makes—and HRT using synthetic hormones, which are drugs made from pregnant mares' urine and formed into a "one-pill-fits-all" type of therapy that has been proven to be harmful to our health. This is information that I shared with readers in *The Sexy Years,* but I want to share it again with you now as we go through my program for weight loss and optimum living. The information makes even more sense as part of this program!

BIOIDENTICAL VS. SYNTHETIC

In 2002 the Women's Health Initiative abruptly stopped the study of hormone replacement, saying that HRT increased the risk of breast cancer, heart attacks, and blood clots. No wonder women all over America (and the globe, for that matter) dumped their synthetic hormones down the toilet. Justifiably so, I might add. The study on Prempro, a drug that millions of American women had been taking, was supposed to be an 8-year study, but they stopped the study after 5.2 years, concluding that it would be better for women not to take anything at all than to take this drug. Yet as I write, doctors all over America are still writing prescriptions for this dangerous drug. The word is not yet out on Premarin, although it has not yet proven to be of any benefit.

Prempro is a synthetic drug. It is a combination of Premarin (an estrogen substitute made from pregnant mares' urine) and Provera (a progesterone substitute). Aside from the dangers this drug imposes by creating a state of hormonal imbalance, and the fact that you are not putting a REAL hormone in your body when you take this drug, taking hormones this way mimics pregnancy. During pregnancy you have high levels of estrogen and HIGHER levels of progesterone. Remember in pregnancy that your ankles, breasts, stomach, and wrists were swollen and bloated? If you have been on synthetic hormones does this sound and feel familiar? Normally when we are young and pregnant we are at our healthiest, so our bodies can tolerate being in a high-insulin state for nine months, but to put a middle-aged woman on combined hormone therapy, meaning high levels of estrogen and higher levels of progesterone, which causes a high-insulin state, is dangerous to her health.

Most women who have been on these synthetic hormones have been on them for years. There are long-term negative consequences for a woman being in a high-insulin state for so long. The connection has already been made between obesity, which creates a high-estrogen effect, and type 2 diabetes. To intentionally put a woman into false pregnancy is dangerous to her health. This is just one of the reasons that the Women's Health Initiative advised women to stop taking these drugs.

These synthetic so-called hormones were able to give women a measure of relief from a few of the nasty symptoms of menopause, namely hot flashes and night sweats. There are many symptoms this drug does not take away, such as depression and weepiness. For these symptoms, women are routinely given prescriptions for antidepressants to take the blues away. That's the state of HRT for women in this country! Treat the symptoms, not the problem. Load us up with drugs. It's time for all of us to wake up and realize that we are on our own during this very difficult and confusing passage.

As our men lose their hormones, they are also left adrift, uninformed, and too embarrassed to be proactive, which prevents them from finding a doctor who understands their lack of vitality, lack of energy, shrinking muscles, grumpiness, and impotence. None of this has to be this way, but unfortunately most of our doctors do not understand the hormonal system, even though in medical school our doctors have had twelve weeks of endocrinology. Twelve weeks may sound substantial, but it's hardly enough time to understand this complex subject. This is especially true when you realize that of those twelve weeks, only four hours (approximately) are spent in learning how to prescribe HRT. No wonder most of our doctors have opted for the synthetic "one-pill-fits-all" type of therapy. Only a doctor (usually an endocrinologist) who has chosen to specialize in bioidentical hormone replacement therapy can assist you during this time.

Synthetic hormones such as those mentioned above have been the standard of care for women for the last fifty years, and they are not working. Women are getting sick and some are dying as a result of these drugs. These drugs have nothing to do with anything we make in our own bodies. Here is the irony and the tragedy: Fifty years ago menopausal women were given bioidentical hormones to help them through the nasty effects of menopause. Bioidentical hormones are natural; they are not a drug. Because of this, they are not patentable, and therefore not profitable. About fifty years ago the pharmaceutical companies realized that around the year 2000, all the baby boomers would be going into menopause. They took the essence of bioidentical hormones, pharmaceuticalized them into a drug, patented them, and created a one-pill-fits-all type of therapy for women that has become the standard of care ever since.

Remember when we were told that formula was better for our babies than breast milk? This, again, was the drug companies at work. Now we realize that NOTHING is better than breast milk. When it comes to hormones, NOTHING IS BETTER THAN THE ACTUAL HORMONES YOUR BODY MAKES. A synthetic replacement cannot be better. How can anyone possibly think that all women are the same, and that our hormonal needs are exactly the same? Hormones fluctuate constantly throughout the day. How could a "one-pill-fits-all" type of drug possibly work? Well, the answer is that it doesn't.

This has been a real tragedy for women. We trust our doctors, and if they give us a pill to take away the symptoms of menopause we feel they know what they are doing. Let me state right here that I am NOT against pharmaceuticals, and I LOVE my doctors. I would not want to live in a world without drugs and doctors. We need them and want them. But why take a drug (and every drug has a consequence) when we can take something that is an exact replica of what our bodies make naturally, and works better?

Bioidentical hormones: Estradiol and progesterone are exactly what our own bodies produce. They are made from yam and soy extracts synthesized in a lab to exactly mimic our own hormones; synthetic hormones are made from pregnant mares' urine. Do not confuse "synthesized" with "synthetic." Bioidentical hormones are natural. You can see how by using bioidentical hormones, we are giving our bodies the levels we need, *when* we need them.

The diabetic analogy makes my point. Everyone knows that a diabetic's need for insulin varies from patient to patient. Insulin is a hormone and every body has different requirements. All diabetic patients know that they need to constantly check their blood for insulin levels. Some test daily, some test hourly, depending upon the severity. Imagine giving a diabetic a "one-pill-fits-all" form of insulin. The concept doesn't make sense. Every diabetic patient has different needs relative to the hormone insulin.

Women at perimenopausal and menopausal age have to think of themselves as if they were operating like a diabetic; the dosage of bioidentical hormones that is right for you today may change because of various stresses in your life. If there is a death in the family, that trauma (stress) will affect your hormone levels. If you have a fight with your husband in the morning, that stress will affect your hormone levels. So you can see how impossible it is to think that synthetic hormones such as Premarin or Prempro can fit your needs.

We all lose hormones as we get older. You can measure the exact extent of this loss by undergoing a simple test, either a blood test or saliva test (some doctors think that the saliva test is more accurate). Then you can take bioidentical hormones, which are a replica of what we make in our own bodies, to replace these lost hormones. Because you are replacing just the amount you need with hormones that are like the ones your body has lost, you will feel normal again and have no menopausal symptoms. Think how good you will feel! It is so difficult to try to "tough out" menopause and not relieve the extremely uncomfortable symptoms. When you lose your hormones your body is thrown out of whack—you basically are trying to manage every moment of every day, trying to get through the hot flashes and mood swings and discomfort. Who wants to live like that?

In contrast, bioidentical hormones, as I explained, are synthesized in a lab to exactly replicate the hormones we make in our own bodies. Don't think that because these hormones are made from yam and soy extract that you can eat these foods and replenish your lost hormones . . . not so. Our bodies have no way of turning these foods into usable hormones. These foods may have other nutritional benefits to your overall health, but only bioidentical hormones made from these foods will actually *replace* what you have lost in the aging process. Do not confuse synthetic hormones (Premarin, Prempro, and others) with these bioidentical hormones *synthesized* in a lab.

LOSS OF HORMONES AND WEIGHT GAIN

One of the most debilitating symptoms of hormonal imbalance is weight gain. Since your doctor may not understand the hormonal system, he or she isn't looking at your hormone levels as the reason you are gaining weight. When your hormones are imbalanced, YOU WILL GAIN WEIGHT! When you are taking synthetic hormones, you have an imbalanced hormonal system. That pill will not be exactly what your body needs so there is no way you can find bal-

ance; therefore you will gain weight. If you are not taking any hormones at all, be it synthetic or bioidentical, you are imbalanced and you will gain weight.

When you are young and making a full complement of hormones, bone loss is not an issue. As we age and lose our hormones we lose bone mass. Estrogen protects bones, but the body now realizes that without balanced hormones your bones will become more and more brittle. Your insulin levels are now imbalanced (remember, when one hormone is off, all the hormones are off), but the weight gain that comes as a result of imbalanced hormones (namely insulin) pads you up. In case you have a fall this extra padding will keep you from breaking those now brittle bones. Nature has thought of everything, but balanced hormones will prevent this entire scenario.

When you are on bioidentical hormones, your bones remain strong and intact. When I first started on HRT seven years ago, I had a bone density test that already showed some bone loss. My last MRI this year showed no bone loss, which means, for me, that in the seven years of replacement, I have not lost any more bone, and that the bioidenticals actually restored lost bone. That in itself is reason to go this route. The other great advantage in taking bioidenticals is that the combination of eating properly (the Somersize way) and bioidentical HRT has me at my perfect weight. Food is not my enemy and I have hormones coursing through my body throughout the day that keep me feeling good and keep my weight exactly where I want it to be.

This is not only for menopausal women. Young women who are having trouble losing weight would be well served to have a blood and/or saliva test to get a clear picture of their hormone levels. Young women in their thirties are so stressed trying to be all and do everything, and that stress is blowing out their hormone levels. Short-term or long-term replacement restores balance and then the weight gain is brought under control.

Hormone replacement is an awesome new tool we all have at our disposal to tweak our body chemistry. The problem is a lack of understanding among our doctors, and an inconsistency from doctor to doctor. Unfortunately, I have not come across many doctors who are willing to do the work to learn something new. The important factor to understand is that eating right at this age is not enough. Proper eating combined with balanced hormones is the formula for maintaining your ideal weight.

SOMERSIZE AND BIOIDENTICAL: A ONE-TWO PUNCH!

As I have mentioned, replacing hormones lost in the aging process is the key to keeping your weight in check, along with good dietary habits. The fact that you are reading this book means that you are open to trying to lose weight the sensible, healthy, Somersize way. The missing element for those of you who are finding that you are eating properly but still can't get rid of those extra pounds is hormone imbalance. As I have said over and over in all of my Somersize books, hormonal imbalance leads to weight gain. When one hormone is imbalanced, then all of your hormones are imbalanced. Hormones are a language. All hormones communicate with one another, and if one is out of balance that will also mean your other hormones are out of balance. Insulin is a fat-storing hormone, so you don't want that to be imbalanced. Somersizing balances your insulin levels, but if you are of menopausal age, or if you are younger and live a high-stress lifestyle, then bioidentical replacement is also for you.

Now, sometimes if you are extremely hormonally deficient, as I was when I finally found help, your doctor won't be able to give you all that you need at first. It took a long time to lose these hormones and you have to build them up gradually. You don't want too much or too little, but if you are starting at zero, then giving you a blast of say, three milligrams a day of estrogen will make you feel like you have very bad PMS. Hormones are to be taken very seriously. Over time, in talking with your doctor and reporting any symptoms you might have, she or he will know from blood testing that you need a little more or a little less. It's new medicine administered by our Western-trained doctors who have chosen to be cutting-edge.

The first and most difficult step in bioidentical HRT is finding the right doctor. It's not the fault of our doctors that they are not versed in the hormonal system. As I said earlier, our Western-trained doctors do have twelve weeks of endocrinology in medical school, but only four hours of that are spent learning how to prescribe hormones. Four hours is not sufficient to understand the complexities of our individual needs, and the result has been that most doctors are influenced by the drug companies and prefer to prescribe synthetic hormones. Prempro and Premarin are two of the most commonly prescribed so-called hormones, but here's the problem with synthetic hormones: They are not really hormones. They are a pharmaceutical drug made from horses' urine. What does horse urine have to do with our bodies?

Because these synthetic drugs are not really hormones, they do nothing to replace lost hormones. The key to good health and weight loss is replacing the hormones you have lost in the aging process. Remember when you were younger and you didn't gain weight with everything you ate? That's because you were naturally hormonally balanced. The result of proper replacement will be a return to your normal weight (providing you are eating sensibly), and an overall good feeling. It's called quality of life.

The combination of Somersizing and replacing lost hormones bioidentically is the key for optimum living. The two go hand in hand. The combination is a winning one and one that you can follow for the rest of your life.

HORMONES AND STRESS

As I said earlier, stress has a big impact on hormones. No matter what age you are, stress blunts hormone production. So if you are planning a wedding, or taking care of a sick parent, or traveling on a nerve-racking plane flight, you are going to be stressed and your hormones will need a little adjusting. You will know because if you are menopausal, you will start to have symptoms again, even if you have already been balancing your hormones with bioidentical HRT. My first sign that stress is interfering with my hormonal balance is an itch on my arm. In my first years it was an itch on my leg. The longer I let it go, the more intense the itch. Recently this happened to me and it required increasing my dosage of estradiol (as determined by my doctor).

Another sign that stress is blunting my HRT is weight gain for no reason. I can put on five pounds in a week without any change in my usual diet. When stress interferes with my hormones, my insulin rises, and then comes the weight. This is how I made the connection between balanced hormones and weight gain. I always Somersize, thank goodness, because if I weren't eating properly I would easily put on a lot of weight. This age takes more handling and managing than any other passage. Truly, you get out of life what you put into it and it's never more obvious than at this age. All the bad eating, drinking, smoking, and unresolved problems start catching up. Without hormones you have nothing with which to battle the damage from these choices you have made in your life. The good news is that there is a solution. You can reverse the damage by eating the Somersize way, exercising regularly, and replacing lost hormones bioidentically. You will be the recipient of a new, healthy life and a beautiful body.

HOW TO GET NATURAL BIOIDENTICAL HORMONES

Your challenge is to find the right doctor. If you are gaining weight even though you are eating well, and have other menopausal symptoms (hot flashes, sleeplessness, moodiness, lack of sex drive) and suspect you are menopausal or perimenopausal, start with an endocrinologist, but first ask if he or she has chosen to specialize in bioidentical hormone replacement therapy. If not, try another doctor and another until you find one who does. Some gynecologists are now much more open to discussing and prescribing bioidenticals since the release of my book *The Sexy Years.*

Here is what will happen with the right doctor. He or she will order a blood test or a saliva test, or both. When the results come back, your levels will indicate to your doctor the amount of each hormone in which you are deficient. The doctor will then prescribe bioidentical hormones exactly tailored to your individual needs. Doesn't that make more sense than giving you a "one-pill-fits-all" drug?

Hormones are not to be played around with. You can't go to the health food store and get them. Bioidentical hormones are made up at a compounding pharmacy. They actually make the pills, gels, troches, drops, or creams while you wait. You and your doctor will find the right method of transport for you. I was not absorbing capsules very well, so my doctor switched me to drops. Then I started absorbing them too much so she switched me to troches, which

are a lozenge I let dissolve under my tongue twice a day. (The good news is that I love the way they taste.)

Your hormones are prepared just for you. Each one of us has a different chemical makeup, so it may take time to find the right balance. You will know you have the right dosage when you look and feel great. You will also know when it is not working because you will have symptoms (those Seven Dwarfs of menopause: Itchy, Bitchy, Sweaty, Sleepy, Bloated, Forgetful, and All Dried Up). It takes some trial and error with your doctor to find just the right amount for you. Be patient and stick with it. The results are worth it!

In the back of this book I give the names of the doctors I have gathered across the country, and you might find the right one for you there. I encourage you to do whatever possible to visit a doctor or an endocrinologist who specializes in bioidentical hormone replacement. If you cannot find one in your area, please look for other solutions. Save your money to make a trip to a doctor in another area. It's worth the money. If you cannot do that, many doctors will work with you remotely. You can have your blood tested at a local lab (per the doctor's instructions) and then send the results to your doctor. It is possible to have appointments over the phone and then the doctor can prescribe the bioidentical cocktail that is best for you.

If this becomes impossible, my doctor has given me the tools to pass on to you so you can obtain this balance for yourself.

HOW TO GET BIOIDENTICALS FOR YOURSELF

If you can't find a doctor in your area, and if it is impossible for you to drive or fly to another city to find this treatment, here is how you can access bioidenticals through your own doctor even though he or she may not know anything about bioidenticals.

First you say to your doctor that you want bioidentical hormone replacement. You must be firm so he or she won't try to talk you out of it because of embarrassment of not knowing anything about bioidenticals. Tell your doctor that you want to be prescribed bioidentical estradiol and progesterone from a compounding pharmacy. You do not want synthetic hormones!

You need your doctor to establish a hormone baseline level through prescribed lab work (blood test and/or saliva test). You want to have your levels of estradiol, progesterone, follicle-stimulating hormone (FSH), testosterone, dehydroepiandrosterone (DHEA), and human growth hormone (HGH) tested. This lab test is usually taken on Day 21 of your menstrual cycle, if you are still getting a period.

If you don't have a good compounding pharmacy in your area, check the back of this book for compounding pharmacy references. If your doctor does not know how to use the compounding pharmacy, ask her to prescribe an estradiol preparation such as Estrace or Gynodiol, which are available in local pharmacies. Estrace and Gynodiol are noncompounded bioidentical hormones and can be prescribed or obtained over the counter. There is also a noncompounded form of bioidentical progesterone known as Prometrium. Your doctor will start with the lowest dose and raise it slowly until you are feeling right.

Doctors generally suggest that one take the estradiol twice a day. Estradiol is in and out of the body very quickly, so most doctors feel that you really need to take smaller amounts more frequently to achieve the best balance. It is taken twice a day about twelve hours apart because you want to mimic a steady stream, as if your own body is still making it. The progesterone may be taken once a day or sometimes twice a day if needed.

To replace your hormones properly you need to take the hormones in a cycling manner. Estradiol is taken every day of the month twice a day, and one pill of progesterone is added for fourteen days out of each month. The easiest way to do this is on calendar Days 1 through 14 every month. For perimenopausal women who are still cycling naturally, the schedule will be determined by the start of your period.

My doctor suggests that one start with 0.5 mg of estradiol twice a day and with 100 mg of progesterone a day, and then track symptoms and levels to determine if a higher or lower dose is needed. On the fourteenth day of progesterone, you will get your period. If you have breakthrough bleeding early, then you are probably taking either too much progesterone or not enough estradiol. This can be tracked by taking another blood test.

Now some women would like to be on 50 mg of progesterone twice a day, not 100 mg once a day. Unfortunately, few drugstores have progesterone in anything but 100-mg units. That is why working with a compounding pharmacy is best, because they can individualize it for you. I am just trying to get you access in any part of the country, and noncompounded bioidentical hormones are better than nothing at all—and certainly are better than synthetic hormones.

TO HAVE A PERIOD OR NOT TO HAVE A PERIOD

I know what you are thinking. "Hey, she sort of blew by that whole issue of bleeding on Day 14. Does this mean I'm going to have a period for the rest of my life?" There is a lot of controversy about this issue. Of course the choice is yours, but let me explain what my research has shown and what I have learned from Dr. Schwarzbein as to why she feels it is essential to mimic normal physiology, which would mean having a period.

According to Dr. Schwarzbein, many doctors who are prescribing bioidentical hormones deliver it through "combined therapy." This means that the patient receives high levels of estrogen and higher levels of progesterone by taking progesterone every day along with the estradiol. Doctors do this when a woman does not want to have a period. This is not the way our bodies worked when we were making hormones. Here is what happens with combined therapy: Your body thinks it is pregnant. When your body thinks it is pregnant, you are in a high-insulin state. Then come

the swollen ankles, bloated stomach, and weight gain. By the way, synthetic hormones (in the one-pill-fits-all dose) are combined therapy, so not only are you not replacing lost hormones, but you are in a constant high-insulin state, so you will gain weight, among other problems. Also, prolonged periods of a high-insulin state can bring on type 2 diabetes, heart attack, stroke, pulmonary embolism, or high blood pressure, to name a few. Many women in this country have been on synthetic hormones for ten, twenty, thirty years. These women are at high risk for serious and even fatal disease. The doctors I have interviewed feel the long-term consequences of combined HRT *whether it be synthetic or bioidentical* are dangerous and therefore do not recommend doing it this way. From my own personal research, I agree.

Besides, if we are mimicking "normal," then normal for a woman who is making a full complement of hormones is to have a period. The fact that we are putting back what we have lost means we want to do it correctly. Our bodies never made hormones this way. Does it make sense to put them back incorrectly? We all know that when we were younger if we missed or skipped a period it meant something was screwy or that we were pregnant. If we were not pregnant, then it probably was the result of severe stress. Stress blocks hormone production and leaves you imbalanced.

Since my book *The Sexy Years* came out I have been challenged by doctors all over America. Dr. Schwarzbein is a leader in this field who has chosen to specialize in bioidentical hormone replacement therapy.

After talking extensively with her, and doing more research on my own, I believe that having a period is essential for me to maintain this beautiful balance and the payoff is that I feel great. Having a period is a lot easier on the body than having my body think it is pregnant and being in a high-insulin state, which creates more hormonal imbalance and other problems.

When you are standing in front of your doctor and he is telling you that this concept is crazy and questioning why you would want to have a period, please remember this chapter. Reread it and do what you think is best for you. It's your life and your body. I happily get my period each month. I know I am operating at maximum.

To me, having a period is a small price to pay for great health, increased vitality, and a slim figure. Now here's the question I get all the time: Is having a period at your age natural? Well, is hip replacement natural? Is heart bypass natural? Is a liver transplant natural? As a society we now have the ability to alter ourselves through technology and advancements in science. If we need a new hip, we do it. So if we have lost our hormones in the aging process, why not replace them with real hormones? Also consider this: Why do young people not get the diseases of aging? Because they make a full complement of hormones, which are coursing through their bodies in a steady stream. I know a lot of women who are toughing it out and doing nothing, thinking that it is the healthiest and safest way to age. Balanced hormones prevent disease, so having no hormones leaves you open to various diseases of aging. Soon comes the high

blood pressure, then heart irregularities, then joint pain from bone loss, then stiffness, wrinkling, and so on and so on.

I gladly take my hormones every day, not only because they make me feel great and look great, but because I consider them the best way I can fight the diseases of aging. I don't want to be thirty anymore, I am really enjoying my age, but I do like having my internal body operating like a thirty-year-old.

In *The Sexy Years* read the chapter called "Eve." Eve is an eighty-three-year-old woman on bioidentical hormones who has a regular period and is feeling great, thinking clearly, and in great health. She is inspiring, and for her, having a period "comes with the territory." She also feels it is a small price to pay for her good health and mental attitude.

PERIMENOPAUSE

Yes, perimenopause is real and in many ways it is a more difficult passage than menopause. With menopause there is a gradual decline and loss of hormones in your body. With perimenopause, there are surges. One day you are balanced, then the next day your estrogen is down, then the next your progesterone surges. All of this leaves you feeling confused and on an emotional roller coaster. Plus, your weight becomes difficult to control.

Once again you have to find a qualified doctor, have a saliva and/or blood test, see where your levels are, and be vigilant over your symptoms. Perimenopause needs close tracking, meaning that as the fluctuations happen you need to be in constant contact with your doctor. The doctors who have chosen to specialize in bioidentical hormone replacement therapy are patient and kind. They are progressive and sympathetic and understand that chemical (hormone) imbalances are real and uncomfortable. These surges affect your quality of life. Perimenopausal women are usually raising children, and, for the most part, working. On top of that they are car-pooling, on school committees, buying their first or second houses, trying to be all to everyone and do everything. The result of this lifestyle is stress. Stress messes with your hormones, so the right doctor is crucial. Perimenopause can be a blissful passage as long as you find yourself a doctor who is compassionate and who understands how to replace hormones in the right way.

This happened to my daughter-in-law Caroline. She has two little girls and, of course, she wants to be the perfect mother. In addition, she runs my Somersize weight-loss, food, and appliance business. Plus, she is a wife (to my darling son, Bruce) and wants to take good care of her husband. It's a constant juggle of kids, work, and loads of stress. On top of it, she is a perfectionist, whether she is remodeling the house to throw the perfect garden wedding for her brother, entertaining friends with fabulous al fresco dining, making homemade cupcakes for the school birthday, or creating a nutrition committee at the school to teach kids and parents about the importance of proper nutrition. She does it all. She has it all. And yet, it takes its toll. Last year, at only thirty-nine, she started having perimenopausal symptoms.

She thought she was way too young to have hot flashes, gain weight, skip periods, and have no time or energy for romance. This is a perfect example of how stress blunts hormone production.

Caroline is like many women. You give it your all and you end up with nothing left for yourself! This is no gift to your kids, your husband, your family, or your community of friends. When we were doing the recipe testing for this book I headed home at the end of a long day and when I spoke with Caroline she was on her way to soccer practice and timing the leg of lamb in the oven for their Tuesday-night dinner. Too much stress! No more hormones!

Fortunately, Caroline sees Dr. David Allen, who wrote the foreword for this book. He is a great doctor who specializes in anti aging medicine and through a blood test he detected that Caroline was low in estrogen, progesterone, testosterone, and DHEA and slightly low in thyroid. With bioidentical hormones, Dr. Allen was able to build her up again and bring her back to balance. It took a while to find the right doses, but when she did, her symptoms disappeared because she fixed the root of the problem by replacing the hormones she had lost due to stress.

The important point to note is that you can replace what you've lost with bioidentical hormones, but you also need to look at your lifestyle and find ways to reduce your stress. It's so easy for me to see it in other people. I look at Caroline and I want to tell her to slow down and take time for herself, yet I keep the same frenetic pace! These are tough habits to break, but it is essential to your health. You can read more about this in the next chapter on adrenals.

WHAT ABOUT MEN AND ANDROPAUSE?

Men also lose their hormones—not as quickly as we do, but nonetheless andropause is a real passage and men too are affected by this loss. Men suffer from loss of vitality, grumpiness, fat bellies, prostate problems, heart problems, hair thinning, and so on. All of this can be avoided or diminished through hormone replacement.

Men don't like to admit this because they think hormones are for women only, and they also feel it is an admission that they are no longer the sexual tigers they used to be. Bioidentical testosterone replacement is the best defense against disease and weight gain for men if they are eating sensibly. Testosterone is the greatest protection for the heart and brain for both men and women. As men lose testosterone, their estrogen rises. It is when they reach the point that they are making more estrogen than testosterone that they begin to have difficulty or are unable to have erections. Look around you at all the men in midlife and notice how many of them have big fat bellies. That is insulin run amok. A balanced diet (Somersize) and hormone replacement (testosterone, DHEA, and whatever else is missing) can bring back the guy he used to be.

My husband has been on bioidentical hormone replacement therapy for a few years now and the difference in his vitality is astounding. He sings the praises of bioidentical hormone replacement therapy (BHRT) to all

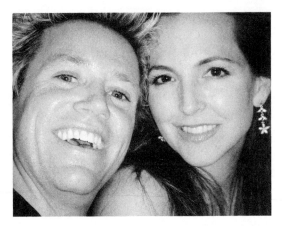

My son, Bruce, and my daughter-in-law, Caroline . . . their happiness makes me happy.

his friends; he wouldn't want to live without its benefits. He looks better and feels better, his muscles are more defined, his skin glows, his heart is in perfect working order, his thinking is clear, he has energy, and he is on the go all the time. Before BHRT he was literally fading before me.

He wasn't convinced of this until he saw how well I was doing and feeling. As usual, we all learn by example. Men need examples of the effects of this therapy. Once they get on bioidenticals they can't stop exclaiming how much better they look and feel.

Bioidentical hormone replacement has given me a life I never thought possible at this age. My weight is where I like it, I have never felt better. I like the way I look and feel, and I treasure the wisdom and perspective I have gained. This is my best passage yet. Every aspect of this passage is harder and takes more work, but the work is so worthwhile. My book *The Sexy Years* goes into more depth on the subject, so if I've gotten you interested so far, I think you would also enjoy reading that book.

CHAPTER 2

The Importance of the Adrenal System

Weight is highly affected by the adrenal hormones. Adrenals are your most important hormones. This is an area that most of us are familiar with since we've all experienced an "adrenaline rush." It's that surge of energy that helps you sprint to the finish line. It's the excitement you feel when your grandchild scores a goal in soccer. It's the rush you get when the doors finally open and you are finally allowed into a show or sporting event you've been dying to see.

Adrenaline is our engine. It pushes us forward. In order to understand the importance of our adrenals, this simple explanation will help. Adrenals are the orchestra leader of all your hormones. If your adrenals are functioning properly, they can successfully lead all the other hormones in your body; however, without the orchestra leader the rest of the musicians (the other hormones) play discordantly.

ADRENALINE JUNKIE

How does this affect our lives? If we are leading a balanced life, our bodies release adrenaline when we need that surge of energy, then we return to a calmer baseline. This is the balanced lifestyle we all hope to achieve. Problems arise when we get addicted to adrenaline and put ourselves in situations that continually feed our bodies more and more. I call these people "adrenaline junkies" and I am the biggest junkie of all! This is my vice and something I have to monitor daily so that it does not get out of hand.

Being an adrenaline junkie means that you live in a high-energy state at all times. You know the type: Every minute of each day is filled with activities, responsibilities, and piles and piles of things on the to-do list—with lots of checks ticking off completed tasks. You know what they say: "If you want something done, ask the busiest person you know." There is truth in that statement. The busy, busy people are running on adrenaline and it's as though they have superhuman energy. It's akin to a caffeine high or even a drug high. And, just like those stimulants, adrenaline can be just as addictive and just as dangerous to your health.

Adrenaline junkies are the ones who keep filling their plates with more and more: work full-time, start a remodel on the house, volunteer for charities, attend all the grandchildren's school functions, and still find time to cook and give the perfect dinner parties for family and friends. They are the overachievers who can't say no to anyone—especially themselves. It's an exciting state in which to live since you literally buzz through each day energetically, ticking things off your list and adding new ones all the time. Sounds like an efficient way to live, right? The problem arises when we live in this state for too long.

I know a little about this since I am the worst offender. For thirty years I have lived in an almost constant state of high adrenaline. I love it. I crave it. I am a wife, mother, and grandmother first, plus I work, I travel, I entertain, I lecture, I run seven businesses, I remodel, I decorate, I write, I perform, and oh, yes, I still cook and give the perfect dinner parties for family and friends. Alan will watch me go like the Energizer Bunny, and he tells me to slow down, but my body does not want to slow down. If I have some time off it's hard for me to relax. I move furniture late at night. I clean the house. I organize a closet. I answer e-mail.

Each month for the last twelve years I have appeared on the Home Shopping Network to sell my jewelry, apparel, beauty, fitness, and Somersize products. I am usually on the air for about twenty-two hours over the course of three days. The adrenaline is amazing! I'm on the air, describing the products and having fun with the host, and cooking and laughing and talking to callers. It's live TV and the rush is addicting. It's not tiring while I'm doing it since I am thriving on adrenaline.

After appearing on HSN, I may have to travel to New York if I am promoting a book or working on my Broadway show. There are meetings with the heads of my departments to keep new and exciting products coming down the pipeline. Looking at the latest jewelry designs, tasting new Somersize foods and developing recipes, making adjustments on new fashions for my line, sampling new beauty products, shooting an infomercial for a piece of exercise equipment. There are interviews with doctors to stay on top of the medical news. Then there is my social life—part business and part personal. I am on the go all the time! In fact, I'm tired just reading about my wonderful and interesting life!

I am not alone in this type of schedule. It doesn't matter if you're writing a book to be published or putting together a silent auction for a fund-raiser. It doesn't matter if you're cooking for celebrities or making food for the church picnic. If you are a person who likes to keep superbusy, you are probably an adrenaline junkie.

Adrenaline junkies don't have much of an appetite. You are so buzzed on the rush of hormones that you skip meals or just nibble here and there. You may have a cup of coffee, a few bites of salad for lunch, and a decent dinner. Or you could be an adrenaline junkie who eats junk food on the run. You probably don't think it matters what you eat, since in this phase you tend to be thin. Yes, adrenaline junkies can get quite skinny.

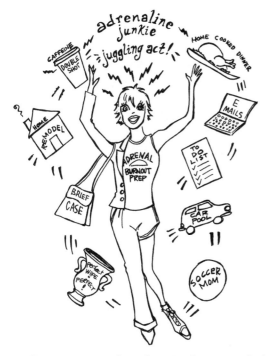

If you are an adrenaline junkie, you feel great. You have a ton of energy from your body's natural stimulant production. You get a whole lot done and you get skinny! What's not to want here? Wouldn't everyone want this? The problem is that you cannot sustain this state indefinitely. Eventually you will fall off the cliff and crash. When the crash comes, you will reach adrenal burnout—and let me tell you, it's not pretty.

There is no adrenal hormone supplement. When your adrenals are burnt out, essentially, you must change your life. Burnt-out adrenals mean that the stresses of your life have overburdened your body's ability to function successfully. Let me tell you my own scenario with burnt-out adrenals.

ADRENAL BURNOUT

Near the end of last year, I was on workaholic overload. Result: adrenal burnout. Flatline. Serious. Bad thing to do to myself. I know this. It is something I have done several times over in my life. I know the severe consequences of doing this to my body, yet I get caught up just like the rest of us, and that is when I get into trouble. Every time I do this to my body I absolutely know that I am shortening my life span. That is why I want to go through this scenario with you, so you can look at your own life to see if you are running yourself into the ground, as I tend to do sometimes, and what it means to your health and your weight.

I have always prided myself on being able to "outwork" everybody. It's an ethic I learned through being raised by a father for whom nothing was ever good enough. When I got straight A's in school I was reprimanded for the one A−. My room was never clean enough; the job I had just finished was never done well enough; and I was never working hard enough or fast enough or just enough, period. (Don't worry, I have had massive amounts of therapy and today I see the role my father played in my life as my greatest teacher. Through him I learned who I was, albeit the hard way. All lessons are hard-won.)

In December of 2003, I found myself, once again, in a familiar state. I had worked so much for so long. I went for extended periods without sleeping or eating enough and then came the crash. It was Christmas vacation. The offices were closed. I had no commitments. I was not entertaining. Finally Alan and I had some time to just relax and enjoy our desert home. This should have been a glorious time, a well-deserved break from the grind. I was so looking forward to it and yet, when it hit and I slowed down, I started weeping for no reason. I had reached adrenal burnout.

After a couple of weeks of being in this state I called Dr. Schwarzbein and said, "I know this is physical and not emotional because I love my life and my marriage, and my kids, and I love what I do. So I know this has nothing to do with reality, but I am very, very depressed." I expected my good doctor to be sympathetic and nuturing, but instead she said to me, "Well, what did you expect?" She continued, "How do you think you can keep on working at such a pace and not give your body any time to build up what has been broken down from all this stress? Your body is a finely tuned machine and like all machinery it needs constant tuning. You can't run an engine night and day continuously without EVER stopping to give your machine a tune-up, so how do you think your body can do this?"

In my heart I knew she was right; after all, I have made this part of my life about learning and understanding about my body so I can be in control of how it is working and how I am feeling. It has been one of the greatest things I have done for myself. It is empowering to have an understanding of how my body works. Yet here I was again, in this all too familiar state. I guess the messenger does not always live the message.

Unfortunately, it is estimated that 85 percent of all American adults are walking around with burnt-out adrenals. Most of them deal with it by drinking coffee and taking Prozac. Why would we drink coffee when we are burnt out? Because coffee is a stimulant and makes us feel like we have energy, and when your adrenals are shot, so is your energy. Also, like me, when you have adrenal burnout, you feel a "racing" inside that makes sleep impossible even though you are dog tired and sleep is the one thing you need and crave the most.

It is also for this reason that your doctor may give you an antidepressant. Most doctors know nothing about the hormone system, and they will prescribe the antidepressant to slow you down and turn off your brain so you can sleep. Once you are on the antidepressant merry-go-round, forget it. Now you might be sleeping a little better, but you still spend your days working like a maniac, causing further adrenal burnout, and this goes on and on until you are severely sick. Also, antidepressants are very difficult to discontinue, because once your body gets accustomed to them it's hard to feel good without them . . . thus addiction. Addictions develop because the antidepressants initially cause the release of a lot of serotonin into your brain, making you feel calm and happy. This is how we all want to feel all of the time. The irony is that these same toxic chemicals that give you an immediate release of serotonin also cause you to use up MORE serotonin. Then you start craving anything that will make serotonin levels rise, even if it is only temporary. Many people go to carbohydrates and refined sugars or self-medicate with caffeine, alcohol, and recreational drugs to feel good, but what you are really doing is using these substances to raise your serotonin levels. When serotonin levels are correct and balanced for you, you feel good, calm, and happy. Unwittingly you are now addicted because you want to continually recapture that calm happy feeling, but because your diet is so bad, the only way you can now produce this happy effect is by continuing to use your antidepressant. So you are on the merry-go-round, and now you are going to start gaining weight, which is going to make you unhappy, so you will probably start abusing your antidepressants by using them more often. Yes, antidepressants will make you fat (now you're listening, aren't you?).

It's not just junkies who get addicted. We are all driven by our deficiencies. We crave feeling good and we will do anything to achieve that, no matter what the consequences. It's not about willpower or intellect. Deficiencies cause craving. Better to start working on eating well, sleeping an adequate amount, managing stress, and keeping your body hormonally balanced, than to get on the Prozac wheel. It's time to think long-term. Think of the consequences of stress and bad diet and harmful lifestyle habits—they will affect *everything*: your mood, your body shape, your weight, your internal health, your quality of life.

Almost everything and anything raises adrenaline levels in your body because adrenaline is one of the hormones needed to access your biochemicals for use in the activities of daily living. When your adrenals are not working correctly, you won't be sleeping well, or eating well, or managing your stress. Overexercising (believe it or not, overexercising causes higher adrenaline levels) or ingesting too many stimulants, coupled with other hormone imbalances, further exacerbate the problem. Unfortunately you still need to function on a daily basis, so your adrenaline levels go higher and higher as your body secretes, uses, and breaks down its biochemicals to keep you functioning as best it can, given the stressful circumstances.

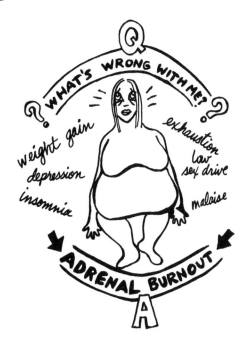

Be on the alert for any number of things that can blow out your adrenals, such as overwork; anemia; stress (good and bad); sleeplessness; fight-or-flight syndrome; hormonal imbalance such as high DHEA levels, high progesterone levels, high testosterone levels, high thyroid levels, high protein intake, hypoglycemia (low blood-sugar levels) and low estrogen levels; inflammation; infections; dietary imbalances; not eating; low-estrogen or high-progesterone birth control pills; overexercising; pain; skipping meals; and stimulants such as caffeine, nicotine, marijuana, ginseng, ma huang or ephedra, Dexedrine, cocaine, ephedrine, and pure white sugar.

As you can see, this highly responsive hormone is easily affected. If your adrenals are burnt out, then every other hormone in your body is unbalanced. When you see what causes burnout, you realize that most American adults are living in a state of burnt-out adrenals. No wonder we are sick as a nation. It seems these days and at this age that everyone has something wrong with him or her. It truly takes work, handling, and management to stay thin and healthy and hormonally balanced from middle age on, but to do so is to give yourself the gift of a long and healthy life (and I mean long; technology is going to keep us alive for ninety or one hundred years). I love the fact that we will be alive longer, but I do not want to be a sick old person. I want to be vital up until the very end. This can only happen if I remain vigilant and don't let myself fall into the workaholic trap of flatlining my most important hormones.

How do we heal from burnt-out adren-als? It's a long process. It took a long time to get to this state and it takes a long time to heal. If your adrenals are not working properly, you will not have the energy to get through the day. This is a foreign feeling to junkies. Suddenly we cannot even get out of bed. We can't tick things off our list and it could take a whole day just to buy one stamp and mail a letter. Remember, adrenals are the leaders of the hormone system and when the leader is out of whack the entire system is out of whack. To add insult to injury, when you reach burnout, YOU WILL GAIN WEIGHT! Great; now you have no energy, you can't seem to get anything done, you're depressed, and you're fat. How can you ever get out of this hole?

It is possible to crawl out, but it's not an overnight solution. There's no magic pill we can take to heal us. We need to act sensibly and slowly get back on course. We must eat good food, real food, and amounts that are required by our particular body's needs. We must get plenty of sleep to rebuild all the used-up energy and to rejuvenate. These things are essential to rebuilding what has been broken down by high stress levels for extended periods of time. With the combination of a good diet of real food and balanced hormones, you will not believe the difference in your quality of life. This is the optimum way of getting slim and staying slim . . . the healthy way. Not as easy as Prozac, synthetic hormones (Premarin, Prempro), and foods laden with trans fats and refined sugar, but the results of doing it right are good health, good mood, a slim body, happiness, a renewed, vibrant sex life, and a daily feeling of joy.

Sleep is the most important component of rebuilding burnt-out adrenals. When I was having a hard time sleeping, my doctor gave me a low-dose prescription of the drug trazadone (without the antidepressant effect), which triggers the sleep mechanism. This is to be used short-term to retrain your body to sleep. I was getting up at 3:30 every morning for the past few years to get my writing done in the quiet, which resulted in writing several books but left me sleep-deprived and led to my burnout. I now look at my rationale with amazement . . . How did I expect to operate at maximum with so little sleep at night? I was averaging four to five hours a night. Not enough for me. That is why I found myself in a heaping pile of tears that December in a very depressed state. My doctor was right: What DID I expect?

You have an ability to rebuild burnt-out adrenals by reinstating good dietary habits and sleeping properly. If you continue to keep yourself stressed, continue to use stimulants, and keep eating improperly, you will most likely end up with burnt-out adrenals and the effects, which include osteoporosis (bone loss) among other things. Now does it make sense that many female marathon runners are experiencing bone loss? Their adrenals are burnt out and they don't have enough energy to rebuild what has been broken down by long-distance running.

It's not easy to put out the effort to take good care of yourself, but what choice do you have? NO one in his or her right mind would choose anything but optimum living, but every time you abuse yourself in the ways described above, you are making the choice to live fat, unhealthily, and unhappily.

CORTISOL: THE STRESS HORMONE

Now that you understand the adrenals, you also need to know about the other major hormone in your body: cortisol, your stress hormone. You cannot live very long without your major hormones (adrenals and cortisol). The main minor hormones are estrogen, progesterone, DHEA, testosterone, HGH, and pregnenolone. You will die without your minor hormones, but it will take longer (and most of the time the connection is never made that today's heart attack is the result of a low estrogen state over the past several years).

If adrenaline is your engine and gives you a rush of energy, cortisol will similarly give you energy, but more in response to stress. For this reason, cortisol is often called the stress hormone. When you encounter a stressful situation, cortisol will be released by your adrenals. If you are swimming in the ocean and see a shark, your body will mobilize energy and increase your blood pressure to send more blood to your cells so that you can quickly swim away from the shark. This response is life-giving. We've heard of superhuman qualities that some experience in panic situations—a child is trapped under a car and a woman is somehow able to lift the car to help her child. These are examples of cortisol in action. This is the right use for these biochemicals. Your body releases these hormones so that you can swim away or lift a car to save a life.

However, the problem is that your body will secrete cortisol for whatever stress you encounter. It does not differentiate between a shark attack or a good berating from your boss at work. Either way, your adrenals will secrete more cortisol. In a situation in which the stress is self-induced—for example, if you let all the piles on your desk make you stressed and crazy—you will secrete more cortisol, which will raise your blood pressure and use up your energy reserves without much benefit to you. Using up your biochemicals like this is a waste because they are being released when there is no threat to your life. Stress is a wasted emotion that takes its toll on every part of your body, emotionally and physically. Stress is a killer, and we must work our hardest to eliminate unnecessary stress and save our cortisol reserves for when we really need them, as in life-threatening situations.

CORTISOL AND WEIGHT GAIN

You can't turn on the TV these days without seeing a host of advertisements for cortisol-related diet pills. What is the cortisol-fat connection? And why does stress make you gain weight? Simply, stress creates high levels of cortisol, and high levels of cortisol create insulin resistance. Insulin resistance makes us gain weight since the sugars and carbohydrates we eat are converted to fat rather than burned as fuel. You will learn about this in detail in the next section. This fat is most commonly stored around the midsection. Not only do we need to eliminate sugar and

bad carbohydrates, but we must reduce our cortisol-inducing stress if we are to control our insulin resistance.

An interesting point about cortisol is that it can help you in times of true famine. Your body needs food for clear thinking. When there isn't enough food to feed your brain, your body mobilizes its biochemicals to be used as brain food as well as for other important body functions. Feeding your brain will keep you alive longer, since brain function can contribute to a solution to obtain food. If cortisol were not working, your brain would simply shut down with the rest of your body from malnutrition. This is a benefit of cortisol in an extreme situation.

Like stress, skipping meals or undereating can also create a cortisol connection. If you diet, skip meals, restrict calories, and eat improperly, your body will perceive this as famine. So guess what? The body secretes cortisol to help you through this famine. Now you are using up your biochemicals when there really is not a problem for you to find food, leading you to age faster.

So many people think that by skipping meals they will lose weight faster. People also cannot understand why they are gaining weight when they live in a constant environment of stress with little appetite. Because of cortisol this scenario will actually cause you to gain weight. You are making it harder for your body to lose weight in the long run and in the process you are creating cortisol surges. Here's why. Every time you miss a meal, cortisol levels go up to take care of the perceived famine, and the body readjusts to survive on fewer calories. It no longer needs the same food requirements because it has learned to survive on less food in the false state of famine. When you return to normal eating you will gain weight, since your body has adjusted to eating less food. To try to lose more weight, you may eat even less. This will increase cortisol further and now you are on the merry-go-round. That is why some people hardly eat at all and they are still gaining weight. Somersize will help you solve this problem.

If you didn't get it the first time, please reread this section above. It is crucial to understand the physiology of your body. Our bodies work like finely tuned machines. The more you understand how your body functions, the easier time you will have understanding the effects of food and stress. Everything in our bodies has to work in balance. Trying to lose weight but having hormonal imbalance is very self-defeating. You will lose some weight because you are eating properly, but until your hormones are in balance you are not going to get your desired effects.

Stress is going to have the same effect. You can eat right, you can have balanced hormones, but stress is going to blunt your hormone production, and that will lead to hormonal imbalance. Hormonal imbalance ALWAYS LEADS TO WEIGHT GAIN. See how it works? Everything works in concert. To keep adrenal and cortisol levels working at optimum, you must live a balanced life. You must sleep, eat right, balance your hormones, and eliminate stress. I know, I know, it sounds like a lot of work, but now is the time when you must ask yourself how important it is to stay healthy, eliminate disease, have a great sex life, have a

slim figure, be in a happy mood, and manage your stress. This is optimum living. You can have it. Excuses are just that.

REDUCING STRESS FACTORS

It has been a year since I flatlined my adrenals. It has taken all year to rebuild what I had destroyed. I have had to say no to a lot of invitations, I have had to stop being Supermom, Supergrandmother, Superwoman. I cannot be everything to everyone anymore. I set limits on the hours that I will take calls from the office. I set boundaries with work and schedule my down time in the same way I schedule my appointments. That is the concession I have made to aging. My body requires more rest and less stress than it once did to work at optimum. I now take burnt-out adrenals very seriously. I now know that it is my job to keep my life in balance . . . whatever that takes.

Funny . . . the world is spinning quite nicely without me burning it at both ends. Instead of me hosting all the birthdays, the dinners, the family events, I pick and choose and let the other family members host the rest of the events for the year. It gives my kids a chance to be all that they are capable of being. I now have time to sit and play with the grandchildren rather than always being the one in the kitchen doing everything. Then when it is my turn, I can go full out.

Another way I am limiting my stress is by turning off outside stressors. I don't know about you, but I am a news addict. I have Fox News on at all times in the house like a radio. If I am not watching Fox I switch to

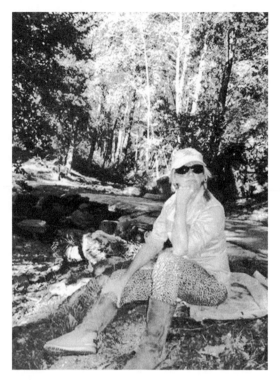
Soul-searching at Solstice Canyon.

CNN. The constant updates from Iraq keep me in a state of constant agitation. This releases cortisol to deal with the stress I feel from the news. And then, as I said, this cortisol breaks down the body to use up biochemicals in order to process all this information. I am now working on my addiction to news and limiting myself to an hour a day, soon to be a half hour, and then fifteen minutes.

We must find the time to calm ourselves and adequately take care of ourselves. Otherwise, the end result is that we are using up more biochemicals than we are rebuilding. This leads to hormonal imbalance, which causes us to seek comfort behaviors (overeating, carbos, alcohol, marijuana,

excessive exercising, or no exercising at all). These behaviors may make you feel better in the short term, but they do not lower your cortisol levels. Because of this, you will start having symptoms that include anything from acne, bloating, lack of sex drive, grumpiness, decreased energy, and forgetfulness to bruising, fatigue, hair loss, headaches, high blood pressure, high cholesterol, increased appetite, increased blood-sugar levels, sugar craving, nicotine and alcohol cravings, increased facial hair, insomnia, impotence, irritability, loss of lean muscle tissue, loss of bone mass, lower back problems, muscle weakness, weight gain, and the problems inherent with these conditions—all of which lead to disease or dis-ease.

I will say this to you over and over: You get out of life what you put into it. You must eat good, real food; avoid chemicals and stimulants; manage your stress, think good thoughts; and balance your hormones. You don't have to be a fanatic, but you can't be stupid about it. Use your common sense. You are old enough to know what your body reacts to and what doesn't seem to affect it. If you get heartburn and nausea from a single glass of white wine, what does that tell you? Probably you have inflammation and the effect of the wine on your esophagus is your body talking to you. Remember to listen! Acid reflux is now an epidemic. Drinking late into the evening is one sure way of creating the inflammation that causes reflux.

We have an epidemic of sickness in our country. It has become normal for us to see people who are very much overweight (though notice you don't see many old overweight people; our bodies just can't make it to old age with such excess weight). It has become normal for us to see people suffering from the effects of burnt-out adrenals who are popping Prozac, or who are suffering the diseases of aging. It has become so common for people to be sick that we have accepted it as normal. What an irony. Technology and science have progressed to the point where we can now see inside our bodies with full-body MRIs and CAT scans to check for any abnormalities before they can kill us. We have saliva tests and blood tests to accurately measure our hormone balance. Either we ignore what is available to us, or we take the tests, we have the scans, we go to all the new doctors and follow the fads, yet still are sick, because the true remedy to illness is simple: take good care of your precious body.

I encourage you to seek out medical professionals who are interested in preventing disease, rather than just treating symptoms. You can learn to manage your stress. You can learn to eat right. You can learn to take care of your body. You can learn to lose weight the healthy way. And you can learn to balance your hormones, your life-giving hormones that will help you stay slim and fight the diseases of aging.

AN INTERVIEW WITH DR. MICHAEL GALITZER

Dr. Michael Galitzer is another of this country's leading physicians. His specialty is natural hormone replacement and antiaging medicine, and he treats men and women of all ages who are looking for an edge relative to their health.

SS: Thank you for giving me this time. I know how busy you are. Especially since I interviewed you for my book The Sexy Years, *I know that you hardly have time to breathe. But I think people resonated with you and the other doctors in my book as the "new thinking," cutting-edge doctors, and, frankly, who doesn't want to be in on that?*

MG: Well, thank you. It's a pleasure to speak with you again.

SS: I'd like to get right into it. I don't think any of us ever realized the importance of the functioning of the adrenals. We've all heard of an "adrenaline rush," but most of us never have understood just how relevant adrenal balance is to our health, and the effect it has on our bodies and their ability to function properly. Let's talk about decreased adrenal function and why it's important to understand this major endocrine gland.

MG: I have to start by saying that adrenal burnout is epidemic in our country. In traditional medical practices adrenal failure is recognized as a disease called Addison's disease. In fact, John F. Kennedy had Addison's disease and treated it with cortisone for years. We're not talking here about adrenal failure, but about adrenal fatigue, which occurs when the adrenals are depleted. This is definitely not being detected in most medical practices. Physicians don't look for it. They don't properly diagnose it, and they don't treat it correctly. When people are under enormous and prolonged stress, they will experience adrenal fatigue.

SS: Where are the adrenals located, and how does stress affect them?

MG: The adrenals are two small glands that sit on top of the kidneys. The adrenals are highly affected by different forms of stress. You can have emotional stress from marital problems, or you may not like your job or your employer. You can have chemical stress resulting from mercury leakage from silver dental fillings, chronic exposure to other heavy metals and pesticides, and food allergies. And you can have physical stress from overtraining, working sixty-plus-hour weeks, or having an infected root canal.

The first stage of stress is called the alarm reaction. At this stage, there is increased secretion of the hormone cortisol, in order to adapt to the stress. High cortisol causes insulin resistance, and insulin resistance causes high cortisol. When you have insulin resistance, you gain weight, you crave sugar, and you are constantly hungry. You also get fatigued after eating a high-carbohydrate meal because lots of insulin has been secreted, while the cells are no longer responsive to insulin. The body converts carbohydrates into fat, which requires energy and which accounts for the fatigue after meals.

Another symptom of high cortisol is that people are unable to fall asleep. They also frequently have symptoms of low thyroid function. When you have low thyroid, your hair falls out, you are constipated, your skin feels very dry, and you feel cold most of the time.

Increased cortisol contributes to high blood pressure. For men, high cortisol will cause a man to lose his testosterone down

the road, because cortisol will block testosterone from working at the cell receptor sites. A man will lose his sex drive and be thirty pounds overweight. He will frequently have high cholesterol and high triglycerides. It's a perfect setup for a heart attack.

SS: So there is a domino effect starting with adrenal burnout.

MG: Yes, but there's even more. The brain becomes less sensitive to estrogen when there is high cortisol, resulting in hot flashes in women who had previously been in perfect hormonal balance. Whenever a major stressor occurs, a woman will call and ask me, "Why am I having hot flashes?" The reason is that the stressor causes the cortisol to go up, which makes the cells less sensitive to estrogen.

Increased cortisol also occurs as a result of chronic inflammation and chronic pain. The liver has a reduced ability to detoxify, promoting a leaky gut, with consequent autoimmune reactions within the body. Increased cortisol can cause ulcers in both the stomach and small intestine. Bone density can go down.

Additionally, high cortisol will suppress the pituitary's ability to release LH. LH is essential for ovulation. So if cortisol suppresses ovulation, you're going to get infertility and no progesterone.

Students who pull all-nighters, who study, study, study and do great on tests, often find that two days later they get an upper respiratory infection. That's because there's no more cortisol around to protect them and, therefore, they get sick. Cortisol is a major player in our health.

Older people are in a more difficult position because they have additional stressors associated with aging that make it more difficult for them to achieve balance. They sleep less, they drink more alcohol, and they take more prescription drugs. There is a greater incidence of death among their friends and relatives. They have a greater sense of helplessness, and they often become caregivers to their spouses who may be sick.

SS: So stress produces high cortisol, which starts a chain reaction of bodily malfunctions, all of which have serious effects on our bodies' ability to operate and function properly. Sounds like high cortisol is not where we want to be.

MG: You are correct because as a result of prolonged stress, this person is at the second stage of adrenal fatigue (the resistance stage). Left unchecked you will quickly progress to the third stage when the effects of cumulative stress are so great that the adrenals are completely burnt out, and this is called the exhaustion stage. At this point the adrenals are unable to respond to any stressor, and you will see low levels of cortisol and DHEA in the body. You don't want to be here.

SS: So how can a person know how to fix this problem? We live in a society in which stress is part and parcel of our daily lives. If a person comes into your office and says, "I want to live a perfect life and avoid the diseases that seem to automatically accompany our everyday lives," what do you do for this person?

MG: Changing one's lifestyle is number one. You can't be drinking six cups of coffee during the day. You can't be drinking three glasses of wine every night. You can't be smoking cigarettes. You can't be drinking several twelve-ounce colas a day.

This person has got to get in touch with his/her purpose in life. Why am I on this planet? You've got to let that purpose guide you as opposed to anything else. Find out why it's important for you to be here. We all need purpose.

Frequently, when I talk with patients, they say their purpose is their children, and that is fine. There isn't only one right answer, the key is for that person to align themselves with that purpose, and let that purpose guide them. I think that's the most important thing that anybody can do. Then you have to stay on top of it. Pay attention to your body. If women and men would follow everything you are telling them to do in this book, from supplements to nutrition, to exercise, to relaxation to meditation, and then balance their hormones bioidentically, everyone would be in much better shape.

The best thing you can do for a woman or man with burned-out adrenals is to balance their hormones. Then I question them about sleep. If you have too much cortisol you can't fall asleep. High cortisol turns off melatonin, so consequently you toss and turn to no avail.

If you wake up in the middle of the night, and can't get back to sleep, that's a sign that your adrenals are fried . . . burned out. You see, when we are sleeping our cells are working. Our cells need glucose to live.

That's the job of cortisol, to tell the liver to keep glucose going to the cells. If the cortisol isn't working, the body says "Hey guys, we need sugar." Well, if your cortisol levels are very low, your body will go into the emergency mode, and go to the adrenal medulla (the inner adrenal), which secretes epinephrine and norepinephrine. It's like the fireman breaking the glass to get to the fire extinguisher. When that epinephrine gets secreted your blood sugar goes up, you wake up, and now you have an adrenaline rush. You can't go back to sleep. This is what happens in third-degree adrenal stress, adrenal burnout, adrenal fatigue.

SS: What do you do for this person?

MG: I would give them B complex injections, 1000 mg of vitamin B_5 daily, 25,000 mg of intravenous vitamin C weekly, and put them on 4,000 mg of vitamin C daily. I would give them adrenal cortex extract injected deep into the muscle. The herb licorice root increases the half-life of cortisol. Licorice is also an antiviral and great for respiratory infections in those who have adrenal fatigue. The hormone pregnenolone, which is produced in the adrenals and the brain, is the precursor of all the adrenal hormones, and also improves memory. DHEA helps with third-degree adrenal fatigue. Lastly, bioidentical progesterone strengthens the adrenals.

SS: Yet, is it at this stage that most people are usually given a sleeping pill and/or an antidepressant?

MG: Yes, which does not fix the root of the problem. Also, sleeping pills like Ambien can become highly addictive. There are certain things that are critical for the adrenal-fatigue people to do to get better. They have got to avoid refined sugar. They must avoid caffeine because it raises your blood sugar. When your blood sugar is raised your insulin gets triggered to drive your blood sugar down. When the blood sugar goes down, cortisol is supposed to bring it back up, but since these adrenal-fatigue people don't have enough cortisol, they become very hypoglycemic. So drinking caffeine is probably the worst thing they can possibly do.

SS: How does all of this affect weight gain or loss?

MG: The people who are adrenal-fatigued are usually pretty thin. The people with high cortisol are the ones who gain the weight. Adrenal-fatigued people must have protein at each meal. It's mandatory that they don't skip breakfast. A muffin and a piece of fruit would be the worst possible thing for breakfast. If they are going to snack, they should snack with low-glycemic foods like seeds and nuts. Fruit juices should be avoided because of the sugar, and if you're going to eat high-glycemic foods, always have protein with it.

SS: What about exercise when you are adrenal fatigued?

MG: The general rule is any exercise that makes them feel okay one to one and a half hours later, and that they don't feel worse the next day. Walking, slow jogging, slow cycling are okay. Running quickly on a treadmill would be the worst thing for an adrenal-fatigued person.

SS: *When the adrenals are shot like this, how does it affect all the other hormones?*

MG: Nothing works right. They really need to take it easy because there isn't enough cortisol to normalize blood sugar.

SS: *It seems crazy that as a society we have chosen to live such stressful lives that we are putting this kind of stress on our bodies' ability to function properly. How do we get back on track?*

MG: We need to look inside of ourselves and realize that there are three main causes of chronic stress:

1. When we have long-term unhealthy beliefs that cause us to perceive life events as "dangers," and thus trigger an alarm response.
2. When we have persistent deprivation of our emotional need for "bonding" or closeness.
3. When we don't get enough of our psychological needs met, in our daily lives, that are unique to our specific personality. Some of us need to have fun and excitement; others need

acknowledgment of our values; others need acknowledgment of our ability to think clearly and logically; other people need solitude; and some of us need to be richly stimulated.

Instead, we work too much. People are driven by this desire to make more and more money. That puts us in a defense mode. One of the things we have to do is slow down. I try and tell my patients to breathe deeply, to try meditation, to do yoga, to take vacations. Laughter is important as a de-stressor. Rest. Go to bed early. All of these things are very simple but at present, antithetical to the way we are living our lives. I think people work because it's an area where you can define yourself and you can find satisfaction. It's great to do something you are really good at doing. It gives you a feeling of worthiness. But at the same time, overworking is not honoring your body. In the end, you don't win because it keeps you in a very closed, locked-out mode that is ultimately not in your best interest. The goal in life, in every aspect, is balance. And always remember that life is not measured by the number of breaths we take, but by the moments that take our breath away.

SS: *Thank you for this fine information.*

MG: Again, my pleasure.

Part Two

BALANCE YOUR DIET

Understanding Obesity

Now that you have heard the dramatic effects of hormonal imbalance, you can come to understand how this translates into the state of our health in this country. In case you've missed the covers of every major newsmagazine, such as *Time, Newsweek,* and *National Geographic;* in case you've had the TV off when every station reported on the problem; in case you haven't picked up a newspaper, maybe you haven't heard that we are in the middle of an obesity epidemic like this country has never seen. According to the National Institutes of Health, the Centers for Disease Control and Prevention, and the American Heart Association, we are in a state of national crisis. One out of every three people is obese and two out of every three are overweight. One in every six kids is overweight, with more than two million in the clinically obese category. Even one out of every four dogs and cats is pudgy! One of the fastest-growing indus-

tries is the oversize coffin business. Standard size is 24 inches wide. The new trend is toward the double oversized model—a full 38 inches. And since the diseases of obesity killed 400,000 in 2000 alone, of course the demand for supersize coffins is on the rise.

People are worried, and they should be. Yet we are growing and growing with no end in sight. In 1951, 27 percent of people said that they wanted to lose weight. Now that number is 58 percent. One in three Americans is obese—that's more than double the statistics of thirty years ago. That's right: In 1971 we had a 14.5 percent rate of obesity. Now it's at 30.9 percent. As for kids, 15 percent are overweight. That number has tripled since 1980. The problem is so pervasive that the Centers for Disease Control and Prevention has declared it an epidemic.

How do you know if you're just heavy or actually obese? A clinical calculation of your body mass index will tell you. The body mass index (BMI) is a measure of body weight relative to height. Here's how it works.

$$\frac{\text{weight in pounds}}{(\text{height in inches})^2} \times 703 = \text{BMI}$$

Multiply your height in inches by itself. Then divide that number into your weight in pounds. Then multiply by 703 and you have your BMI. Or simply identify your height and weight on the table and you will locate your BMI.

The BMI is a more accurate measurement than simply weight and height since it takes into account that shorter people tend to weigh less than tall people. (Not that it's a perfect calculation; very muscular people can actually appear in the obese range because muscle weighs more than fat.)

Why is it important to know if we are clinically overweight, obese, or morbidly obese? It's not just a vanity issue and about looking good in your clothes. If it were, we could all do some soul-searching and realize that God gave us each a different body and we have no choice but to live in it and love ourselves. We could get used to the fact that the average dress size in the 1950s was a size eight and that today it's a fourteen. Unfortu-

Weight in pounds

Height	90	100	110	120	130	140	150	160	170	180	190	200	210	220	230	240	250	260
4'11"	18.2	20.2	22.2	24.2	26.3	28.3	30.3	32.3	34.3	36.4	38.4	40.4	42.4	44.4	46.4	48.5	50.5	52.5
5'0"	17.6	19.5	21.5	23.4	25.4	27.3	29.3	31.2	33.2	35.2	37.1	39.1	41.0	43.0	44.9	46.9	48.8	50.8
5'1"	17.0	18.9	20.8	22.7	24.6	26.4	28.3	30.2	32.1	34.0	35.9	37.8	39.7	41.6	43.5	45.3	47.2	49.1
5'2"	16.5	18.3	20.1	21.9	23.8	25.6	27.4	29.3	31.1	32.9	34.7	36.6	38.4	40.2	42.1	43.9	45.7	47.5
5'3"	15.9	17.7	19.5	21.3	23.0	24.8	26.6	28.3	30.1	31.9	33.7	35.4	37.2	39.0	40.7	42.5	44.3	46.1
5'4"	15.4	17.2	18.9	20.6	22.3	24.0	25.7	27.5	29.2	30.9	32.6	34.3	36.0	37.8	39.5	41.2	42.9	44.6
5'5"	15.0	16.6	18.3	20.0	21.6	23.3	25.0	26.6	28.3	30.0	31.6	33.3	34.9	36.6	38.3	39.9	41.6	43.3
5'6"	14.5	16.1	17.8	19.4	21.0	22.6	24.2	25.8	27.4	29.0	30.7	32.3	33.9	35.5	37.1	38.7	40.3	42.0
5'7"	14.1	15.7	17.2	18.8	20.4	21.9	23.5	25.1	26.6	28.2	29.8	31.3	32.9	34.5	36.0	37.6	39.2	40.7
5'8"	13.7	15.2	16.7	18.2	19.8	21.3	22.8	24.3	25.8	27.3	28.9	30.4	31.9	33.4	35.0	36.5	38.0	39.5
5'9"	13.3	14.8	16.2	17.7	19.2	20.7	22.1	23.6	25.1	26.6	28.1	29.5	31.0	32.5	34.0	35.4	36.9	38.4
5'10"	12.9	14.3	15.8	17.2	18.7	20.1	21.5	23.0	24.4	25.8	27.3	28.7	30.1	31.6	33.0	34.4	35.9	37.3
5'11"	12.6	13.9	15.3	16.7	18.1	19.5	20.9	22.3	23.7	25.1	26.5	27.9	29.3	30.7	32.1	33.5	34.9	36.3
6'0"	12.2	13.6	14.9	16.3	17.6	19.0	20.3	21.7	23.1	24.4	25.8	27.1	28.5	29.8	31.2	32.5	33.9	35.3
6'1"	11.9	13.2	14.5	15.8	17.1	18.5	19.8	21.1	22.4	23.7	25.1	26.4	27.7	29.0	30.3	31.7	33.0	34.3
6'2"	11.6	12.8	14.1	15.4	16.7	18.0	19.3	20.5	21.8	23.1	24.4	25.7	27.0	28.2	29.5	30.8	32.1	33.4
6'3"	11.2	12.5	13.7	15.0	16.2	17.5	18.7	20.0	21.2	22.5	23.7	25.0	26.2	27.5	28.7	30.0	31.2	32.5
6'4"	11.0	12.2	13.4	14.6	15.8	17.0	18.3	19.5	20.7	21.9	23.1	24.3	25.6	26.8	28.0	29.2	30.4	31.6

Height in feet and inches

BODY MASS INDEX CHART

Below 18.5	Underweight
18.5 – 24.9	Normal
25.0 – 29.9	Overweight
30.0 and above	Obese

nately, the negative physical effects of being overweight and obese reach far beyond dress size. Being overweight significantly increases the risk of heart disease, high blood pressure, stroke, diabetes, osteoarthritis, and many forms of cancer.

The August 2004 issue of *National Geographic* magazine took an inside look at how obesity affects internal organs. Using a state-of-the-art open scanner to get a high-resolution MRI, they compared a morbidly obese woman with a woman of healthy weight. Here are the astounding results. The diseases of obesity may include any one or more of the following conditions.

Liver Disease: Many obese people develop deposits of fat inside the liver, a condition that can progress to cirrhosis in about 10 percent of cases, and occasionally to liver failure.

Colon Cancer: Obese people are at greater risk of colon cancer. Abdominal fat appears to increase risk more than fat elsewhere, which may explain why men who tend to store fat in their abdomens have a higher risk.

Osteoarthritis: Being overweight places additional strain on the spine, hips, and knee joints, causing loss of cartilage. As the cartilage deteriorates, joint space narrows and bones grind together.

Stroke: Risk is two to four times higher in people with type 2 diabetes, 90 percent of whom are overweight. Stroke occurs either when a blood vessel ruptures or when a blood clot blocks an artery to the brain, causing damage to the nerve cells.

Type 2 Diabetes: People with excess body fat, especially in the abdomen, often become resistant to insulin, a hormone that helps the body store glucose. When glucose levels soar, diabetes results. One side effect is damage to blood vessels in the retina, which can lead to blindness. The number of Americans with diabetes in 1980 was 5.8 million. That rose to a shocking 13.3 million in 2002.

Heart Disease: Obese people tend to have elevated cholesterol, which can lead to plaque buildup in the arteries. They are twice as likely to have hypertension.

Additionally, the obese commonly have varicose veins along with pain and swelling in their feet and ankles. On the emotional side, there is a pervasive amount of psychological pain, including depression. Let's face it; it's embarrassing to be obese and it makes it extremely difficult to survive in our culture. Many cannot fit into the seats at the movie theater or make it up a few stairs. Many cannot fly on airplanes. They may have to buy two seats. Then there's the humiliating moment of asking for the seat-belt extender. As for your love life? Try dating as an obese person in this country. It's not easy for people to look beyond the physical to get to the beautiful person inside. In fact, one study at Michigan State University showed that undergrads would select an embezzler or a cocaine user over an obese person as a potential candidate for marriage. We live in a shallow world!

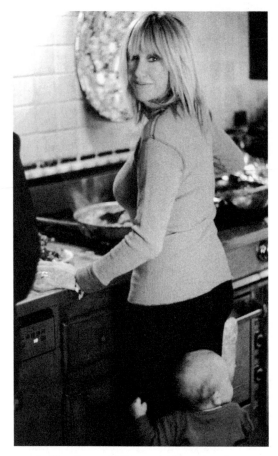

Cooking dinner with the grandchildren at my knee.

After many failed diets, an increasing number of obese people are selecting gastric bypass surgery as a solution. It's a major operation that reconfigures the small intestine and dramatically shrinks the size of the stomach. After surgery, many patients get two-thirds of the way to their goal weight within a year. Since it reduces the patient's stomach, he or she literally cannot eat as much. In most cases if the patient eats sugary or fatty foods, it can cause nausea and sweating. Overall, the results are astounding. (Although it works for most, the operation

fails for about 15 percent. The results can also be reversed, in a small number of cases, by continuous snacking.) We've all watched Al Roker on the *Today* show lose a whole person!

Sounds like a good solution, right? Perhaps, but the risks are enormous. In 2003, 7 percent of these cases included complications such as blood clots in the lungs, pneumonia, infection, intestinal leakage, and, in a shocking one out of a hundred cases, death. Yet even with all the risk, this surgery is becoming more and more common. In 1992 there were 16,200 surgeries of this kind. By 2004 that number was estimated to reach 144,000. Yes, gastric bypass is dangerous, but so is being morbidly obese. Again, when last calculated in 2000 the number of deaths associated with being overweight was a staggering 400,000.

What about the cost of obesity? With so many people who are uninsured or underinsured, the diseases of obesity create not only a personal strain on the health of individuals, but a national strain on the country and the taxpayers to support these enormous costs. Our total medical tab for illnesses related to obesity is $117 billion a year. That's billion, with a "b." Think of what we could do for the education system with that kind of money! Think of what we could do for environmental conservation with that kind of money! Think of the number of police and fire workers we could put on the street for that kind of money!

We are in a state of crisis, but we have nobody to blame but ourselves. Repeat after me, "Responsibility starts with me." When I hear of people suing McDonald's for their obesity problem, I think to myself, "Did you really think your cheeseburger with fries and a shake was a healthy meal?" I doubt it. We eat fast food because it's fast and convenient and because it tastes good. And we eat it because we have not prioritized healthy eating *and the time it takes to do so* into our schedules. I will give you a road map to change those habits in this book.

Let's face it, most of us have weight problems because we eat the wrong kinds of food and we eat too much of them. We have weight problems because we eat too much and move too little. We have weight problems because we overindulge. When the *Journal of the American Medical Association* tells us that poor diet and physical inactivity will soon overtake tobacco as the leading cause of preventable death in the United States, it's time to say, "Responsibility starts with me." When obesity ranks with heart disease, cancer, AIDS, and drug abuse as the nation's most pressing public health issue, it's time to say, "Responsibility starts with me." (There are exceptions to every rule, and I am well aware that many people out there trying to lose weight are still not getting results. There may very well be obstacles beyond willpower that are standing in your way, such as certain health conditions or medical treatments that lead to weight gain, or, as I have discussed, if you have hormonal imbalance, even though you may be eating and exercising properly you still may not be getting results.)

Why has the obesity problem ballooned so out of control? As American experts at overindulgence, we have created a breeding ground for weight gain. We expend as little energy as possible to feed ourselves more food than our bodies need. We sit in front of the TV watching commercials for processed foods that we have to have to feed our imagined cravings. This scenario plays out all over the United States and it becomes very clear how it affects our weight when we watch people from poorer nations move to this country and join the throngs of overweight Americans as they forgo their native foods and eat our processed and refined food. If you don't believe it, consider the native people who still live like their ancient ancestors; they grow their own food, grind their own grains, and hunt or fish for their protein. In these cultures there is virtually no obesity at all. These people, as did our ancestors, forage and hunt for food in a race to stay alive. Can you find enough to eat to stay alive? That is no longer our question. In our industrialized nation, the question is, *Can you limit what you eat to stay alive?*

We now consume 150 pounds of sugar or sweetener every year (half of that is high-fructose corn syrup). Sweets are everywhere and most prominent in processed foods such as bags of cookies, candies, cereals, chips, crackers, breakfast bars, and more. In earlier times if you wanted something sweet, like cookies, you had to chop the wood to create the fire for the stove, churn some butter, make the dough, then bake your cookies and enjoy. *Little House on the Prairie* is a thing of the past as we buzz through convenience stores filling up with loads of processed sweets that we end up downing with a swig of soda.

Another huge reason for our growing

problem is portion size. We have become like dogs. "Hey, here's a plate of food. Guess I'd better eat it." We simply eat what's given to us. In doing so, we have increased our idea of a normal portion. Plates get larger at the buffets so we can literally PILE food and carry as much back as we can balance. Restaurants make names for themselves with "all you can eat" specials or huge portions that are enough for two adults. We pay little attention to the actual need for food. In Somersize, I tell you to eat until you are full, but you must use your common sense and break these bad habits.

Look at the difference in the portion sizes over the years.

A hamburger in the 1950s: 2.8 ounces
A hamburger today: 4.3 ounces

McDonald's French fries in 1955: 2.4 ounces
McDonald's French fries today: 7 ounces

Hershey's chocolate bars in 1900: 2 ounces
Hershey's chocolate bars today: 7 ounces

Coca-Cola in 1916: 6.5 fluid ounces
Coca-Cola today: 16 fluid ounces

Movie popcorn in the 1950s: 3 cups
Movie popcorn today: 21 cups

When my son, Bruce, was young, I used to take him out for ice cream at Baskin-Robbins. He would pick a flavor and I would watch his eyes light up as they formed a perfect scoop on a cone. He loved it and so did I. A couple of decades later we

were introduced to Ben & Jerry's. Wow! This was great ice cream with lots of extra chunks of cookies or candy mixed in. And the single scoop was much bigger than the one at Baskin-Robbins. And so the cycle continues . . . I recently had my granddaughters spend the night and Alan and I offered to take them out for ice cream. Baskin-Robbins? Ben & Jerry's? "Cold Stone Creamery!" they screamed. I had never been. I walked down the street and passed right by Ben & Jerry's—there was not a soul in the store. Down the block I approached Cold Stone Creamery and saw there was a line all the way out the door! No wonder. The smallest size is ridiculously huge, but it's not just about the obscene portion size. First you select your flavor of ice cream. Then they scoop it out onto a cold marble slab and add in "extras" to your liking. Here are the nutrition facts for one of their Cold Stone Creamery Original creations called Birthday Cake Remix as calculated from their Web site. It's a combination of Cake Batter Ice Cream, rainbow sprinkles, hot fudge, and brownies. So far you're thinking it doesn't sound much different from a regular ice cream sundae, right? Check out the portion sizes and the correlating nutrition facts. There are three sizes, Like It, Love It, and Gotta Have It. Gotta Have It—that's so American, isn't it? "I have got to have an obscene amount of ice cream." Then you add the mix-ins.

In this creation you add rainbow sprinkles, hot fudge, and brownies. The reference amounts say one ounce of rainbow sprinkles and one ounce of fudge, but that does not necessarily indicate the amount they add at the store. I have calculated the Like It and the Gotta Have It sizes and for these purposes I will estimate two ounces of fudge for the Like It and three ounces for the Gotta Have It. For each I will also estimate one ounce of sprinkles and one piece of brownie. Actual portions may vary.

BIRTHDAY CAKE REMIX—LIKE IT

Calories	845
Calories from Fat	320
Carbohydrate	119 g
Sugars	87 g

BIRTHDAY CAKE REMIX— GOTTA HAVE IT

Calories	1515
Calories from Fat	620
Carbohydrate	201 g
Sugars	150 g

Shocking? Yes. But it's no surprise that Americans are eating it up. New franchises are popping up around the country. WE ARE EATING IT UP! To be fair, they do carry several fat-free selections and also one made with a sugar substitute (tastes good, but watch out for the gas). The problem is the portion size. They have a kid's size, but only for those under twelve. I don't believe in telling lies, but in this case, if you're going to indulge I would say it's for a kid and get the child's portion for yourself. A true kid's size should be half of what it is.

Sugar overload! It's no wonder we are obese. This is a typical case of America's love of everything in excess. Too much of everything is just enough, right? People in other countries find this excess disgusting. Can you imagine the French eating that portion of dessert?

A report in 2004 from the Centers for Disease Control and Prevention shows that, indeed, we are eating way more food than we did in 1970. In 1970 we consumed approximately 1,497 pounds of food, whereas today we eat about 1,775 pounds of food. Although the study showed we are eating more fruits and vegetables, over one-third of that category is made up of iceberg lettuce, French fries, and potato chips! That's hardly a healthy addition of fruits and vegetables. In the 1980s, the USDA Food Pyramid encouraged everyone to eat more grains. Americans loaded up on all the wrong kinds—processed and refined flour products such as white bread, tortillas, and pasta. All of these foods turn directly to sugar upon ingestion and carry the same nutritional value: none. The food pyramid told us to avoid fats and eat more grains, so we replaced real fats with processed fillers and loaded up on starches instead of whole grains. Today we are in the worst shape in human history and it's time for a wake-up call.

RICH AND THIN?

There seems to be a correlation of socioeconomic class and the size of your waistline. Studies show that the higher the paycheck, the thinner the waist. Can you believe it? Yes, it's true. The less money you have in America, the more likely you are to be overweight. For those below the poverty line, one in four is obese, as compared with one in six for those who make at least $67,000 a year. For our youth, it's even more severe. One in three are obese among low-income African Americans.

Most people think that if you are short on cash you have less to spend on food and are less likely to overeat. Actually the reverse is true. The cost of quality food is too high for those in poverty so they tend to fill up on cheap, mass-produced foods that are loaded with sugar, fat, and refined carbohydrates. Bottom line, it's cheaper to fill your tummy with inexpensive food. It's not just that processed foods are cheap, tasty, and filling. They are also more accessible. Twenty-eight percent of Americans live in virtual nutrition deserts where a large supermarket is at least ten miles away. That's a twenty-minute drive and for those without a car it's a bus ride. Many people with limited access end up buying the majority of their groceries at convenience stores or gas stations. The food selection is the worst of what we have to offer: canned pastas filled with starches, sweeteners, and fillers; boxed macaroni and cheese; chips; white bread; and plenty of candy.

It is harder to eat healthy food when you don't have access to good grocery stores and when you work such long hours that the last thing you want to do is make a salad and grill some chicken. But the alternative can kill you—and it is killing thousands of people. We have to make finding healthy food a priority. We have to make healthy food for the kids a priority. We have no other choice. The alternative is a lifetime of obesity and the life-threatening diseases that accompany it.

How has our health spun so out of con-trol? How did we get so far off track so fast? How is it that we now have as many over-weight people on this globe as we do under-fed people? The answer is processed foods. We have gotten far away from real food and we are paying the price. It's the sugars and the refined carbohydrates. Bad food is cheap, heavily promoted, and loaded with chemicals that make it taste really good. Healthy food is harder to get (you have to drive to the market, shop, and cook), not promoted, and expensive. We have soft drinks and vending machines at schools and offices. We eat out more and cook less at home. Our portions are too large. Mom has stripped off her apron and grabbed the car keys to get to the closest fast and inexpensive restaurant to grab a quick bite to eat. We fill ourselves, and our families, with foods that are processed and refined, with all the nutrition being sucked out. Even our soil has been leached of its nutrients, rendering our fruits and vegetables less nutritious than ever before. Add to all these things the overabun-dance of food in prosperous nations, with TV video games and an intensive marketing campaign to get kids to buy chemically sweetened products, and you have a perfect recipe for an epidemic.

Do sugar and processed foods really take enough of a toll on our bodies to have cre-ated the mess in which we now find our country? The answer is a resounding yes, and I will explain how and why in the next chapter. After identifying sugar as public enemy number one, I will explain how to reverse the situation with a recipe for improvement, a recipe for delight, a recipe for health called Somersize!

CHAPTER 4

Public Enemy Number One: Sugar

After all the terrifying information about the dangers of obesity, I'm sure you are eager to learn how to get on the right path. I will tell you in one simple sentence: The best thing you can do for your health and your body is to eliminate sugar. I know what you're thinking. "Sugar? C'mon, Suzanne! We all need sweets. How can I give up sugar?"

I know it is not easy, but I promise to give you alternatives that will make you think you are eating the real deal and that will not damage your cells and make you gain weight. Sugar addiction is serious in this country and giving it up takes commitment. The average American eats over 150 pounds of sugar and sweeteners (like high-fructose corn syrup) every year! That's a 20 percent increase since the 1970s. We all know the obvious sugar carriers, like candy and cookies, but these days manufacturers put sugar or hidden sugars into just about everything.

We have sugary cereals that are advertised as part of a nutritious breakfast, only because they are fortified with vitamins and minerals so that they can be called "healthy." That's like putting vitamins into candy and calling the candy healthy! Look at the sugar content in breakfast bars. They are about as nutritious as doughnuts for breakfast. We are tricked by low-fat, supposedly healthy alternatives like Nutri-Grain bars, granola, and muffins. These things are better than Cocoa Puffs, but they still have a lot of sugar and refined carbohydrates. There is sugar in peanut butter and pasta sauce and salad dressings and marinades. It's everywhere! Plus, many processed foods contain plenty of chemicals and preservatives.

After many decades of being a sugar fanatic, I can actually say that I have lost my incredible sweet tooth. I used to crave the evil white villain. Now I am one of those people who says things like, "That's too sweet for me." I never thought those words would come out of my mouth! I believe the love of sugar is a conditioned love. The more we have, the more we need to satisfy our craving. Since I have cut way back in the last ten years, my sweetness quotient has diminished. When I do my recipe testing for these books I have my friends and coworkers taste the foods. Years ago I was the one saying, "It needs to be sweeter." Now I'm the one backing off. I just don't need that intensity of sweetness anymore.

For those who know me well, my diminished craving for sugar is nothing short of a miracle. I am an absolute freak for cake. Yeah, yeah, I may love the couple, but for me the reason to go to a wedding is for the cake! And I may enjoy party games, but I would never leave before the birthday cake! My affection for cake is how my sugar addiction began. At a young age I used to bake with my mom and I was quite good at it. At the time, I was so skinny, I could eat whatever I wanted and stay slim. My body had no trouble metabolizing sugar or any other foods. Then I hit forty and suddenly the party was over. I started noticing a thickness in my midsection. My hips were rounder than ever and I had a hard time holding my stomach in. I would eat a meal and then feel bloated and uncomfortable.

Along with everyone else in the '80s, I bought in to the fat-free craze and tried cutting back on fats. There was a certain logic to the fat-free movement; if you eat fat you will get fat, if you cut out fat you will get thin. It's no wonder we all fell for it hook, line, and sinker. It was an easy link to make that fat would clog arteries. You could easily

imagine Crisco inside your arteries or adding a layer of fat on your stomach and butt. I believed it, so I really tried to watch those fats. That meant that I ate less meat with those incredible cream or reduction sauces. I ate less pork—all that grease! I ate less cheese and used only the egg whites— all that cholesterol. I switched from my beloved butter to margarine.

What was left? Lots of pasta. Yeah! At least I loved my pasta. I could whip up incredible meals as long as I had some pasta in the house. I still used olive oil, cheese (I had to have some fats), and some vegetables or nuts. I missed my meats, but the pasta was great! I could also make a meal out of my coveted potato with vegetables and salads. I loved potatoes! So I missed my meat with gravy. I missed my full-fat salad dressings. I missed my eggs and bacon. But at least I got pasta and potatoes and at least I would lose weight and stay healthy, right?

The biggest problem with the fat-free movement was that it didn't work! Eating all that pasta and potatoes, my weight did not improve; in fact, it got worse. At the time I had not connected the fact that those carbohydrates may have been fat-free, but they were all sugar. White pasta is a fat-free food, but like all refined carbohydrates, it turns right to sugar upon digestion.

It was not until I started doing research for Somersize that I learned how sugar affects the body. Like most of us, I was still convinced that fat was the problem. It's hard to imagine sugar clogging your arteries. It's hard to imagine a potato raising your cholesterol. How could I have known that these were the foods causing dips in my energy

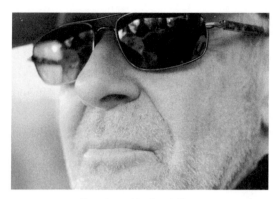

My very cool husband, Alan.

level? How could I have known it was sugar that was making me hippy? How could I have known the addictive mechanism was created by my affection for sugar? Eating sugar made me crave even more and more sugar. When I uncovered the research, I learned that SUGAR IS THE BODY'S GREATEST ENEMY!

Sugars and starches are carbohydrates. Carbohydrates are one of the body's main sources of fuel. The other is fat. In order to understand why some carbohydrates can cause weight problems, let's look at what happens when you eat carbs. Just like sugar, when you eat carbs, they break down into glucose, which causes your blood sugar to rise. When the blood sugar is elevated, it is the job of the pancreas to secrete a hormone called insulin. Insulin balances the blood sugar by carrying the glucose to the liver, where it will be converted to fat. If everything is working as it should, the fat is then stored in the muscle cells, where it will be burned off for energy. By storing the converted sugar away in the muscle cells, your blood sugar level becomes balanced. This scenario plays over and over again for those who have a metabolism working at optimum. When your system is working as it should, you eat carbohydrates and they get burned off as fuel.

INSULIN: THE FAT-STORING HORMONE

If you have read my earlier Somersize books, you know that insulin must be present in our bodies for food to be stored as fat. That's why it is called the "fat-storing hormone," because insulin is solely responsible for determining whether food will be burned off as energy or stored as fat. It is vitally important to identify the foods that cause our bodies to secrete insulin, because if we can control our insulin levels, we can control our weight.

Now that you understand what happens when we eat sugar or carbohydrates, you can begin to see what happens when all does not go according to plan. We say people are "insulin resistant" when their muscle cells will not accept any additional sugar. When these cells are closed and do not accept the converted glucose, the blood sugar level does not decrease, initiating a further release of insulin from the pancreas. This leads to even higher insulin levels and higher blood sugar levels. If the blood sugar is not accepted into the cells to be burned as fuel, it will instead be stored in the fat cells, especially around the midsection, where it will be saved for later use. *Even fat-free carbohydrates, such as sugar and white flour, can be converted to fat if we do not need the energy at the time we eat,* demonstrating how the elevation of our blood sugar can lead to weight gain if we eat too many carbohydrates at one time.

As we get older our metabolic processes slow down and we do not need as many carbohydrates as we did when we were young. That's why we gain weight as we age—we are becoming more insulin resistant. If we don't change our eating habits, those carbohydrates we used to burn off as energy start to get converted to fat, and we start to get fat around the middle!

NAKED MIRROR TEST

If you have read my earlier Somersize books, you know that Dr. Diana Schwarzbein, our country's leading endocrinologist, advocates the "naked mirror test." Take off your clothes and stand naked in front of the mirror. If you are thick through the middle—a man with love handles and a pot belly, or a woman with extra padding around the

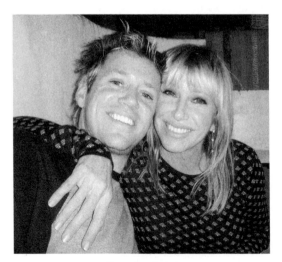

Me and my baby!

reproductive areas, such as stomach, hips, thighs, and buttocks—then you have raised insulin levels and your cells are full of sugar. If you eat more sugar—a potato, bread, cake, anything—it will be converted into fat and stored for later use.

Too much of the hormone insulin in our bodies throws off our entire hormonal balance, because one hormone out of balance affects the other hormones and leads to weight gain, increased cholesterol, and disease. A great battle has been waged over the past few years between people who support fat-free diets to lose weight and those who believe that high-protein programs are more effective for losing weight and improving cholesterol than low-fat/high-carb programs. Well, recent studies have shown that fat really isn't the enemy; carbohydrates and sugar are. New studies on high-protein programs were commissioned to protect consumers from people (like me!) who make "outrageous claims" about eating fats and losing weight. Surprise, surprise, the medical community was wrong. With all this new information, it's no wonder the nation has swung from a country obsessed with fats to a country obsessed with carbohydrates.

As I have said, overeating sugar and carbohydrates can lead to insulin resistance or what many doctors call Syndrome X. Many of us have varying degrees of insulin resistance leading to weight gain and disease. Even some children have a genetic predisposition to insulin resistance and can't help but gain weight, while other kids pig out on junk food and never gain a pound. But the majority of weight gain among kids is due to the fact that they are living on sugar and processed foods.

Whether you're an adult or a child, a few pounds overweight or obese, it's never too late to improve your health and appearance from the inside out. Public enemy number one has been identified—sugar—and that's why the crux of this program is to teach you how to keep your pancreas from oversecreting insulin, which will keep your blood sugar and your hormones balanced. With balance come weight loss, lowered cholesterol levels, decreased risk of heart disease and cancer, and longevity. When you heal your insulin resistance, your body will unload the sugar stored in your cells. That's when "the melt" begins. First your body will release all that stored sugar, then it will turn to your fat reserves and break them down to use as an energy source. The result? You get thinner and thinner while your body is being fed a constant source of energy.

SUGAR . . . AND ITS MANY DISGUISED FRIENDS

Now that we understand the importance of controlling insulin, let's look at the foods that cause our bodies to secrete insulin. The amount your blood sugar is elevated depends upon the amount and the *type* of sugars you are eating. Sugar is not only the granulated white stuff you use to sweeten your coffee. Potatoes are sugar. White pasta is sugar. Rice is sugar. Bread is sugar. Alcohol is sugar. Cereal is sugar. Milk is sugar. Fruit is sugar.

However, some sugars cause more of an insulin release than others. Carbohydrates in their refined form are much harder on our systems than those in their natural form. In the last century we have refined most of the nutrients out of our foods. White rice is simply brown rice without the nutty exterior. Brown rice has a wonderful flavor and is loaded with fiber you won't find in white rice. Fiber is essential when we are eating carbohydrates because fiber helps lower insulin levels. Breads and pastas are no longer made with natural whole grains but white flour. As the grains became more refined throughout the years, we as a society gained more and more weight.

We can all improve our health by replacing these processed foods with their whole-grain counterparts. This is part of the Somersize program and is the reason my program differs from others on the market. I allow, in fact I encourage, the addition of whole-grain carbohydrates. A moderate amount of carbohydrates is essential for hormonal balance. While I will ask you to eliminate all the refined carbohydrates in Level One, some of these will be reintroduced when we get to the maintenance portion of the program.

Let's look at why refined carbs are so hard on our systems. Complex carbohydrates (such as whole grains and vegetables low in starch) cause moderate to minimal increases in our blood sugar, meaning less insulin is needed to balance the blood sugar. But simple carbohydrates (such as sugar, white flour, and pasta) cause a sharp increase in blood sugar. This surge of blood sugar gives us a "sugar rush" or a "sugar high." After the sugar rush, our blood sugar drops below its starting point and we feel tired or artificially hungry for more sweets.

Here's what happens to us physiologically

CORN: THE WORLD'S CHEAP FILLER

My husband, Alan, is a huge corn lover. In fact, he tells a story from his childhood about going to the Jolly Green Giant cornfield, where he could fill his entire trunk with fresh corn for a nickel. He's told the story so many times that our kids call it the "Corn Story," which is a phrase that has now become synonymous with a story they've heard over and over and over. Fresh corn is delicious and sweet and a wonderful summer treat. It does, however, have a high glycemic index, and it causes a surge of insulin to balance the increase in blood sugar.

Corn is so inexpensive it is used as feed for livestock. In France they think we are crazy for eating corn. Corn is used to fatten up cows! In the United States our consumption of corn has grown at an alarming rate. We consume not only corn on the cob, frozen corn, and canned corn, but also corn in its most processed form, called high-fructose corn syrup. This corn derivative is cheaper and sweeter than sugar and is just as pervasive in processed-food products. Because of the low price, food manufacturers use it as a filler to replace more-expensive ingredients. Ever wonder why your peanut butter contains high-fructose corn syrup? It's not needed for flavor, but it's cheaper than an all-peanut product. Same with spaghetti sauce. Who needs all that sugar? But it reduces the cost of the product because it's cheaper than tomatoes, so manufacturers will save a buck at the expense of your health. Then we, as a society, become accustomed to the sweeter profile of these foods. When we go back to eat them in their pure form, they don't taste sweet enough to us and so the cycle for cheap, processed food begins.

We are producing more sugar and high-fructose corn syrup than ever before. In 1972, only 1 percent of the sugar in our food was high-fructose corn syrup—now 50 percent of the sugar we eat comes from corn syrup. Watch for these hidden sugars! They are just as dangerous to your health as sugar and will sabotage your weight-loss goals.

when we eat sugar or carbohydrates that convert to sugar upon digestion. As we now know, when we eat sugar our blood sugar spikes. When the blood sugar is elevated to such a high level, insulin is released and the sugar is carried to the liver, where it is converted to fat. If the insulin is successful, the fat will be burned off as fuel; however, if our cells are filled with sugar, they will not accept any more. When our cells are filled, it's like the doors are closed and the insulin has nowhere to store the blood sugar. Then the pancreas secretes even more insulin to attempt to balance the blood sugar. This results in an excess amount of insulin in the bloodstream, which causes a condition called "hyperinsulinemia." The insulin must find a place to store the blood sugar. If the cells are filled with sugar and won't accept any more, the insulin will then go to the fat cells and store it there. However, because we had more insulin than necessary to balance our blood sugar, our blood sugar will actually drop below its starting point. This is when we feel the sugar low and may feel tired or artificially hungry for sweets or caffeine. These cravings are ways to heal our low blood sugar. Give me more sugar! Now you can see how the cycle is created over and over again. If you give in to the craving, the roller coaster begins again.

Insulin must be present for food to be stored as fat. This very powerful hormone is the sole decision maker as to whether sugar gets burned as fuel or stored as fat for later use. You may be one of those people who can eat a ton of sugar and you just keep burning it off. That means your cells get filled with sugar, then you burn off that "energy" and the cycle repeats. You're lucky now, but eventually it will probably catch up with you. With a perfect metabolism, sugar will be converted to fat, then sent to the muscle cells, where it will be burned off as energy. Over time, if you consume too much sugar you will become insulin resistant; your muscle cells will become filled with energy and will not accept any more. At this point, the converted sugar is stored in the fat cells, particularly around the midsection, and we start to gain weight.

Syndrome X—or insulin resistance—is serious because it is a precursor to type 2 diabetes. Here's how the less serious insulin resistance can escalate to its more serious counterpart. The next progression of insulin resistance is type 2 diabetes. If the muscle cells are filled, and the fat cells are filled, the liver cannot convert the sugar to fat, so it remains in the bloodstream and the blood sugar does not become balanced. This is type 2 diabetes—a disease becoming more and more prevalent in our society, even among children. This is just one of the ways in which we are killing ourselves with sugar.

The biggest culprit to insulin resistance and type 2 diabetes is sugar and refined, processed foods. Here we go again with the effects of our industrialized nation. Our lack of real foods and our overconsumption of processed convenience foods are creating weight gain and poor health like we've never seen before. Tricky labeling makes these foods even more desirable, since manufacturers make us think we are doing our bodies good by eating them. This phenomenon follows every trend in the dieting world. It used to be that everyone was getting duped into buying fat-free items even though they were loaded with sugar and carbohydrates that make insulin levels go through the roof. This made me crazy! All of these fat-free cookies, cakes, and potato chips were marketed as "healthy" since they were fat-free. Fat used to be blamed for everything. Now, the trend is toward limiting sugar and carbohydrates. That is a step in the right direction, but it still doesn't make manufacturers any more trustworthy. Beware of buying foods just because they are labeled "low in carbs." You must look further! You must become a label reader! You must return to real food! Avoid eating a bucket of chemicals just because it

Of all the products I have developed in my lifetime, I am most proud of SomerSweet. This delicious low-glycemic sweetener has solved such an enormous problem for me. When I reached the second half of life, I had to choose between sweets and health. I had to choose between the desserts I loved and the dress size I wanted to wear. What a horrible dilemma! How could I give up my favorite sweet treats? Then again, how could I not, with my figure and my health at stake?

Now I don't have to make any tough choices. I have my health and my figure AND I GET TO HAVE MY SWEETS! It's all thanks to SomerSweet. SomerSweet is five times sweeter than sugar. It has a wonderful flavor with no unpleasant aftertaste. It's blended with natural, sweet fiber—fiber your body needs. This pro-biotic fiber source actually increases the healthy flora in your colon. And unlike other artificial sweeteners, SomerSweet stands up in the heating process so it cooks and bakes like a dream!

Clearly this is the most exciting product I have ever developed, since now you can have something sweet while you Somersize down to your goal weight. I love the clean, sweet taste. It's perfect to sweeten your coffee or tea. SomerSweet is five times sweeter than sugar, so a little one-gram scoop is about the same sweetness as a teaspoon of sugar. It's sold in 150-gram cans, which is the equivalent of one and a half pounds of sugar. SomerSweet is also available in individual packets. I keep them in my purse.

Controlling your sugar and carbohydrate intake is the key to my Somersize weight-loss program. With less than one gram of carbohydrates and zero sugars per serving, SomerSweet is a great choice for anyone who understands the health benefits of a low-sugar diet. SomerSweet has been specially formulated for individuals who want to control their sugar intake and normal blood sugar levels. SomerSweet is a delicious blend of oligofructose, inulin, fructose, sprouted mung bean extract, and acesulfame K. Let me tell you about these wonderful ingredients. Oligofructose and inulin are sweet fibers derived from chicory. A bit of fructose is naturally occurring in these sweet fibers; we do not add it to the blend and it's such a small amount that our nutrition label boasts zero sugars per servings under the FDA guidelines for labeling. Acesulfame K is a nonnutritive sweetener that is fed to a mung bean plant along with water. When the mung bean plant sprouts, the leaves become sweet, with only a touch of acesulfame K in the sweet extract that is used to make SomerSweet. In the digestive process, the acesulfame K leaves the body virtually unchanged. It does not break down in the system and is eliminated 99.2 percent intact. This incredible com-

bination of ingredients adds up to a product that tastes amazing, that bakes beautifully, and that you can feel good about using.

Many diabetics ask if SomerSweet is safe for them. If you are diabetic, please check with your doctor to see if SomerSweet is right for you. We have many diabetics who use the product and love it, but it takes millions of dollars in clinical studies to say that a product is safe for diabetics. Please put your health before your taste buds and make sure SomerSweet is approved by your doctor.

I have developed many incredible desserts using SomerSweet. You will find several in this book, along with my previous Somersize books. For you serious sweets lovers, make sure to grab a copy of Somersize Desserts and Somersize Chocolate! Plus, I have an expansive line of dessert mixes, candies, chocolates, and more on my Web site.

You really can have your cake and eat it, too! SomerSweet is available in cans, in packets, and by the case at SuzanneSomers.com.

---

says "low in carbs." Remember that FAKE FOOD IS HARMFUL TO YOUR HEALTH. YOUR BODY IS HAPPIEST WHEN YOU GIVE IT REAL FOOD. SUGAR TURNS RIGHT INTO FAT!

Sugar begets sugar, begets sugar, begets sugar. You know the routine. You eat sugar or carbohydrates. After the insulin has been converted to fat and denied in the muscle cells, it gets stored in fat cells, but not before your body has released too much insulin. This extra insulin lowers your blood sugar even below its starting point. That's when we feel the letdown or the "sugar low." This sugar low leaves us feeling tired, listless, and artificially hungry. You've all seen a kid an hour or two after the birthday party ends—it's not pretty. During this time we often feel like taking a nap, or we reach for something sweet or caffeinated to give us more

energy—then the vicious cycle repeats. Sugar goes in, blood sugar goes up, pancreas secretes insulin, then blood sugar drops and we feel tired and hungry again, causing us to eat more and more without ever satisfying our nutritional needs.

Now you are beginning to see the importance of insulin in determining whether the broken-down sugar will be burned as fuel or stored as fat. As I mentioned, some complex carbs cause smaller insulin responses (whole grains, green vegetables) and will usually be burned off from the sugar cells as readily available fuel. Other carbs cause larger insulin responses (sugar, white flour, potatoes) and will often be stored as fat because they contain way more energy than our bodies need for immediate use. A single potato is so high in starch it provides us with more energy than most people need in an entire day. Think about how many excess carbohydrates you eat in a normal day and imagine how much your body actually needs for fuel and how much gets stored as fat. Unless you're a marathon runner, you're probably storing an ample supply of fat reserves from overindulging in the wrong kind of carbohydrates.

You may be thinking to yourself that you know people who live on bad carbs and sugar and they seem to contradict what I just told you. It's those skinny people who live on fries, chips, and candy bars without gaining weight. Some people have a perfect metabolism that will always burn the food they eat as fuel—even if it's bad food like refined carbs—rather than storing it as fat. Other people start out with a perfect metabolism and as they get older their metabolism changes and suddenly they find themselves with a weight problem (this is what happened to me). But nothing is free. Those seemingly "lucky" friends can be hurting their health by eating poorly, and setting themselves up for heart attacks, decreased energy, mood swings, and possible early death from poor nutrition.

Whether you have an imperfect metabolism and want to lose weight or your weight is fine and you want to achieve maximum health, Somersize is the answer! By eliminating foods that cause large fluctuations in our blood sugar and by properly combining nutritious, delicious foods, we are able to lose weight and gain energy while achieving our maximum health. Most of us do not have a perfect metabolism, but Somersizing can show you how to *get control* over your metabolism. This program can actually heal your ailing metabolism. It's never too late to change, and, especially in the second half of life, it is essential that we adapt our eating habits since we will have to deal with loss of hormones during the aging process that can disrupt our metabolism like never before. First, we will replace the lost hormones as we lose them so that we can live life at optimum. Secondly, we must eat the Somersize way.

THE SOMERSIZE SOLUTION

Now you are beginning to see the importance of eliminating sugar and refined carbohydrates while we Somersize. In doing so, you will lose weight and gain energy. When your body needs energy, it will first look for the sugars and carbohydrates that you eat to burn as fuel. If there are no carbohydrate sources available and your body needs energy, it will break down your fat reserves and convert them to fuel. You can see that if you constantly eat a steady source of sugars and carbs, your body will have more energy than it needs for immediate use and it will store that extra energy as fat. Conversely, by cutting back on sugar and highly starchy foods, you force your body to find another energy source. The next place it looks for energy is in your fat reserves. Your fat reserves are converted to fuel. Bottom line, you get the energy you need and the weight begins to melt away.

That's the key to Somersizing. We convert our bodies from carbo-burning machines into fat-burning machines. By limiting our sugars and starches, we force our bodies to break down our fat reserves to use as a constant source of energy. No sugar highs and lows—just an even source of energy to get through the day as we watch our fat melt away.

The good news is that you don't have to say good-bye to sugar and starches forever. While you are on the weight-loss portion of the program, Level One, the built-up sugar is being emptied from your cells. When you reach your goal weight, you will advance to Level Two, the maintenance portion of Somersizing. In Level Two you may incor-porate some sugar and starches back into your eating plans (in moderation). Because your cells are no longer filled with sugar, they can handle moderate amounts without becoming overloaded. On Level Two some previously forbidden sugars and starches are permitted because they will be burned off rather than stored as fat.

Speaking of fat, let's take a closer look at your newest Somersize friend.

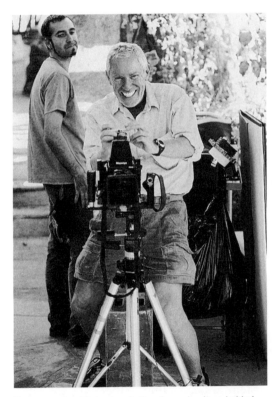

My funny, adorable husband, Alan, hamming it up behind the camera.

CHAPTER 5

Protein and Fat: The Good, the Bad, and the Triglycerides

Remember when "fat" used to be a bad word? For many people fat equals fear. Eating fat has been synonymous with gaining weight and increasing your risk of a myriad of diseases. After many years of heated debate, the pendulum has swung to the other side. Now the mainstream seems to understand the role of sugar in creating weight gain and disease. Still, it's hard to undo years of conditioning about the dangers of eating fat. Cheese is not a dirty word. Meat is not the enemy. Butter is not a bully. Pork is not the devil—and even cream will not kill you.

In my Somersize program I put protein and fats in the same category since many of the foods that contain protein also contain fat. Most of us know why protein is important. Protein is made up of amino acids, which are building blocks for the human body. Proteins help facilitate virtually every cellular function: They help our muscles move as they should, they help produce antibodies, and they help to regulate normal blood pressure. Protein is critically important to our diet since it supplies us with amino acids that are needed to make these different proteins.

The human body needs 9 grams of protein for every 20 pounds of weight. So if you weigh 140 pounds you need 63 grams of protein. In the face of low-carb mania, many are asking how much protein is too much. And are some kinds more dangerous than others? Certainly, there is not much controversy over lean sources of protein, like chicken and fish. We also know that animal protein is a complete protein—meaning that it contains complete amino acids. This type of protein contains everything you need to make new proteins and keep the body's systems running properly. Other sources of protein from nuts, fruits, vegetables, and grains are incomplete proteins and lack all the amino acids that the body can't make from scratch. For vegetarians it is important to eat a wide variety of foods with protein each day.

Some people say that too much protein puts a strain on the kidneys. A report from the *Archives of Internal Medicine* followed thirty subjects eating more than 100 grams of protein a day compared with vegetarians who ate only 30 grams of protein per day. The results showed that with healthy subjects experiencing normal aging, the kidney function was equal in both groups.

Most of the controversy does not come from eating protein; it's the fats that are often found in protein. Somersizers know that fat is our friend. We know that we can enjoy delicious, rich foods and get results. We have read the information in previous books and now understand how we can enjoy fats and still lose weight. What you will find in this book are new studies that have even convinced the skeptical medical community that you can lose weight in a healthy way by including fats in your meals. If you are new to the program you will soon understand this as well. Eating fats is sensible. Fats support healthy cellular function and healthy cellular reproduction. Fats can help you lose weight . . . and they taste incredible! It's true; when you Somersize, you may eat fats and still lose weight. Fats are your friend for life. The key to incorporating fats into your lifestyle is to choose REAL fats, not the fats found in fake, processed foods.

I've spent a great deal of time defending my position on fats. There are still many in the mainstream medical establishment who do not share my opinions about fat, but they can no longer refute the medical studies that prove the contrary. Even still, some believe that dietary fats are the primary cause of weight gain, obesity, and poor health. I don't agree. I watched the fat-free movement come into play. As I have said, I got sucked in and cut back on the fats and started to gain weight. I was not alone! Then I watched the entire nation literally balloon from giving up real fats and loading up on sugar and refined carbohydrates. The results are staggering.

I have done my homework—countless hours of research reading medical journals and having long discussions with leading doctors in the field. Wait until you see the research from the top medical establishments in the world. We've been led to believe that eating fats will make us gain weight, increase our cholesterol, and eventually make us die from heart disease. If you accept that as the truth, then how do you explain the following facts?

When I wrote the first Somersize book in 1996, I quoted the following statistic: "The percentage of adults who are overweight has increased by 10 percent since 1980. Over 37 percent of females and 34 percent of males are now overweight. Obesity is rampant in our country, and everyone thinks fat is to blame." By the time I wrote my last book, *Fast and Easy,* the number of overweight Americans had climbed to 54.9 percent. Just a few years later that statistic is 65 percent, double the percentage from my first book! I believe the fat-free movement started the trend of obesity that is now out of control.

When you Somersize, you may eat double cheeseburgers as long as you do not include the white-flour bun. You may eat eggs fried in bacon fat as long as you pass on the white toast. You may eat chicken with mushroom cream sauce as long as you hold the potatoes. You may pour full-fat dressings on your salads as long as you nix the croutons. You may freely snack on cheese as long as you do not layer it on a cracker. Protein and fats are not the culprit here—it is sugar and refined carbohydrates that are to blame.

Let me recap what Somersizers who have read my previous books already know, and what you may already have guessed if you are new to the program but have read the previous chapters. Go back to what we learned about insulin. Insulin is the fat-storing hormone. Insulin is solely responsible for deciding whether food will be burned as fuel or stored as fat. Insulin must be present for food to be stored as fat. Eating dietary fat causes virtually no secretion of insulin. Without the presence of insulin, food cannot be stored as fat. Regardless of how much fat you eat, the pancreas will not secrete insulin, which is the only way fat can be stored as body fat. As long as you are eating in Somersize combinations, you may eat fat and still lose weight.

If you eat a protein or fat alone, like a piece of meat, your body will break it down easily. These foods will not cause weight gain when eaten alone because they trigger virtually no increase in your blood sugar levels, so there is not a significant insulin response. Proteins and fats can also be eaten in combination with vegetables low in starch (which are also foods that cause little to no insulin production). Therefore, eating eggs, meat, cheese, and butter will not make you fat when eaten in the suggested Somersize combinations.

Let's say you eat proteins or fats with carbohydrates, like meat with potatoes. If your body is in perfect balance, it should use the carbohydrates in the potato for energy, extract the protein and healthy fats from the meat, and discard the remainder. However, if your cells are filled with sugar and will not accept any more, the carbohydrates in the potato will trigger an insulin response that can lead to both the potato and the meat being sent to the fat cells. That is why we save the combination of meat with potatoes for Level Two, when our bodies are back in balance and can handle a secretion of insulin. For the weight-loss phase we will eliminate combinations of meat with potatoes, white bread with cheese, and turkey with yams. I know this may sound difficult, but there are so many other things you can eat in the right combinations that you won't even miss these foods. Once your body is back in balance you may enjoy the pro/fats–carbos combination in moderation.

As I have said all along, fat is not fattening when eaten alone. You can eat fat with other fats, with proteins, or with vegetables in Somersize combinations and still lose weight. What a decadent way to drop the pounds! Forget the dry, skinless chicken breasts—leave on the skin and bring on the sauce! Forget the plain steamed vegetables—bring on the cheese! Forget the sugary, starchy, fat-free desserts . . . bring on the SomerSweet Crème Brûlée made with real cream! Does this information give you a license to live on protein and fats? Of course not. I do not advise you to gorge on fats or any of the Somersize foods. Somersize promotes balanced eating filled with essential nutrients from several food groups.

In addition, fats give you a feeling of being full. Your body will signal you when you've had enough. (Of course, you have to listen!) Unlike refined carbohydrates that you can eat and eat without ever feeling full (yes, we've all downed an entire bag of potato chips!), with fats you can eat only so much and then you just don't want any more. What a thrill it is to know that I can enjoy a piece of Brie without guilt. That does not mean I eat the whole wheel. How wonderful not to feel deprived when you're trying to lose weight! I think that's the main reason Somersizing has been so successful with everyone who has tried it. You can incorporate rich, flavorful foods into your diet and still lose all the weight you want; that helps people stick to the program.

Once again, fats in combination with sugars create the problem. Remember the Cold Stone Creamery ice cream with 620 calories from fat, 150 grams of sugar, and a whopping 201 grams of carbohydrates? The combination of fats with sugars is a recipe for disaster.

FAT AND HEART HEALTH

If you are new to Somersize, you may be thinking to yourself, "Okay, so now that I understand the insulin connection, I see how if I eliminate sugar I can eat fat and still lose weight, but what kind of damage will I do to my cholesterol and heart by eating fats?" I know it is difficult to take years of information and reverse it by reading a few chapters in a book written by the former Chrissy Snow. I may not be a doctor, but I have done my research and the facts are plain to see. That's why I want to share with you the clinical studies that support healthy fats as part of a heart-healthy lifestyle.

We've all been told that a diet low in fat will help improve our cholesterol levels, our risk of heart disease, and our risk of developing certain types of cancer. I'm going to change your thinking about this as well. I am going to replace one word in that sentence. It is a diet low in *sugar* (and refined carbohydrates) that will help improve our cholesterol levels, our risk of heart disease, and our risk for certain types of cancer. When you Somersize, you may eat fat to your heart's content . . . and I mean that literally.

When I first wrote about Somersizing, I had medical reports from twenty-five years that connected high insulin levels to heart disease. It was easy to make the leap that eliminating foods that cause high insulin levels would improve heart health, but for many this information was not enough. Fortunately, there are now several medical studies that support losing weight by cutting sugar and refined carbs. It happened because many concerned physicians set out to prove how dangerous it is to eat fewer carbs if it means consuming more dietary fat. We have the controversy over Dr. Atkins' program to thank for this. As his very-low-carb program grew in popularity, the medical community decided to take matters into their own hands and prove to everyone how dangerous it was to eat proteins and fat without restriction. They launched expensive clinical studies so that they could prove, once and for all, how dangerous fat is for heart health. And the results? Well, what do you know? The doctors were wrong! In study after study, the results were clear. People lost more weight eating high-protein over low-fat and they kept the weight off longer. And even more shocking to the medical establishment: They improved their cholesterol levels and triglyceride levels.

Here are just a few of the studies that support cutting back on sugar and refined carbohydrates to lose weight and improve health.

In 2004 the *New England Journal of Medicine* published a study called "A Randomized Study Comparing the Effects of a Low Carbohydrate Diet and a Conventional Diet on Lipoprotein Subfractions and Reactive Protein Levels in Patients with Severe Obesity." The study set out to compare the effects of a low-carb diet with a conventional diet (restrictive in fat and calories). At the six-month mark, both groups of dieters had similar results in decreasing LDL levels (bad cholesterol) and improving HDL (good cholesterol). Here is where the differences became apparent: The low-carb dieters lost more weight, had a greater decrease in triglycerides, had in increase in insulin sensitivity, and experienced a greater decrease in very-low-density lipoprotein (VLDL) levels. Overall, the study concluded that severely obese individuals on a low-carb diet

may experience benefits with decreases in insulin resistance, blood lipids, and marked inflammation.

Another recent study in the *Journal of the American College of Nutrition* compared women on a low-carb program with women on a low-fat diet. The low-carb women lost more weight and showed improvements in their insulin sensitivity.

One hundred twenty overweight volunteers with high cholesterol participated in a study, published in the *Annals of Internal Medicine*, in which half the group followed a low-carb program and the other half followed a low-fat, reduced-calorie program. Researchers cited the low-carb group had lost significantly more weight (20.7 pounds vs. 10.6 pounds). As for risk factors of cardiovascular disease, both triglyceride levels and cholesterol levels were improved on the low-carb program. In addition, those on the low-carb program, encouraged by their results, were better able to stick with the program.

Harvard researcher Walter C. Willett, M.D., Dr.PH recently published an article in the *Annals of Internal Medicine* stating, "We can no longer dismiss very-low-carbohydrate diets. The findings raise important questions, foremost being the long-term effects on weight." Studies have shown that at the six-month mark, those on low-carb diets lost more weight and were able to stick with the program longer than those on conventional diets. Though conventional wisdom holds that low-fat diets reduce risk for heart disease and cancer, Willett claims there is no evidence to support this notion. Citing four recent studies, Willett showed that low-carb programs reduced harmful triglycerides and increased good cholesterol.

For decades, low-fat diets have been recommended as the common course to lose weight and lower the risk of heart disease. The *Journal of the American College of Nutrition* recently set out to confirm whether low-fat diets actually accomplish this. They launched a study concerning the effect of dietary fat on selected cardiovascular risk factors of healthy yet sedentary men and women. Data showed that a diet that severely restricts fats is not necessarily beneficial to plasma lipoproteins. In addition, the low-fat, high-carbohydrate diet did not show improved serum cholesterol. Plus, this restrictive diet is not easy for the participant to adhere to, thus long-term compliance is poor.

A recently published study in the *American Journal of Clinical Nutrition* examined the correlation between consumption of refined carbohydrates and increasing occurrence of type 2 diabetes in the twentieth century. Researchers found a distinct correlation between obesity and the prevalence of type 2 diabetes, both of which increased proportionally with the consumption of refined carbohydrates. Researchers found no correlation between protein and fat consumption and type 2 diabetes. Rather, it was sugar and high-fructose corn syrup that were associated with the disease. In conclusion, the American diet has gone through dramatic changes in the last twenty years, especially with regard to refined carbohydrates. This consumption has increased the risk of obesity, glucose intolerance, and type 2 diabetes, which has reached epidemic proportions.

A study in Framingham, Massachusetts, has followed the diets and health of a large test group of the city's residents. In the early years this study supported the notion that saturated fats increase our risk of cholesterol. However, Dr. William Castelli, who was the director of the study, changed his tune. In 1992 he said, "In Framingham, Massachusetts, the more saturated fats one ate, the more cholesterol one ate, the more calories one ate, the lower people's serum cholesterol. . . . We found that the people who ate the most cholesterol, the most saturated fat, ate the most calories, weighed the least, and were the most physically active." Most of the women who had better health reports got their fats from eating creamy salad dressings two to three times per week. The moral of the story is: Bring on the blue cheese, creamy Italian, and Caesar dressings and stay away from the tasteless fat-free dressings with ingredient lists that no one can pronounce.

I could go on and on citing scores of studies, but the results are clear. Eating dietary fat does not raise your risk of heart disease. Rather, it is sugar and refined carbohydrates that are to blame for these medical ills. Eating in proper Somersize combinations helps control your insulin levels, which subsequently helps improve your cholesterol. I've heard it time and time again from all of you who have seen the results for yourself. I cannot count the hundreds and hundreds of testimonial letters from people who tell me how their cholesterol profile is improving while they are eating the richest foods of their lives. Their doctors are stunned!

FATS: POLY, MONO, UNSATURATED, SATURATED, AND TRANS

Now that I have eased your concerns about eating fats, I have to give some clarification about what types of fat are recommended and what types should be avoided. A balanced diet, including fat, is essential to life. When I say fat, I don't mean the fat you give your body in the form of cake, or fat from a candy bar, or fat from French fries. There are several different types of fat. Some are good, in fact essential to your health and well-being. Other fats should be eliminated from your diet. There are two main types of fats: saturated and unsaturated. Saturated fats include animal fats, butter, lard, coconut oil, and palm oil. These types of fats are usually solid at room temperature. Unsaturated fats are generally liquid at room temperature. These liquid types of fat are categorized as monounsaturated—such as olive oil, canola oil, and nut oil—or polyunsaturated, such as corn oil or safflower oil. All of these fats are included in the Somersize program.

Trans fats are the fats that come from polyunsaturated fat, such as partially hydrogenated oil. These trans fats are the most unhealthy kind because they are completely unnatural. Margarine is an excellent example. We've been led to believe that margarine is a healthier choice than real butter, because butter is saturated and margarine is unsaturated. But margarine is made by taking a vegetable oil and stripping it of its essential fatty acids. The remainder is processed by forcing hydrogen atoms into it.

When complete, margarine, which comes in a solid state, is actually more saturated than its original liquid form. Trans fats also occur when we heat polyunsaturated fats (such as vegetable oil) to high temperatures for frying. I know it sounds ironic, but you are actually better off frying food in saturated fat—such as butter, lard, or palm kernel oil—or in monounsaturated fat—such as peanut oil—than you are frying it in polyunsaturated oil such as corn, safflower, or vegetable oil. We've been led to believe these polyunsaturated oils are a healthier choice, but beware of frying foods with them because when heated too high, they become the most unhealthy types of fats—trans fats.

In response to the fat scare, many restaurants and food chains boast that they fry only in "cholesterol-free" oils, such as vegetable, corn, or safflower oil. These "healthy" oils in their natural state become dangerous trans fats when heated to high temperatures for frying! Don't be duped by fat-free propaganda. Eating foods filled with these trans fats is bad for our health. Trans fats are rampant in the processed foods we eat. It's not just the fries at restaurants. They appear in almost every snack food that comes in a bag or a box at the grocery store—cakes, cookies, crackers, breads, chips, margarine, bottled salad dressings, and more. Even many of the low-fat varieties of these foods are filled with trans fats.

And why are trans fats so bad for us? They raise your bad cholesterol (LDL) and lower your good cholesterol (HDL). Plus, they muck up your cells with these fake fats and actually block your body from accepting the good fats it needs to produce healthy cells. Sadly, people are eliminating saturated fats, like eggs, cheese, butter, and red meat, thinking they are the culprits for raised cholesterol and heart disease, when in actuality raised insulin levels and trans fats are the problems. Since the introduction of fake foods into our society, we have been on a fast road to weight gain and disease. When I was a child, my mother baked me cookies made with real butter. That was considered a treat. Now cookies are prepackaged in the grocery store, depleted of any real fats and filled with unhealthful trans fats.

Get back to eating real fats like butter, cream, cheese, sour cream, and eggs. Most doctors will tell you that eating foods high in saturated fats is a recipe for weight gain and a heart attack. They will tell you these types of "fatty" foods will raise our cholesterol. They advise us to stick to unsaturated fats in minimal amounts. So how can I share with you my program with a clear conscience when Somersizing supports eating saturated fats to your heart's content? Because I have done the research and have seen that the majority of the medical community is wrong! Finally, we have the mainstream medical establishment sitting up and taking notice of the health benefits of low-carbohydrate programs. Saturated fats are good fats and essential to life. They must be included in our daily meals.

After years of talking to Somersizers and reading the success stories in their moving testimonial letters, it makes more sense to me than ever. People are bringing cheese, cream, and bacon back into their lives, and they have healthier cholesterol levels than ever before. Plus, they're losing weight. This is a dramatic turnaround.

If you can't bring yourself to eat fat because you're still worried about the negative health impact, at least give up the sugar and the refined carbohydrates. If you are giving up fat and still not seeing your cholesterol drop, you must also try giving up the sugar and starches. When you see your cholesterol begin to drop, perhaps you will believe me that you can begin to eat fats and watch your numbers further improve. Then you will be the one writing me a letter to tell me of your success!

Even the die-hard medical conservatives telling us to limit our fat intake and replace real fats with fat substitutes can no longer ignore the evidence. Some still adhere to the low-fat diet, but they are recognizing the need to limit sugar consumption as well. Everyone should have this critical information.

Your body cannot produce fats on its own; therefore, two essential fatty acids must come from the food you eat. The two important essential fatty acids that we must include in our diets to enjoy health and longevity are omega-3 and omega-6. Omega-3 can be found in egg yolks, fish (salmon, tuna, herring, mackerel), nuts, soybeans, canola oil, and flaxseed oil. Omega-6 can be found in egg yolks, dark green leafy vegetables, whole grains, and seeds. (I take a supplement called borage oil that is an excellent source of omega-6, and it also helps tremendously to reduce the symptoms of PMS and menstrual cramps.)

Eggs are a great source of protein and

these healthy fats. Omega-3 and omega-6 essential fatty acids are appropriately named "essential"! I eat as many eggs a week as I want. I often eat three eggs for breakfast and it really keeps me satisfied. I am perfectly content until the next meal. Eating cereal or pancakes won't make you feel that way; an hour or so after eating, you will start craving more sugar or caffeine to make up for the dip in your blood sugar levels. Eat your eggs. The campaign does not lie; they are incredible and edible and a great way to get your protein and healthy fats.

Real fats are necessary for healthy cell reproduction. We need fats to make hormones, and hormones are essential for breaking down old cells and making new ones. "Why is healthy cell reproduction so important?" you ask. The human body is made up of cells. We must produce healthy cells to thrive. When we deny our bodies the nutrients they need for healthy cell reproduction, we will start producing abnormal cells. That's when disease sets in. You should care about healthy cells, because if you don't, your health is at risk. We must have sufficient hormones to make healthy cells, and we must have healthy cells to make more hormones. The health benefit comes from eating real fat in its natural state, like butter, oil, cheese, sour cream, eggs, or fat found in meat or fish.

So make sure to get enough protein and eat your healthy fats! But while you are losing weight, please do not eat them with carbohydrates so that you avoid the release of insulin. Once you get to your goal weight, you may bring back whole-grain carbohydrates in combination with your proteins and fats—in moderation, of course.

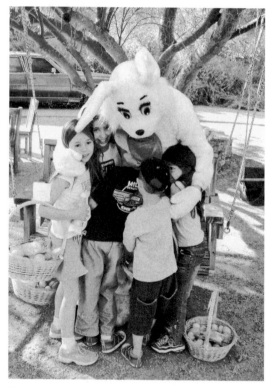

The Easter Bunny lives!

CHAPTER 6

Carbohydrates: Good Carbs That Make You Fit, Bad Carbs That Make You Fat

No food group is more front and center right now than carbohydrates. Before the 1980s we didn't think much of carbs—they were a side dish; some potatoes with our meat, some rice with our chicken, some toast with our eggs. Then we were barraged with the fear of fat and we were told to reduce our intake of protein and fats and eat more carbohydrates. Yes, eat a whole lot of fat-free carbohydrates and you will lose weight and protect yourself from high cholesterol, heart disease, and cancer. What a crock that turned out to be!

For twenty years the fat-free movement swept the nation and we cut out all the real foods and replaced them with anything labeled "fat-free." We counted our fat grams and passed on the butter, cream, bacon, and steaks, yet oddly, none of us were losing weight. Instead we started putting on the pounds. You can see for yourself how the obesity crisis has blossomed in the last twenty years.

Now the pendulum has swung all the way over to the other side and carbohydrates have replaced fat as the evil villain that will make you gain weight. Once again, you have a society of overweight people looking for answers. You start counting again and watching those carbs, but how low is too low?

Ever since Somersize began I have encouraged you to eat carbohydrates. I simply specified what kind of carbohydrates to consume, and what foods to eat with them. Carbohydrates are an important part of any diet because they give us fuel and also because they provide fiber, vitamins, and minerals. Most important, you need all the food groups to have a balanced, healthy diet. This is essential for weight loss, health, and hormonal balance, which, as you know, affects both weight and health.

Carbohydrates are sugars, fibers, and starches: cakes, pies, cookies, breads, cereals, pastas, potatoes, rice, corn, and more. A common way to divide carbohydrates is to call them simple carbohydrates or complex carbohydrates. Simple carbohydrates are sugars, such as white sugar, white flour, and potatoes, and complex carbohydrates include everything made of three or more links of sugars, such as whole grains and vegetables low in starach. Many people will say that we should eliminate simple carbohydrates and include complex carbohydrates, but it's more complicated than that.

The body accepts all carbohydrates as sugar, and you know from earlier reading that when we eat carbs, the body breaks the carbs down into single sugar molecules and absorbs them into the bloodstream. Then the digestible carbohydrates are converted into glucose and used as an energy source. Fiber is the only exception here, since it cannot be broken down into sugar molecules. It actually passes through the body undigested. Plus, fiber slows the release of sugar molecules into the bloodstream. For these reasons, you will see "Net Impact Carbohydrate" claims on my Somersize products and other low-carb products. The net impact carbohydrates are the only carbohydrates that affect blood sugar. Fiber is a carbohydrate, but since it does not affect blood sugar, the carbohydrates from fiber are subtracted from the total carbohydrates. Similarly, sugar alcohols, such as maltitol and glycerine, are carbohydrates, but they have a minimal effect on blood-sugar levels. Therefore, these are also subtracted from the total carbohydrates.

Anyone who has read my earlier Somersize books knows how much I value the glycemic index, an important tool to determine which carbohydrates affect our blood sugar. For example, a potato is actually a complex carbohydrate, yet it is one of the highest-ranking on the glycemic index, meaning that it is absorbed very quickly into the bloodstream, causing a spike in blood sugar. This helps determine which carbohydrates we include when we Somersize, and which we eliminate in order to keep our blood sugar balanced. Sugar, sodas, white bread, white rice, white pasta, potatoes, carrots, and bananas all are high on the glycemic index. If you do not need the energy they supply your body at the time you eat them (i.e., if your cells are filled with sugar), these will be converted to fat and stored for later use. Processing carbohydrates removes the fiber-rich outer bran and the vitamin- and mineral-rich inner germ. These foods are rapidly digested and so they have a higher glycemic index. When we reach our goal weight and have cleaned out the stored sugar in our cells, we can bring back these foods, in moderation, without upsetting our balance.

While we Somersize, we continue to eat good carbohydrates, which are the complex carbohydrates that have less of an effect on blood sugar. These are the carbohydrates that appear on the lower part of the glycemic index. Whole grains are full of fiber and that's why we include a variety of whole-grain breads, pastas, and cereals. These foods are left in their natural state rather than being refined down to a processed food product.

These carbohydrates, with the bran intact, are digested more slowly into the bloodstream and do not impact blood sugar so much.

Let's revisit our discussion of insulin so you can see how the glycemic index is important for insulin production. As I said, carbohydrates are broken down into sugar, which causes the blood sugar to rise. That signals the pancreas to secrete insulin, the hormone that tells the cells to absorb the blood sugar for energy. As the blood sugar is absorbed into the cells, the blood-sugar levels comes back to balance.

A person who has type 1 diabetes does not make enough insulin, so his or her cells cannot absorb the sugar. Type 2 diabetes was formerly known as adult onset diabetes, but the name has been changed because so many kids are developing it! This type of diabetes starts with insulin resistance, then progresses to type 2 diabetes. When someone is insulin resistant, the insulin is telling the cells to absorb the sugar, but the cells do not respond because they are full. This causes the blood sugar and insulin levels to remain high long after they should. In time, this process wears out the cells and insulin production slows or even stops and you end up with type 2 diabetes.

Insulin resistance has been documented to correlate with a myriad of health problems including high blood pressure, high levels of triglycerides, lowering of good cholesterol, increased risk of heart disease, and some forms of cancer. That's why so many people are finally agreeing to give up their carbs! The important thing to remember is that not all carbs create this scenario. That is why Somersize makes sure to

GLYCEMIC INDEX CHART	
Beer	110
Sugar	100
White bread	95
Instant potatoes	95
Honey	90
Jam	90
Cornflakes	85
Popcorn	85
Carrots	85
Potatoes	70
Pasta (from white flour)	65
Bananas	60
Dried fruit	60
Brown rice	50
Whole-wheat bread	50
Whole-wheat pasta	45
Fresh white beans	40
Oatmeal	40
Whole rye bread	40
Green peas	40
Whole cereals	35
Dairy products	35
Wild rice	35
Fresh fruits	35
Dried beans	30
Dark chocolate	22
Fructose	20
Soy	15
Green vegetables	Less than 15
SomerSweet	approx. 5

include the whole grains that are essential to health, balance, and weight loss.

CARBOHYDRATES AND LEVEL TWO

Finally we have all the studies we want to prove that eating protein and fats is a healthy and effective way to lose weight. I believe that eliminating sugar, refined carbohydrates, and high-starch foods is essential to safe, effective, and quick weight loss. In addition, I think it is vitally important to include whole grains so that we are not eliminating this group altogether. The question is, for how long should we separate our protein and fats from our carbohydrates? When you Somersize, once you get down to your goal weight, you need to add back the carbohydrates with your protein meals.

This is essential for balance and healthy cell reproduction. During weight loss when your cells are filled with sugar it is essential to eliminate the foods that would cause more stress on your overloaded cells. When you have reached your goal weight and cleaned out your cells of the stored sugar, it then becomes just as important to add back a moderate amount of carbohydrates with your protein meals.

Dr. Diana Schwarzbein has been my doctor for many years now. She is a leading, cutting-edge endocrinologist and has an incredible understanding of the hormonal system. In addition, she has been my good friend and teacher. One of the main things I have learned from Dr. Schwarzbein is how

---

QUINOA

Quinoa—pronounced "keen-wa"—is an ancient grain that comes from the Incas. Many call it the world's most perfect food. The Incas called it the "mother grain" because of the plant's ever-bearing qualities. They considered it a sacred plant and used it in rituals. Ironically, although it is categorized as a grain, it is technically a fruit! Cultivation of this tiny, disk-shaped so-called "grain" began about 3,000 years ago in Peru and Bolivia. Just one cup contains a whopping twenty-two grams of complete protein! And it contains calcium, phosphorus, B vitamins, and iron. Perfect for vegetarians looking for nonanimal sources of protein. Plus, the carbohydrates in quinoa are released very slowly into the bloodstream. Quinoa is also low in gluten. Many people have negative reactions to gluten, so quinoa is perfect for them. With its low-glycemic index it's a perfect Somersize grain.

The bonus is that it tastes delicious. This is my new favorite grain. It's not only superhealthy, it also is convenient since it cooks in about fifteen minutes! I use it as a side dish or in salads, and it's delicious in soups. Check out my recipes for it in the recipe section. I just love it. You can find it at some grocery stores and most health food stores. I hope you will experiment with this great new taste!

---

essential it is for our hormones to add back those carbohydrates to the protein meals when we reach Level Two. Diana and I differ when it comes to weight loss. She believes in having protein, fat, and carbohydrate at every meal for a slow and steady weight loss. I believe in eating whole-grain carbohydrates separately, because you achieve weight loss much faster, which makes it easier for people to stick to the program. Then when you get to Level Two, I ask you to add the carbohydrate back so that you can give your body what it needs once it's in perfect balance and your cells are cleaned out of their stored sugar.

The only exception to this rule for Somersizers is when you hit a plateau or when you burn out your adrenals. A plateau or burnt-out adrenals signals a hormonal imbalance, which must be addressed to continue your weight loss. You can read a full explanation of this in Chapter 12.

SEROTONIN: THE FEEL-GOOD HORMONE

As you know by now, if one hormone in the body is off, it can throw off the entire hormonal system. Let me explain how eating too many or too few carbohydrates can affect your serotonin levels and your weight-loss goals.

"STRESSED" IS "DESSERTS" SPELLED BACKWARD

Why do we crave sweets or carbs when we are stressed or feeling down? It's not just a play on words. Eating carbohydrates actually creates a hormone release that makes us feel better—at least temporarily. When we eat carbohydrates, it stimulates the release of the hormone serotonin. Serotonin makes you feel good. It's a soothing hormone. That's why we crave comfort foods or even junk food when we are stressed or feeling down. Eating these foods gives us the blast of serotonin to make us feel good. If you are cutting carbs too low for too long, and there is no ongoing serotonin production in your body, your brain will cry out for carbohydrates (sugar, carbohydrates, or caffeine) to raise your serotonin levels. Bingeing on these forbidden foods will lead to the roller coaster of blood sugar levels to which I referred in earlier sections. Your blood sugar is elevated, then lowered below its starting point, which leads to craving more sugar or carbohydrates. It creates that "sugar low" that leads to cycles of overeating the very foods that cause the problem.

When it feels as though your blood-sugar levels have dropped below normal range, what you are actually experiencing is the side effect of rising adrenaline levels. We have all had this experience when we feel depressed and crave comfort foods like mashed potatoes, macaroni and cheese, or chocolate. This is your body asking for carbohydrates so that it can "cure" your depression with a blast of serotonin.

Unfortunately, "curing" depression wreaks havoc on your diet. Balanced serotonin levels make it more likely that you will be able to eat in a healthy way. Without balanced serotonin levels, the brain sends powerful signals that can make willpower ineffective, no matter how much you want to change. Ironically, overconsumption of carbohydrates creates a low-serotonin state; and similarly, eating very few carbohydrates for extended periods of time will eventually lead to a low-serotonin state. Unfortunately, you can't balance your serotonin levels with a supplement from a health food store; serotonin is produced only by your body and by the foods you ingest.

The way to keep your serotonin balanced is to eat the right ratio of proteins, fats, and carbohydrates. For Somersizing purposes, we eat a variety of these foods throughout the day. Remember, fruits and vegetables are carbohydrates as are the whole-grain carbohydrates we enjoy. This is where my program differs from other "low-carb" diets. My beliefs are based on science and on the premise that we require protein, fats, and carbohydrates for healthy cell reproduction. Balance is the key.

When we eat too few or too many carbohydrates, we may experience hypoglycemia (low blood sugar). The symptoms of hypoglycemia are nausea, shakiness, clamminess, sweating, lightheadedness, irritability, racing heart, anxiety, and carbohydrate craving. If you continue in a low-serotonin state, you will keep craving carbohydrates. On the other hand, if you keep overconsuming carbohydrates, you will never lose the weight you desire, your insulin levels will remain elevated, the cravings for carbohydrates (sugar) will never go away, and the merry-go-round of your weight will continue.

Just remember that continually depriving yourself of carbohydrates is as bad as overconsuming them. I had to go to Dr. Schwarzbein

a few years ago to help me find out why I was gaining weight, even though I was living in Level One and eating almost no carbs. She explained to me that by eliminating the carbohydrates so severely and for such a long time, I had depleted my serotonin levels. Without knowing it, I was craving sugars in some form and cheating on the side. The only way to address this issue was by adding some kind of carbohydrate to every meal, like a small potato, whole grains, or a high-starch vegetable.

At first I resisted; potatoes are the evil insulin raiser and master of all Funky Foods! I had long talks with Diana about this and she tutored me on the importance of the entire hormonal system being in balance. If one hormone is depleted, the entire hormonal system can be disrupted. Sure enough, as soon as I added some carbohydrate to my Protein/Fats meals (even an occasional small potato!), my weight gradually returned to normal.

Please refer to the sections on Level Two for more explanations of how to add back the carbohydrates in a way that will help you to balance your hormones and achieve your goals. When you add back the carbohydrates, you must modify your program to make it work to your advantage. This means eating a moderate amount of carbohydrates with your protein meals and not overdoing it on the saturated fats. Since you have the presence of insulin with the carbohydrates, you don't want to include too many fats that could be trapped and stored. I will explain this in detail in the coming sections.

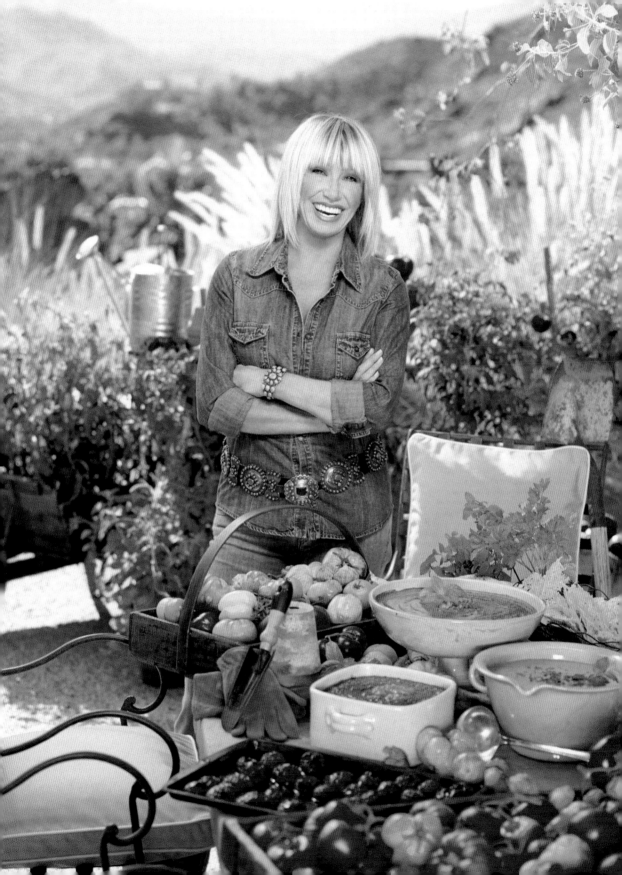

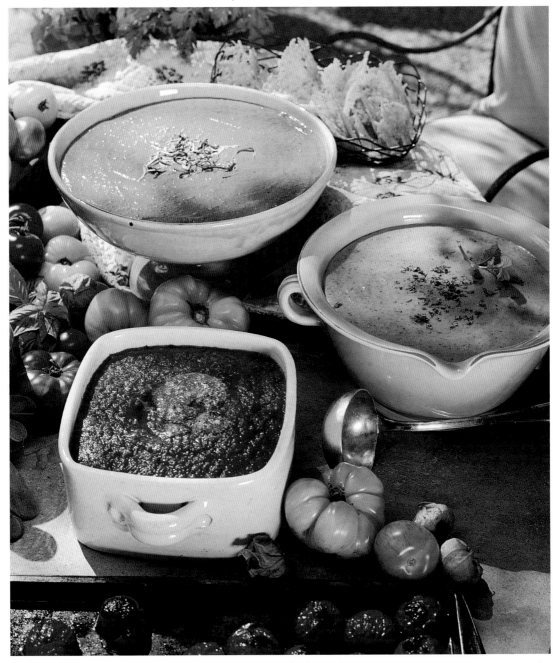

A closer look at my three delicious tomato soups (clockwise from top): Summer Tomato Soup with Black Pepper Parmesan Crisps, Grilled Tomatillo and Red Onion Soup with Fresh Mint, and Roasted Tomato Soup (pictured with Basil Pistou).

PRECEDING PAGE: With a bountiful harvest of heirloom tomatoes I made three soups and a tray of Candied Tomatoes on the baking sheet.

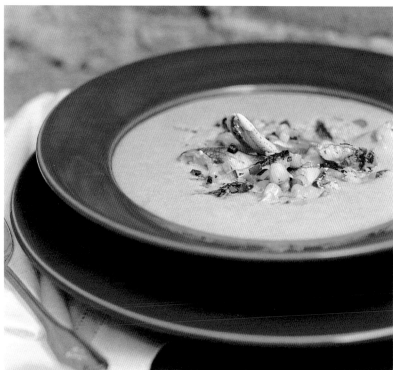

This Crab Bisque with Sweet Corn and Crab Relish will rock your world!

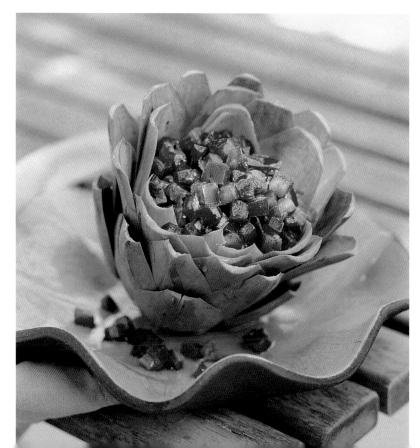

Who says you have to give up bruscetta? I serve it in a beautiful artichoke "flower" and use the leaves instead of bread.

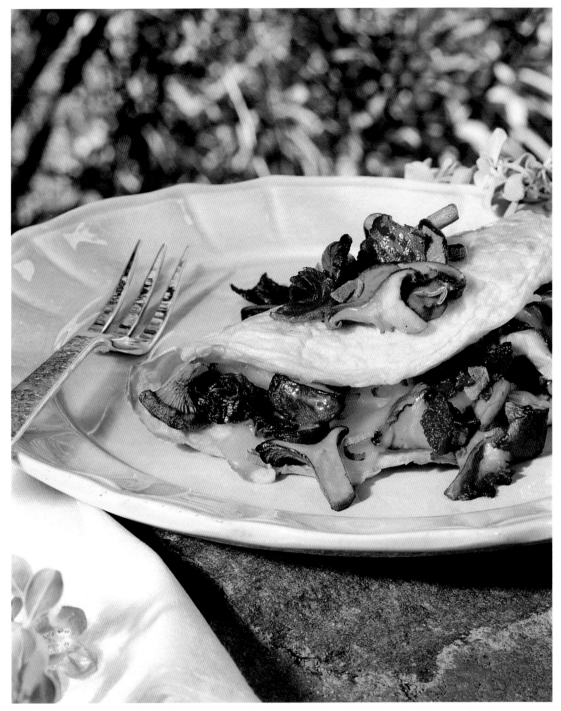

My Omelette with Fontina, Wild Mushrooms, Pancetta, and Sage makes for a perfect morning.

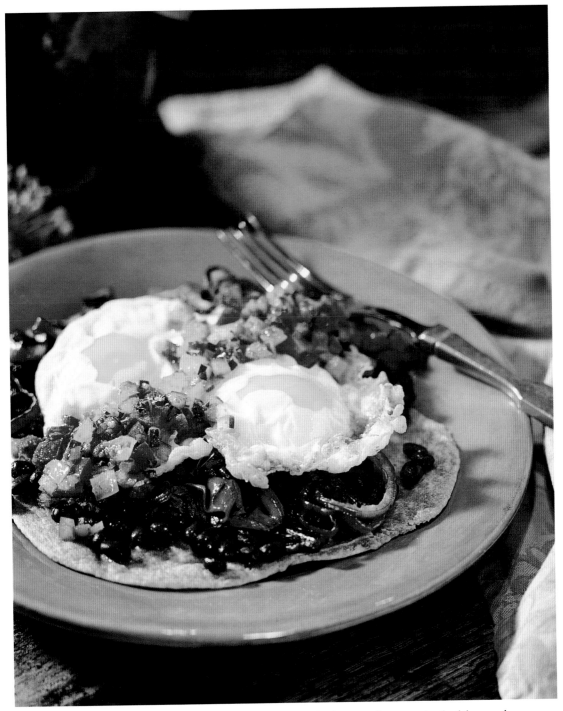

A scrumptious dish of New Mexican Huevos. The key is Alan's method of frying the eggs in olive oil.

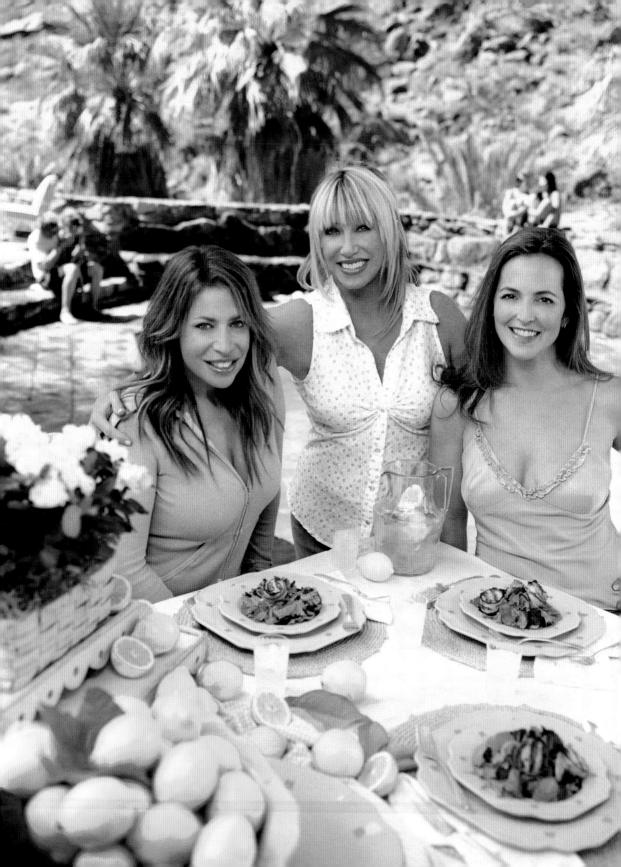

OPPOSITE: A poolside lunch with my beautiful and talented girls—Leslie (who runs the apparel department) and Caroline (who runs Somersize). My son, Bruce, is getting the kids out of the pool to join us for SomerSweet Lemonade and Grilled Scallops Wrapped in Pancetta with Baby Greens.

RIGHT: Grilled Scallops Wrapped in Pancetta with Baby Greens are served on my beautiful Suzanne Somers green dishes with tiny violets.

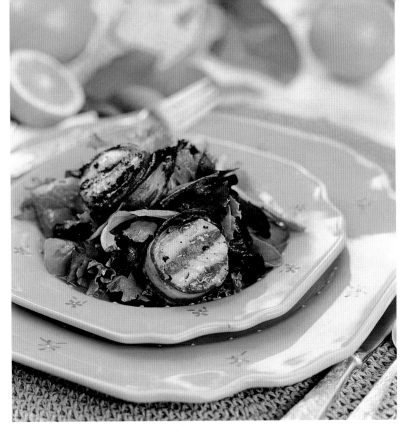

LEFT: Thai Beef with Cucumber Salad served over Asian Greens with Soy Vinaigrette and Soba Noodles. Divine!

FOLLOWING PAGE: Who says fiber can't be delicious? A harvest of whole grain dishes that can make a meal (clockwise from top): Whole-Wheat Fettuccine with Candied Tomatoes, Red Rice, Sautéed Herb Quinoa, Baby Black Lentil Salad, and Quinoa Tabbouleh.

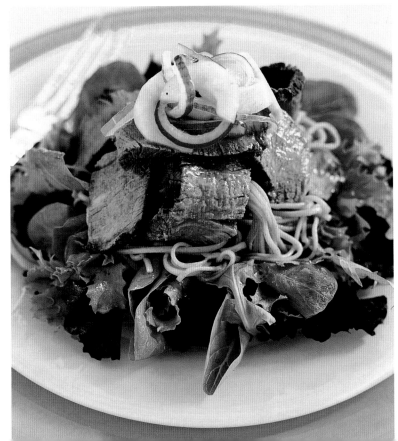

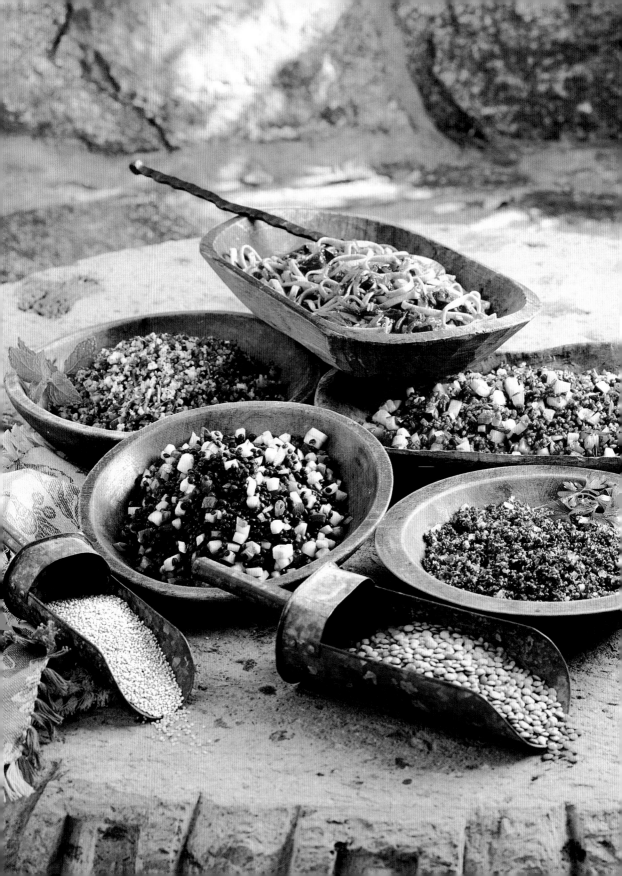

CHAPTER 7

Fruits and Vegetables—Your Best Defense Against Disease

There are a lot of differing opinions when it comes to nutrition, but just about everyone agrees that fruits and vegetables are essential for good health. "Eat your fruits and vegetables!" We've heard it all our lives, and no wonder. They are rich in vitamins, minerals, fiber, carbohydrates (the good kind), and phytochemicals. Eating a diet rich in fruits and vegetables has also been linked to many health benefits such as reduced risk of cancer, stroke, heart disease, and high blood pressure.

Other low-carb programs recommend severely cutting back on fruits and vegetables, lumping them with other carbohydrates. Despite their obvious health benefits, other programs say you should stay away from many fruits and veg-

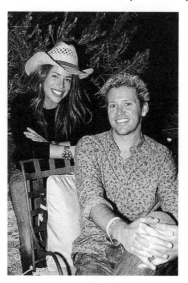

Leslie and Bruce.

etables while you are losing weight. But not with Somersize. I eat fruit and I want you to eat real food. Eating real food helps our bodies to create and reproduce healthy cells. Processed foods and trans fats damage healthy cells by introducing free radicals into the system. Free radicals are molecules that carry an extra electron. Since electrons need to be paired off, these free radicals roam through the system and try to steal electrons from healthy cells. This process damages the system on a cellular level. If you eat processed junk food with trans fats, refined carbohydrates, and sugar, you are introducing free radicals into your system. How do we combat free radicals? Antioxidants, like those found in fruits and vegetables, neutralize free radicals. If we do not have enough antioxidants to neutralize the free radicals, we are accelerating the metabolic aging process.

FRUITS, VEGETABLES, AND HEART DISEASE

Heart disease is one of the leading causes of death in this country. A Harvard study showed that men and women who ate eight or more servings a day of fruits and vegetables had a 20 percent lower risk of heart disease compared with those who ate fewer than three servings a day. Dark green leafy vegetables (like broccoli and spinach) and fruits high in vitamin C were regarded as the most beneficial. Results also showed that even one serving of fruits and vegetables had a real impact on heart disease. For every extra serving, the decrease in risk of heart disease dropped by 4 percent.

Fruits and vegetables are filled with a number of nutrients that help protect the heart: fiber, which helps to reduce blood clots; potassium, which can help with blood

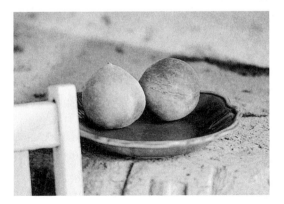

pressure; folate, which can help lower a heart-disease-promoting amino acid called homocysteine. In fact, in a study of 80,000 female nurses, the subjects with the highest intake of folate and vitamin B_6 had nearly half the heart disease of those who were low in both. Foods high in folate include orange juice, eggs, and dark green leafy vegetables. For vitamin B_6 include chicken, milk, fish, and whole grains.

LYCOPENE AND PROSTATE CANCER AND MACULAR DEGENERATION

More and more evidence is showing the benefits of lycopene. Lycopene is a carotenoid found in high concentrations in cooked tomato products. Lycopene is a natural pigment that gives tomatoes their red color. Two major studies suggest that a diet rich in lycopene delivers benefits such as resisting heart disease and prostate cancer. In a 2002 Harvard Medical School study of 48,000 men, it was found that consuming tomato products more than twice a week, as opposed to never, was associated with a reduced risk of prostate cancer of up to 34 percent. For women, the data compiled from the Women's Health Study showed that lycopene may reduce the risk of heart disease in middle age and older women by as much as 33 percent.

Interestingly, cooked tomatoes deliver higher levels of lycopene than uncooked. The lycopene is better absorbed into the bloodstream when the tomatoes have been cooked or processed into ketchup, sauce,

FIBER

Rough it with fiber! Experts agree that fiber is an essential part of a healthy diet, shown to reduce the risk of developing heart disease, diabetes, diverticular disease, and constipation. Most of us know that fiber is good for us, but how much do we need and what is the best source?

Fiber actually refers to carbohydrates that cannot be digested. Fiber is present in all plant material that is eaten as food, including fruits, vegetables, grains, and legumes. In addition to the diseases above, constipation is the most common gastrointestinal complaint in the United States and is of particular concern to older people. Fiber helps to relieve constipation. Wheat bran and oat bran seem to be even more effective than fiber from fruits and vegetables.

The average American eats only fourteen to fifteen grams of dietary fiber per day even though one should consume twenty to thirty-five grams per day, according to health guidelines. Children two and over should consume at least their age plus five grams per day, meaning a five-year-old needs ten grams per day, while a ten-year-old needs fifteen grams per day.

It is important to increase fiber gradually, since taking too much suddenly can cause severe gastrointestinal distress. Also, it's important to drink water, since fiber absorbs water.

What are the best ways to get your fiber? Fresh fruits, vegetables, nuts, legumes, and whole-grain foods. Here are some tips for increasing your fiber intake.

> *Snack on raw vegetables instead of chips, crackers, or candy.*
> *Eat the whole fruit, rather than just drinking the juice.*
> *Replace white rice, bread, and carbohydrates with brown rice and whole-grain products.*
> *Eat whole-grain cereal for breakfast.*
> *Add legumes to your diet—as snacks or as a complete meal with whole grains.*

And don't forget, SomerSweet is blended with natural, sweet fiber from chicory. We don't add maltodextrin like other sweeteners do. We use pure, probiotic fiber—fiber your body needs anyway! And what a delicious way to add it to your diet.

soup, juice, or other products. Lycopene is two and a half times more bioavailable from tomato paste than from fresh tomatoes. There is also evidence that lycopene may halt the onset of macular degeneration, a major cause of blindness in people over sixty-five. My mother suffered from macular degeneration and I am genetically at risk. You bet I am eating my cooked tomatoes!

FOLATE AND COLON CANCER

Folate is found in dark green leafy vegetables such as lettuces, broccoli, spinach, kale, chard, dandelion, and more. The Harvard School of Public Health has linked a decreased risk of colon cancer with high levels of folate. Folate can be eaten in the form of dark green leafy vegetables (which you will be enjoying with vigor on the Somersize program!) or can be taken as a nutritional supplement.

FRUITS, VEGETABLES, AND STROKE

Research has shown that a diet rich in fruits and vegetables may also reduce the risk of stroke. Ischemic stroke, like coronary heart disease, is caused by the blockage of blood vessels. Studies show that those who eat at least five servings of fruit and vegetables every day have a 30 percent lower risk of ischemic stroke. Cruciferous vegetables (like broccoli), green leafy vegetables (like spinach), and citrus fruits and juices seem to

provide the greatest benefit. Unlike low-carb programs that have you count your carbs, I encourage you to eat as many fruits and low-starch vegetables as you like. They taste great, they fill you up, and they are so good for you!

ARE YOU GETTING ENOUGH?

As you can see, fruits and vegetables are our best defense against disease and clearly play an important role in any good diet. It's not only important to get plenty of them, but you need variety to ensure that you get the wide array of nutrients found in different types. Make sure to include dark green leafy vegetables; yellow, orange, and red fruits and vegetables; cooked tomatoes; and citrus fruits. Although the recommended daily allowance is five servings, many experts are suggesting that the number should be increased to nine servings per day.

PLANT A GARDEN

For years I have transported fresh produce to my home in the desert: crates of Roma tomatoes in the spring for making my favorite candied tomatoes, heirloom tomatoes to have with basil and my friend Marco's olive oil, peaches in the summer, cases of fresh persimmons around Thanksgiving—anything in season to capitalize on the flavor of seasonal, fresh, farm-grown, organic fruits and vegetables. All the while I complained that I couldn't get good pro-

KALE: THE GREEN LEAFY MOGUL

Where can you get 240 percent of your recommended allowance of vitamin A? In a single cup of kale! This supervegetable is the king of the dark green leafy vegetables. It also has 71 percent of your vitamin C and a host of other wonderful vitamins and minerals like B_6, manganese, calcium, copper, iron, B_1, B_2, and E. Plus, it contains fiber and a concentrated amount of beta-carotene.

This is your anticancer vegetable. Here's how it works. Cruciferous vegetables, such as kale, broccoli, and cauliflower, contain sulforaphane, which triggers the liver to produce enzymes that detoxify cancer-causing chemicals. These enzymes also inhibit chemically induced breast cancers (shown in animal studies) and induce colon cancer cells to commit suicide. Now a study in the Journal of the American College of Nutrition *shows that sulforaphane also helps stop the proliferation of breast cancer cells, even in later stages of growth.*

Plus, kale is loaded with carotenoids like lutein and zeaxanthin. These act like filters for your eyes to prevent damage from excessive exposure to ultraviolet light. Studies have shown these protective effects reduce the risk of cataracts, a condition in which the eyes become clouded, leading to blurred vision.

Kale is also known to boost the immune system, help protect against rheumatoid arthritis, improve cardiovascular health, and make for healthy bones. You must find a way to include this fabulous food in your lifestyle. And it's delicious! Try it sautéed with garlic and olive oil. It's a great side dish with your protein meals.

duce anywhere but at the farmers' market. So, for all those years, I carried my precious cargo up the hill to my kitchen in the desert to enjoy the most delicious foods in season.

It only took me twenty-seven years to have this next epiphany . . . Duh! What was I thinking? I have a bit of property; I could grow my own garden. Yes! A four-season organic garden filled with all the wonderful fruits and vegetables that I have been trans-porting all this time from Los Angeles. Then I got excited. The possibilities kept me awake at night. I could customize this garden with all my favorite foods: delicious California avocados, the small ones with the creamy texture; heirloom tomatoes, the juicy, tasty, most delicious varieties; Roma tomatoes to dry in the hot desert sun with fresh lemon thyme that I could grow by the bushelful; small baby Japanese tomatoes, just to pop in my mouth while I am busy gathering vegetables. Papaya trees; mango trees, the creamy Manila variety. Strawberries (nothing is as delicious as just-picked strawberries, still hot from the sun), Fuji apples, baby lettuce, romaine lettuce, garlic, onions (the yellow and the red, plus sweet Vidalias), several varieties of basil, watermelons, cantaloupe (the small Israeli variety known for their fantastic flavor), pumpkins, squash, zucchini, peach trees, Mexican limes, Meyer lemons, and on and on and on.

With a little ingenuity any of us can find a place somewhere (even if it is a sunny windowsill) to grow something that we love. It's a different experience to eat something you have grown and nurtured yourself. The French call it *terroir,* which means "of the earth." Ever notice that the produce in France is like nothing we get in our supermarkets here in America? The French feel strongly about the food they eat. It starts with the soil, and the health of that soil; then it's about the sunshine and the love of nurturing that food through the entire growing season. Watering and keeping the soil healthy is all part of the process that eventually leads to that first bite. In that bite you can actually experience the entire process of growing from beginning to the ultimate end when it is in your mouth. It puts you in touch with your food. When you grow it yourself you tend not to gobble it down. You think about the process, and now you are part of the food chain. It's a truly wonderful experience. For those of you who have a decent plot of land to plant an exten-sive garden, you will be able to experience that joy, as I am able, knowing that you were there every step of the way, knowing that the food you are eating has not been contaminated with sprays and poisons, knowing that you are able to give to your family the healthiest, best-tasting, most desirable food. For smaller areas, try potted gardens!

So much of our poor health as a nation has to do with our environment. It takes effort to avoid the pollutants that are part of our everyday lives. Planting your own garden gives you an edge on staying healthy, and the rewards of eating food so delicious go without saying. Think about it. Having your own garden, even if it is only on a windowsill, is a calming experience; it takes the stress out of the day, it puts you in touch with nature. There is a quote by Frank Lloyd Wright that I love: "Nature is the only face of God you will ever see." When you plant your own garden you will get in touch with that. Living our lives is about being in touch with those things that are important. When you are working in your vegetable garden, the desire for that new dress, or that new car, or those earrings you saw at the jewelry store seems to disappear. When you are working with nature, those other material things just don't seem all that important.

Give it a try. Think about your favorite foods, plant in whatever space you have available, and experience the pure joy of the first taste to come. It's better than therapy. Enjoy.

Part Three

SOMERSIZE —
THE PROGRAM

CHAPTER 8

Somersize Scrapbook and Photo Album

I am so knocked out by these success stories. What a fabulous look into the lives of Somersizers everywhere. The results are nothing short of astounding. I am so touched by each and every one of your letters. Thank you for sending them to me at SuzanneSomers.com. I do read them and wish I could send a personal response to each one of you. I am so proud that this program has helped you to make the commitment. Many of you say I changed your life. I didn't do it. You did it! You are the ones who accepted the information and put it to work. You are the ones who resisted temptation for the greater good of health. You are the ones who have made yourselves stronger. You are the success stories!

To those of you reading these letters and wishing it were you, you are next. Let these remarkable people inspire you to soak up this information and make it your new lifestyle. If you are looking for support, go to my Web site. Register with me so that I can send you updates on the program. Then go to Community and join the chat room or read over the posts on the discussion boards. Look through the FAQs and you will find answers to most of the questions you have about Somersize. Go to the Photo Album to see many more postings. We are there to help you and support you.

You are on your way to the new you. Then don't forget to send me your testimonial letter and photos!

December 2004

Dear Suzanne:

I could fill this page with "thank-yous" and it would still fall short of the gratitude I'd like to express. Weight has been an issue all of my life. From early childhood—with my mom dragging me to diet doctors for who knows what kind of pills—to trying every diet imaginable. I'd lose, only to gain it back plus more. I lost almost 60 pounds three years ago on Somersizing, but going through the change it piled back on.

As you can see in my "before" picture, I was miserable! In fact, there aren't many "before" pictures of me. I was always the one taking everyone else's picture . . . or hiding behind someone else if I could. It's tough enough growing old gracefully when you hate what you see in the mirror, but far worse being so despondent that you simply don't care. And my old friend Somersize wasn't working for me either. Then I realized why—my hormones were so out of whack my body wasn't working properly.

Then I saw you on TV discussing *The Sexy Years*—whoa, talk about a lightbulb moment . . . every one of your seven dwarfs was at my house, too! I ordered your book, made my doctor appointment for hormone testing, and found I was totally depleted of estrogen. Within two weeks of starting my compounded natural hormones, I noticed my symptoms diminish and the weight started melting, too!

The "after" picture is still a work in progress, but such a happier person to be around. In just five and a half months of Somersizing, I am 2 pounds from my first goal. I've lost 28 pounds, $11^3/_4$ inches, and 12.60 lbs of body fat. I exercise daily (for the first time in my life), I'm

eating fabulous food (desserts, too), my hormones are back in balance, and my darling husband of thirty-one years is happy to have his vibrant wife dragging him into the bedroom again! I will be a Somersizer and BioId girl for life.

Suzanne, I thank you every day for changing my life! Your books have given me better health, weight loss, and hormonal balance, and I am further blessed with your wonderful online chat room—meeting new friends who offer support and motivation daily as we challenge and encourage each other to be our best. "Who'da thunk" that the funny blonde I loved to watch on TV would grow up to be such a humanitarian? I understand why everyone thinks they are your biggest fan, because you have touched our lives in so many ways. You are my hero!

I truly am a butterfly coming out of my cocoon, and cannot thank you enough for helping me through my metamorphosis. Thanks from the bottom of my heart for helping me find the fun girl I thought I would never see again.

With love,
Sherri Elliott

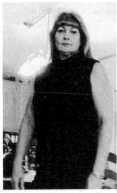
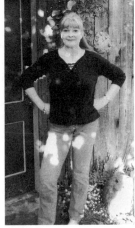

before   Sherri lost 28 lbs!   after

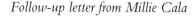

Dear Suzanne:

Grid from our chat room urged me to write and tell you of my wonderful health benefits since Somersizing. I have lost 22 pounds since April 22, 2003, but even more important, as a diabetic, I have gone from a total of 65 units of insulin (three shots a day) to insulin free as of Aug. 20th. Two weeks ago I had a reduction in blood pressure medication. I am on half of the medication, and my cholesterol is down to 153 total and HDL is 91.

Needless to say, my doctor is happy, but not HAPPIER than I am. I really am so glad! Grid said, "Tell Suzanne your age!" I am seventy-two years old and since Somersizing feel so much more energetic.

Your plan is a WOE (way of eating) and I am grateful that you introduced us to this. I am convinced that this will be my way of life.

My daughter started Somersizing a month before me and she is down 45 pounds. She lives in San Diego and will be front row center for your show on January 22nd.

Thank you, Suzanne. What wonderful support!
Millie Cala

Follow-up letter from Millie Cala

July 8, 2004

Dear Suzanne,

This is an update to my e-mail sent in November 2003.

I stated then that I am no longer on insulin shots for diabetes. That is still true, which will be one year in August. More good news, though. I no longer need blood pressure medication and my readings have been perfect.

I joined a health club and have been doing water aerobics two or three times a week. I also use my BodyRow™, not bad for a seventy-three-year-old!! I really don't feel my age.

I owe you great big thanks for this WOE (way of eating). Together with the exercise, I have had so many wonderful health benefits. Somersizing is not only my WOE, but also my way of life.

I enjoy going to your chat room, it really is great for support. When I visit the site, it's like talking to old friends, which they really have become.

The attached picture of me was taken about three weeks ago.

Keep up the great work, Suzanne.

Regards,
Millie Cala

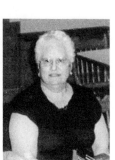

before   after

December 7, 2004

Dear Suzanne:

If only I had learned the concepts of your program over thirty years ago, I could have avoided all the emotional ups and downs that a lifetime of fluctuating weight has caused me. My roller coaster ride began in my late teens/early twenties. I have tried so many of the conventional diet plans, but when something did work, it was only temporary. If only I had known that sugar is the "white poison" and the demon in disguise!!!

I am fifty-four years old and began your plan in May of 2003. By November of 2003, I had lost 30 lbs and had gone from size 14—16 to a size 8. I am so thrilled to report that I have maintained the weight loss, and am now a size 6, and have bought a few 4s. Never have I felt so healthy and so alive!! It is a brand-new way of life and a totally changed state of mind!!

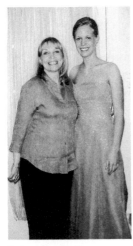

before, size 14-16   after, size 4-6

Everyone around me says "Wow," and wants to know the secret to my success. But what means the most to me is when my twenty-five-year-old son keeps telling me how proud he is of me and my accomplishments!!

Suzanne, I can't begin to thank you enough for turning my life around!!

With heartfelt thanks,
Linda Cohen

December 7, 2004

Dear Suzanne:

When I turned forty years old, I knew I would have to do something to lose weight or else I'd start seeing serious health problems, given how overweight I was. Worse still, my life was a constant hassle with little energy to do things, always having to ask for chairs without armrests in restaurants, and having to ask for seatbelt extenders on airplanes. And oh those poor people that had to sit beside me on the planes!

I tried another plan for a couple weeks, but it was too strict for me. I looked into stomach operations, but they scared me too much and so I did nothing for a couple of years. I was beginning to think that I'd have to get that stomach operation anyway when a friend told me about the Somersize plan. It sounded so simple because there was absolutely no counting to do and it didn't sound strict at all. I figured I'd give it a try and see if it actually worked.

If it didn't, I knew the stomach operation was my only alternative. Believe me, that alone gave me a lot of incentive to take your

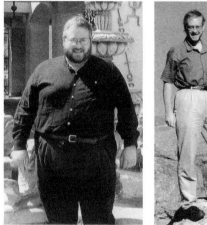

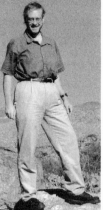

before, 390 lbs   after, 200 lbs

Dean lost 189 lbs!

plan seriously! And that has paid off hand-
somely. I started in June of 2003 at a weight
of about 390 pounds and have now lost 189
pounds in just eighteen months.

Thank you, Suzanne, for helping me
change my life!

Dean Cooper

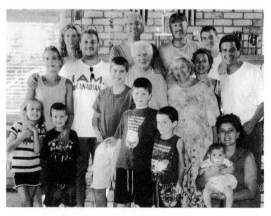

after, the Daley Family—150 lbs. lighter

Dear Suzanne:

I've been Somersizing for two years now,
along with my older brother. It took a while,
but with all the weight loss and great-tasting
food we enjoyed, the rest of the family finally
joined in this past summer!

There are now ten of us Somersizing! We've
lost more than 150 pounds combined, but
more important, we feel great and love our big
family get-togethers, which usually feature a
variety of great-tasting food!

Eating and staying slim has never been so
easy and so enjoyable!

Thanks!

Your fans in Winnipeg,
The Daleys

November 23, 2004

Dear Suzanne:

My name is Heather Fenner. I am a stay-at-
home mom of three. I have been a Somersizer
(even throughout my pregnancy, only gaining
25 lbs) for four years now. I can't thank you
enough for this lifestyle. Thanks to you I am now
past my goal weight. I just had my third and last
baby seven and a half months ago. Because of
Somersizing, I am in a size 6 to 8 ALREADY.

I look great, feel great, and I am healthy. I
love that I get to eat. I do exercise regularly, for
the muscle tone of course! And these days,
there are so many endless possibilities in the
sugar-free market. Actually, after a while you
don't even miss sugar.

I LOVE your sauces and mixes, and I could

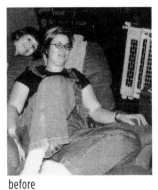
before

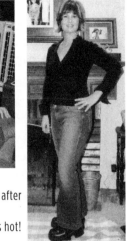
after

Heather looks hot!

not live without your BBQ sauce and ketchup. Oh my gosh, it's better than Heinz and I love Heinz. The recipes that I have come up with are amazing as well, like my artichoke dip with your Parmesan chips.

There have been times when my weight would fluctuate, even when I wasn't pregnant. So I just dove right back in and lost it, fast. It is so easy and fun! I can't imagine my life with sugar right now. You really notice a difference in how you feel if you combine those FUNKY FOODS into your lifestyle, as that's what SOMERSIZE is, a LIFESTYLE.

At one point, I even tried to get into acting because I felt so good. WHATEVER!! That didn't work out, but at least Somersizing gave me the confidence. That says a lot about you. You're a girl's girl. Thank you for that.

Thank you, Suzanne. You are an awesome friend. I am so excited to tell you how appreciated you are. I am pretty hot now; my husband thanks you as well.

Lots of thanks and grace,
Heather Fenner

December 2004

Dear Suzanne:

I am not sure how to begin this, but I guess the best way is to start from the beginning.

When my late husband and I got married on Valentine's Day, 1993, I was a size 4. Now mind you, that only happened because I had just lost 186 lbs. on one of the "little boxes" plans.

I know that you know how this is going to end . . . badly! The minute I started eating "outside of the box," so to speak—back came the weight. First 10 lbs, then 20 lbs, then 50 lbs; and so on and so on.

Fast-forward to 1996. That was the year that I lost my mom. Any motivation that I might have had went right out the window, and by the end of 1997 I was right back where I started.

I had been carrying this weight around for six more years, and it just kept getting worse.

Between the time that I lost my mom and now, I lost my husband, my job of thirteen years, and was out of work for one and a half years, when I decided I couldn't control anything else in my life, at least I would control my weight!!

Enter Somersize. I cannot tell you what a blessing you and your wonderful program have been to me. On May 1, 2003, while watching you on HSN, I had what can only be explained as an epiphany, and made up my mind that I could use your plan to achieve a good, healthy weight loss—something that I could maintain for LIFE!!

I started on that very day. I threw out each and every piece of food that contained any white flour or sugar. I went to the store and bought chicken, turkey, fish, vegetables, fruit, and water.

The simple parameters that you lay out were the easiest thing for me to assimilate.

After one week, I had dropped 5 lbs. By the end of the first month, I had lost 10, the second month 20, and so it went for the next eight months. I pretty much lost 10 lbs per month on a steady basis.

I was lucky enough to speak to you on HSN when I was at the 65-lb mark and then again at 98. It was such a pleasure to speak to you. You said to me, "I can tell from listening to you, you get it, you really get it." That was true. It is a way of life for me now.

I talk about you and your program wherever I am. People are constantly asking me how I did it. I always say one word, SUZANNE!! That is how I feel, truly. I know that it was me doing all the work and staying focused, there is no doubt of that, but it was listening to you and hearing the testimonials of other Somer-sizers that got me started.

I thank you from the bottom of my heart, Suzanne. Thank you for caring enough about your "ladies" to develop this program and all the delicious foods that you have come out with since I started. My kitchen is a Suzanne pantry. That is pretty much all I have in the cupboards, all those cute little colorful boxes.

Everything is so delicious and sat-isfying. I have no cravings for any-thing that you have not provided an answer for, and one thing is better than the next. I take my salad dress-ings and condiments anytime I go to a restaurant. At first people looked

at me like I was nuts when I would pull out my little containers, but now that they have seen the results—they don't think that anymore.

I am the only person who never gains weight over the holidays in my family. I made all my own side dishes with the holiday package you created and took my Gingerbread Cake for dessert. It was delicious, I was satisfied, and I didn't gain an ounce.

So, in closing, I have gone from a size 4X/28, to a size 6!! I lost 160 lbs in fifteen months, and have been maintaining now for about 4 months. And the best part is, I feel fantastic.

If I ever got the opportunity to meet you in person, I would probably give you the biggest hug you ever had—in fact they would probably have to pry me off you—that is how much I want to thank you for saving my life. I believe that is what you did when you inspired me to start Somersizing, because at almost 300 lbs I was a disaster waiting to happen.

I wish you and yours a very Merry Christ-mas and a fabulous New Year 2005.

Sincerely,
Carol Ann Friedman, A Success Story!

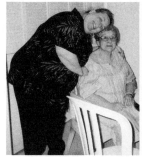
before, size 4X/28

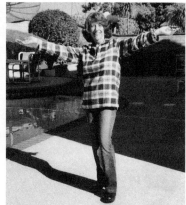
after, size 6
Carol lost 160 lbs!

December 9, 2004

Dear Suzanne:

I started Somersizing with my husband in February 2004 and have had great results. The diet is so easy and fun to follow, and the fact that there is no counting involved, i.e., calories or carbs, makes it simple to stick to.

My husband, Andy, and I have lost 70 pounds each, he is 6 pounds from his target weight, but I still have a ways to go. I started at 287 pounds, and have now reached 217! But unlike other diets I have tried, I know I am going to make it; I have no desire to cheat. This is truly a great lifestyle.

We now have our whole office converted to Somersize, and now work for a much healthier boss, who has lost over 30 pounds himself.

Thank you so much for this great diet and all of your fantastic books. . . . Keep up the great work.

Clare & Andy Gray

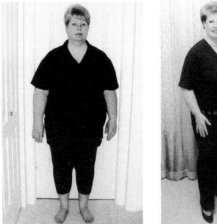

before, 287 lbs   after, 217 lbs

Clare lost 70 lbs!

December 7, 2004

Dear Suzanne:

I am so thrilled about the success I've experienced with your Somersize plan that I just had to write to you.

I started your program on July 31, 2003, and as of today (November 27, 2004) I have lost a total of 60 lbs. For many, many years I suffered from swollen ankles and all sorts of digestive problems. All of these problems are now gone and I feel wonderful. I haven't been this weight since my wedding seventeen years ago.

I had tried Weight Watchers off and on for many years and lost a few pounds here and there, but I always gained it back and more. I tried many other diet programs and, since I didn't lose much weight on those programs, I became totally discouraged and, of course, gave up.

Right from the start, the Somersize Plan was so different. First of all, it was so easy to follow . . . no points to count, no calories to worry about. And the thing that I think really makes me stick with it is the fact that I'm never hungry and therefore I never, ever feel deprived. The program is also the easiest ever to stick with whether you're eating out or eating at home. It's absolutely amazing. I am so thrilled and enthusiastic about your program that I tell everyone about it whenever I'm complimented on my weight loss, which is very often. For the first few months, I didn't even exercise a whole lot and I was still losing weight but now I'm exercising for at least a half hour daily and I can really feel myself toning up. I have 15 more pounds to lose and I am confident that I will make it to my goal.

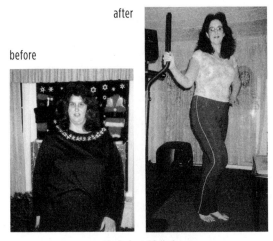

before after

Maria lost 60 lbs!

My brain fog was soon gone. I started to feel better and was up and doing. I love the food, I am able to eat, and I love not being hungry. I have hyperglycemia, and with this way of eating I am able to eat every two hours, keeping my blood sugar level. As I lost weight I began to exercise, and being able to get off the floor after working out without a struggle was a red-letter day. I am able to move and bend again and can tie my shoes without any trouble.

I have lost 52 pounds in twenty-one months. I feel and act twenty years younger than my fifty-three years. This is a wonderful way of eating. It has changed my life for the better and I never ever want to go back to my old ways of eating again.

Thanks, Suzanne, for sharing this wonderful WOE (way of eating)!

Connie E. Hainline

Your program has been such a godsend and I want so much to thank you and let you know how much I appreciate it. You are the best and I can't thank you enough.

Sincerely,
Maria Greenwood

◇

December 8, 2004

Dear Suzanne:

Before I started Somersizing, I was ready to sit down and stay there. When I saw you on TV, I thought, Why not? I have tried almost everything. I would lose 15 pounds and then stall or be unable to stay the course because of hunger.

I started to Somersize and within a week I lost 6 pounds. My acid reflux disappeared.

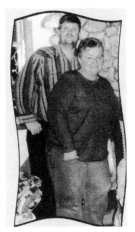 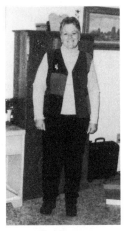

before after

Connie lost 52 lbs!

December 2, 2004

Dear Suzanne,

I just have to say THANK YOU! Somersize has changed my life.

In December 2003, my friend Rhonda introduced me to Somersize. At first, I was very hesitant to try it. I had tried several diets and lost some weight, only to gain it all back and more. Rhonda convinced me to give it a try. So, on December 30, 2003, at 270 pounds, I began Somersizing. I was amazed that in the first week I lost 7 pounds, and by the end of the second week I had lost 13 pounds. The weight has continued to come off.

As of November 27, 2004, I have lost 76 pounds. I feel better than I have for years. People whom I haven't seen for a while don't recognize me. It feels GREAT! Recently I HAD to go shopping for new clothes. Everything I had was falling off me. It felt so good to be able to shop for clothes in the regular women's section, instead of in the plus sizes. I haven't been able to do that since I was a teenager. I feel so much better about myself. I still have about 60 more pounds to lose, but am confident that I will reach my goal.

I found that Somersizing was not as hard to follow as other diets, because you can have so many great foods. I found that after a few weeks, I didn't miss all of the Funky Foods that I craved so much before. People ask me how I have lost the weight. I am quick to tell them, "By Somersizing." I have several friends who are now Somersizing and seeing great results, too!

So once again I want to say thanks, Suzanne, for a great meal plan and a new way of life. Also, thanks to my family and to

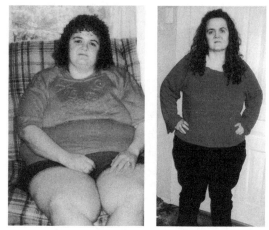

before, 270 lbs   after, 194 lbs

Lisa lost 76 lbs!

Rhonda, who have encouraged me all along the way. I couldn't do it without them.

Forever Grateful,
Lisa McCallister

December 8, 2004

Dear Suzanne:

In April 2001, I saw you on the Oprah show . . . having tried every diet that came down the pike and never kept the weight off, I decided to try your program. For a few years, I had been experiencing extremely painful heartburn and indigestion on a daily basis. I was getting worried. I bought your book and began immediately. By day two the heartburn and indigestion had disappeared and did not return. My energy level zoomed and has continued to do so.

My loss to date is 40 pounds with 15 to go! The thing that still puzzles me the most is how amazed I am when I see pictures of myself. It's like I'm seeing someone else—that this just can't be me. I am so thankful that this has worked and changed my life in so many ways. I have lots of energy for my precious grand-daughter now.

After witnessing my success physically and emotionally, my husband Kevin Pannell also decided to give Somersizing a try. He has lost 56 pounds!

Thank you, Suzanne, from the bottom of our hearts. We sing your praises all the time for sharing this life-saving information.

Bless you!
Debbie Pannell

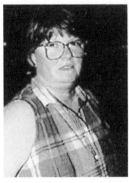 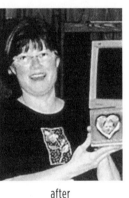

before   after

Debbie lost 40 lbs!

◇

December 8, 2004
Dear Suzanne:

After witnessing my wife's success with Somersizing, I decided to try it for two weeks during my Christmas 2001 vacation. Twenty pounds later, I decided that I never wanted to return to my old way of eating.

Talk about melting—by May, I'd lost 56 pounds.

Kevin Pannell

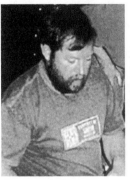 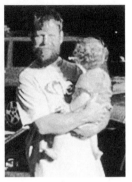

before   after

Kevin lost 56 lbs!

◇

December 9, 2004
Dear Suzanne:

My wife has been Somersizing for years. After Memorial Day, I started to do so, too. I have lost 25 pounds and my love handles! A lipid panel taken from LabCorp® in December 2003 revealed my cholesterol at 176, LDL at 122, and blood pressure 120/80. In December 2004 those numbers are 123, 67, and 101/59, and I am NOT taking any medication! We walk 3 miles, four times a week and up 55 flights of stairs.

These photos are of me in December 2003 and on Thanksgiving Day 2004.

I'm glad I finally listened to my wife's advice! I travel over 75,000 miles per year and am perfectly able to maintain my weight with your plan. Now I tell whoever will listen to me

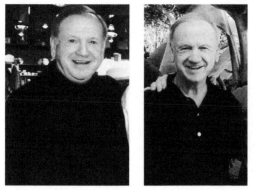

before   after

Ron lost weight and lowered his cholesterol!

about your simple and sensible plan. It works wonders!

Thank you for my new way of eating for the rest of my life!

Dr. Ron Rand

◇

November 28, 2004

Dear Suzanne:

I am a fifty-two-year-old man and 5'8" tall. I was extremely overweight (weighing 230 pounds) and I was as tall lying down as I was standing up. I was disgusted with myself. I have several medical conditions such as a hiatal hernia, asbestosis, a diagnosis of asthma, shortness of breath, and pain in my legs and knees from being overweight. After trying several diets over the last ten years without having any success, I told my wife that I could not stand myself anymore and that I needed her to help me lose weight. About a year ago or so, my wife and I met up with a friend at a car show who we had not seen for quite some time. He looked great and in talking to us he said

that he had been on your Somersize diet for about a year. He told us the diet, or life change as he called it, had helped him with his diabetes and in his business. He said he felt better, had more energy, and had less stress in his life, which had caused him to overeat. I asked my wife to get the book and help me to lose the weight. She did and we both began Somersizing. In fact, she has several of the books because she enjoys making recipes.

We have been Somersizing for about six months now. I have lost over 41 pounds and my wife has lost 15 pounds. (My wife did not need to lose much.) I feel great, I have a lot of energy, I enjoy the food, and I no longer have any problems with my hiatal hernia, asthma, shortness of breath, or the pain in my legs or knees.

Somersizing has changed my life—I have told a lot of my family and friends about Somersizing and several of them are Somersizing and are now losing weight. My wife can't wait for your next book and all of the fantastic recipes.

Thank you.

Rick Ricardy

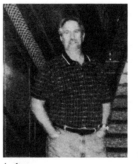

before

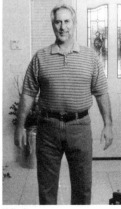

after

Rick lost 41 lbs!

December 8, 2004

Dear Suzanne:

My story is a little different from the other Somersizers but I wanted to let you know about it just the same. I first read *Eat Great, Lose Weight* after literally knocking it off the table in my library with my big fat behind! True story. When I picked up the book, I remembered that I had wanted to read your book so I checked it out. I read it along with all of your other books at the time and it changed my life.

So, I lost 25 pounds Somersizing and enjoyed the way of life so much that I stayed on it for six years. I may have gained a few pounds back, not sure, because I threw away my scale long ago, but I always stayed a size 10 so I knew it was working.

The only reason I had to quit Somersizing is because six months ago, I found out that I have celiac disease and had to go on a gluten-free diet. I couldn't eliminate wheat, rye, barley, oats, rice, corn, bananas, and potatoes, too!

I still use many of your recipes and products even with this gluten-free lifestyle. I always have SomerSweet and the Sea Salts in my cupboard. The flourless brownies and cakes are gluten-free so I get them often. Most chocolate is GF also. Yeah! And I still shop the perimeter of the grocery store, buying real food and cooking from scratch.

As it turns out, Somersize is basically a low-gluten diet and that is why I felt so much better eating this way. You see, in my twenties, I was very sick all the time. I couldn't hold down a job, I was so tired and had so many digestive problems. So in my thirties, I was on a quest to learn about food and eat

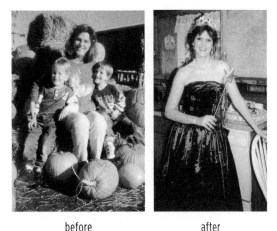

before   after

Shelley lost 25 lbs!

healthy. This led me to you and your attitudes toward food. Many of my digestive problems were eliminated since I was eating less gluten. I didn't know any of this at the time, however, because I was constantly misdiagnosed by my doctors.

I am so grateful to you, Suzanne, for helping me improve my way of life and my health. Most people are grateful because of the weight loss. I am grateful because I followed your plan and, although it was inadvertent, I reduced my gluten intake. Now that I am gluten-free, all my digestive symptoms and chronic fatigue are gone.

Between GF foods I get from the health food store and your products that I can still have, I am doing fantastic! I have never felt better in my life.

Thank you again, Suzanne, for bringing this way of eating to my life. You have made such a huge impact on my life.

Sincerely,
Shelley Rockefeller

◇

December 7, 2004

Dear Suzanne:

You are such a large part of my life, I feel as if I know you.

My weight has been a problem on and off most of my life, but prior to age forty, I'd gain a few pounds and lose a few pounds. After forty, I'd gain many and starve trying to lose only a few. I call them the "low-FOOD diets." That's how it feels; you eat so little and still can't lose much.

Your program allows me to eat all I want and lose all I want. I love to cook and I love my own cooking. I LOVE YOUR BOOKS. You have me eating wonderful food and very fancy sweets. SomerSweet is great. Crème Brûlée and Tiramisu are my number one and two favorites from long before I ever bought one of your books. Now I have either at will.

I really appreciate your continued willingness to share. I know this is how you make your living, but I am certain you no longer

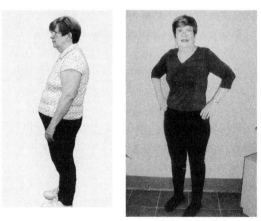

before   after

Fabulous Mary!

need to work this hard. I also appreciate your publication of recipes even when you have the product for sale. Can't think of anyone else that does that and it makes me believe you actually care about us fat and over-forty folks.

My mom and dad were born in Ireland, so I had potatoes at every meal for years. I'll be sixty-two in May and would like to say thank you for helping make this part of my life so much easier.

Mary Duffy Shaw

◇

December 8, 2004

Dear Suzanne:

My husband, Frank's, cholesterol levels were over 200 and our doctor wanted him to try a diet to lower them rather than going straight on medication. The doctor gave us the usual low-fat regimen to follow, but instead, I started Frank on Somersize. I have to admit that I was a little scared to try it since it goes down a different path than what our doctor was suggesting, but I have read all of your books and I had faith in what you said. When he went back for his checkup after six months, his cholesterol level had dropped by 80 points. We were really happy.

At the same time, my sister went on a statin drug for her cholesterol problem. She called to tell me that she had dropped 20 points on the drug. She was pretty happy about it until I told her about Frank's results with Somersizing.

Thanks a lot, Suzanne!

Frank & Sarah Sichra

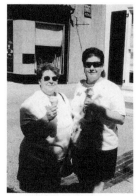 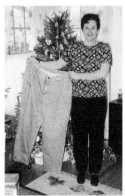

before, size 18–20   after, size 13–14

Dana lost 60 lbs!

I've got my daughter and several relatives on the program, too. I have so much energy, and I love not being hungry all the time. Therefore, I don't sit and think about my next meal like I did on other diets. This isn't really a diet but a new way of eating and thinking. I've been on Atkins before, but didn't like the restricted carbs. I went from a size 18W/20W and now I wear a size 13/14. Thanks, Suzanne, for giving us your secret! Now I find myself saying to others, "Fat is your friend, sugar is your enemy" . . . just like you.

Dana Stuedemann

◇

December 2004

Dear Suzanne,

My story begins in 2002 when I went on vacation to Florida with my family. I had bought your book called *Eat, Cheat, and Melt the Fat Away,* but went on vacation not giving it another thought. Well, after the horror of seeing myself in a swimsuit, I decided to try it out. What did I have to lose? I have been Somersizing now for the past two and a half years and can't imagine my life without it! Also, after five back surgeries and suffering from arthritis it sure helps not having the extra weight on my joints and back!

Thanks so much, Suzanne, for sharing this way of great eating! I've lost a total now of 60 lbs. For the first time in my life, I can actually say I didn't go back to my old ways and gain back all the weight I lost! People say to me, "Oh, you will eat sugar again," and I say, "No way," not when I can have such great desserts and not have to feel guilty!!

◇

December 9, 2004

Dear Suzanne:

I am so glad to finally find an eating program that does not deprive me in any way. I started following your Somersize plan; however, I never went on Level One. I love my sugar and cannot part with it totally. So I food-combine the way that you explain, avoiding eating certain foods together. Even though I still eat some cookies, candy, or ice cream each day, I still lose weight and keep it off. This is the way of life for me forever. When I want more chocolate or some type of sweets, I make the Somersize Ice Cream in the Somersize Ice-Cream Maker and I make other recipes from your books using SomerSweet. By doing so, I do not expose my body to an overdose of sugar, which spikes the insulin levels and can cause a person to feel tired afterward. In addition to the weight loss, my digestive system works much better. No heartburn, belching, or bloating.

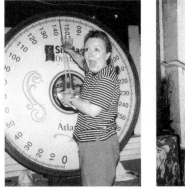
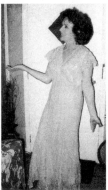

before   after

Connie is loving life!

I am fifty-six years of age, going through menopause, and have managed to lose weight without starving and have continued to keep it off. Hey, and guess what! For once in a long, long time, my inner thighs do not rub together when I walk. It's wonderful.

I highly recommend your plan to all of my friends and relatives. I'm one happy camper.

Thank you, Suzanne.

We love you. God bless you.

Connie Tucker

◇

December 8, 2004

Dear Suzanne:

In March of 2001, I walked into the bathroom and took a long look in the mirror. I was just shocked. My arms were disgustingly flabby . . . I was more than "fluffy." My joints ached and I barely had the energy to pull myself out of bed. At the time I had four children at home to take care of ranging in ages from two to sixteen. I looked at myself and said, "My children already have grandmothers and if I don't do something, they're going to have a third." They needed a "functional" mother.

This began my quest on the low-fat journey. I struggled for a year, exercising and watching everything that I ate. My size dropped from a 16 to a 12 . . . but the weight continually crept back on.

In March you changed my life. I saw you on HSN presenting your "way of eating" (I refuse to call it a diet). When you said we could eat all we want and have fat, I was ecstatic . . . IF YOU COULD ONLY BE TELLING THE TRUTH! I told my children that I was going to take a chance and order your program because I had to do something. Well . . . it came and my life hasn't been the same since.

From March until October, I went from a size 12/14 to a size 4/6 with a 40-lb weight loss!! Everyone kept asking me, "What are you doing? Starving??" To which I replied, "I eat like a HORSE." I would tell all the inquirers about how it was the easiest thing I'd ever tried. My husband, Brian, wanted to try it, if I would cook and send his lunch with him. He dropped 15 lbs. My dear friend Cyndi (who talked me into writing to you) lost 25—30 lbs. My cousin Lisa has lost 50 lbs. Aunt Carol has gone down two to three dress sizes. Both two years and counting! Another dear friend in her eighties has lost over 50 lbs (also over two years ago). My sister-in-law Beverly also was able to lose right before knee surgery. We've taken it off and are all keeping it off!

There came a point and time that even though I was following the plan I was still getting thicker and thicker through the middle!

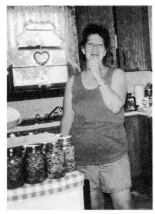
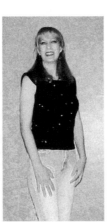

before, size 12–14   after, size 4–6

Sandra lost 40 lbs!

Thank you so much, Suzanne, for allowing yourself to be used to change people's lives for the good.

May God bless,
Sandra Wallace

◇

December 6, 2004

Dear Suzanne:

I had been a fat kid all of my life, trying every weight-loss program. I even worked for one of the weight clubs for five years only to gain everything back and then some.

When I was fifty-two, I was diagnosed with breast cancer, was treated for that and in three years it returned. The doctor put me on steroids and I immediately started gaining weight. I said, That is it, I can't do this anymore, so I let myself go up to 290 pounds. My best friend bought me your book and I thought, Oh well, I have tried everything else, why not try this? That was January 24, 2003. I have been on your program since then and have lost 120 pounds. No one knows me and I am a sexy sixty-five-year-old and loving life.

Here I was, forty years old and pregnant with my sixth child! I started telling people that there were some serious side effects with this way of eating and that they'd better watch out! There must be something to say for eating healthy?!! You cannot believe how much teasing my husband, Brian, and I have taken over this! The whole situation was really funny!

On October 29, 2003, we were blessed with our first boy, weighing over 9 lbs. During my pregnancy, I gained 35 lbs and within a few weeks of delivery, I was in a size 10.

Within 9 or 10 months, I was back in my size 4/6's at the age of forty-one with a new baby. To me, this is amazing even as it happened to me.

It is wonderful to pick him up, crawl around, chase him, and take all of my girls (and boy!) out every week for a fun day. I wake up in the mornings with such energy, remembering to be thankful because I can remember when I couldn't! I can honestly state, "I AM A NEW PERSON."

Mary Ann lost 120 lbs!

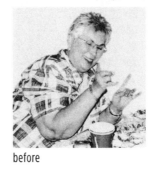

before

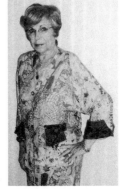

after

Your program has been a lifesaver for me. In the two years that I have been on your program I have not cheated. I never feel deprived and feel healthier than when I was young. My blood work is perfect and the doctors are amazed.

I so appreciate all the hard work that you have done to make this a program that I can LIVE with and never feel hungry. You and your program have changed my life!

Thanks again for all of your hard work.

Mary Ann Ward

◇

December 2004

Dear Suzanne,

My name is Sharon Wilgus, and I started your program May 3, 2004. I had purchased your book in the fall of 2003, read it, and put it on our bookshelf. In May, I decided to start your program and as of December 13, 2004, have lost $81^3/_4$ lbs.

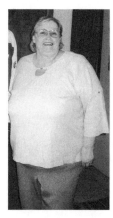 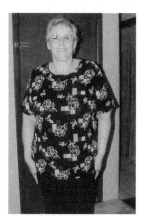

before   after

Sharon lost 81 lbs!

I was very overweight and was having a lot of problems with my knees. Thanks to your program I have lost those 81 lbs. and will continue to follow the program. I have found the program very easy to follow. I discovered that without the sugar, I truly am not hungry. Because the changes in my eating worked so well, I never even ate anything off the program until November when we went to visit our son in Colorado. I had a few things that week, but stayed right on the program and managed to still lose about 3 lbs.

I have been on many programs in my lifetime and have always lost weight, but regained it back very soon. Your program has been the first one that I was not hungry on.

Thank you again for your great program.

Sincerely,
Sharon Wilgus

◇

Dear Suzanne:

I have been overweight most of my life. I have tried every diet and pill introduced to me.

In 1988, I went on a liquid diet for seven months and lost 100 pounds. Not only did I gain it back, I gained 60 extra pounds.

In 1994, I developed gestational diabetes during the pregnancy with my son. The doctor, concerned about my weight problem, warned me that I could easily develop diabetes. Again, I tried diets and pills, again without success.

Out of desperation, in 1997 I decided to have stomach surgery. A portion of my stomach was stapled to prevent me from eating too

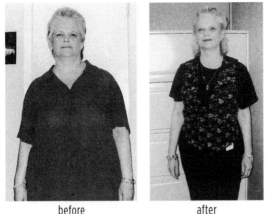

before   after

Vickie lost 85 lbs!

much, to feel full. With the surgery came the warning that if I ate the wrong foods I would not lose any weight and could gain weight. The surgery gave me the incentive I needed and over a six-month period, I lost 105 pounds. By October 2002, I had gained 35 pounds back and began to panic; I had been there before. I was determined not to let my weight get out of hand.

One of my best friends had been on your Somersize program in 2001 and she did great. When Deborah explained the program, I was hesitant. You had to watch the food combination and watch when you eat it. Sounded complicated, but with her encouragement I decided to begin. The program was easy; I had successfully made it through the Thanksgiving and Christmas holidays and by January 2003 had lost 40 pounds. It's not a diet but simply a "lifestyle change," I love it.

It's now June 2003 and I have lost 70 pounds, I like the way I look and I feel great. The new me even joined the gym to firm up and I continue to lose inches and weight. I

have self-esteem and confidence that I have never known before. I tell everyone how great and easy the Somersize program really is. I would also like to tell everyone and anyone, "Don't go through what I did. Join the Somersize Program and watch what happens."

I would like to thank you, Suzanne, for the research you did to make this program possible. Also, I want to thank my boss, Karen Hawkins, my husband Darrell, and my son Tyler. They were and are always there to encourage and help me.

A special thanks to Deborah Penn, who took the time to cook and bake all the Somersize recipes I asked for, especially the ice cream!

Vickie Wright

◇

Update—March 23, 2004
I have now lost 85 pounds and still enjoy my new way of eating. The food is really good. I know that I will be successful in keeping the weight off this time.

Vickie Wright

◇

December 6, 2004
Dear Suzanne:
Two years ago, before the low-carb craze, a friend of mine gave me your book. I was telling her that I didn't really understand what carbs were and she told me that your book would thoroughly explain the differences between carbs, proteins, and fats.

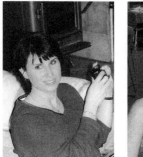 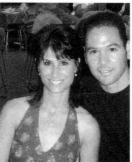

before   after

Shirley lost 15 lbs!

I have always been a healthy person, and I thought that I ate really good foods. I was, however, about 15 pounds overweight at this time. I read your whole book the day it was given to me. I was blown away. Finally, I understood what was wrong. I was a carb junkie. I thought that a bagel and a banana for lunch were really great. I thought that a fat-free muffin and coffee for breakfast was cutting calories. I never understood why I would get the shakes, feel grouchy, and even dizzy around mid-morning. It was a sugar low.

Well, I started your program right away. The first two weeks were hard, but I stuck with it. I had to completely retrain my low-fat/no-fat brain. In just a few weeks the pounds started melting away like magic. I couldn't believe it. I was eating more than I ever had, and every morning I dropped another pound. I had tried many exercise programs and diets in the past and nothing ever worked like this. I had to re-read your book several times over because so many people asked me what I was doing to lose the weight. I became a Somersize spokesperson! What I love the most about the program is that I am never hungry and I never feel guilty about what I eat. I am over my sugar addiction and I can easily say no to muffins, bagels, cookies, candy, and cakes.

It has been two years since I started Somersizing and I just recently had a baby. I am only four pounds over my pre-pregnancy weight and my baby is only four weeks old. I Somersized throughout my pregnancy and my doctor was thrilled with my health. Thank you, Suzanne, thank you for changing my life and my habits. I am healthier and happier than I have ever been. I will never go back to my old way of eating.

Sincerely,
Shirley Yunk

◇

Dear Suzanne:

In 1997, when I heard you speaking about your way of eating and saw your new book on television, I knew this was something I could do.

I bought *Eat Great, Lose Weight* and began my new way of life. I loved it from the beginning.

Now, several years later and 150 pounds lighter, I continue to love eating the Somersize way. I've had no trouble maintaining my weight over the years. Because of my new self-confidence, I've traveled to Australia, New Zealand, and Hawaii; parasailed in Mexico; and flown to see my new granddaughter two times. I was able to sit comfortably in the airplane seat with room to spare. That was a miracle in itself.

I had no trouble sticking to this way of eating last winter when my husband and I went on our first cruise. We are looking forward to another one in a year.

In 2003, my friend and I completed the Columbus Marathon after an extensive training program. That is how I celebrated reaching my goal. Last summer I learned to play golf. None of these things would have been possible with my old body.

I am sixty years old and have never felt better. Going from size 26-28W to size 12 is just unbelievable to me. I STILL love it and will continue this way of life.

Sincerely,
Cheryl Pelasky

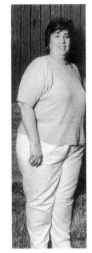 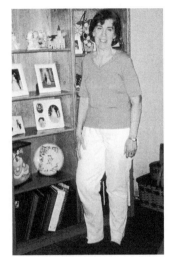

before, size 26–28   after, size 12

Cheryl dropped 14 dress sizes!

CHAPTER 9

The Basics

In this section I am going to lay out the basic tenets of this simple and effective weight-loss plan. This includes everything you need to know about Somersize. I have refined and developed this program throughout the years and I'm constantly updating it as new science emerges. If you are already a Somersizer, you may skim this section, but make sure to pay close attention to the sections on plateaus and carbohydrates, as the information is new and important. If you are a new Somersizer, let's get to it!

Level One is the weight-loss portion of the program. The first step is to eliminate a small list of foods that raise our insulin levels, like sugar, white flour, potatoes, white rice, and alcohol. These foods are called Funky Foods and I promise you will not miss them. After we eliminate the Funky Foods, we separate normal, everyday foods into groups. Then we combine these foods in a way that aids in digestion and weight

control. Here are the four Somersize Food Groups:

Pro/Fats—including meat, chicken, fish, butter, cheese, cream
Veggies—including low-starch vegetables
Carbos—including whole-grain carbohydrates and nonfat dairy products
Fruit—with a huge variety of your favorites

You will find complete lists of the Funky Foods and all of the Somersize Food Groups in the back of the book in the Reference Guide. Once you understand the food groups, you simply follow:

THE SEVEN EASY STEPS TO SOMERSIZING

1. Eliminate all Funky Foods.
2. Eat Fruit alone, on an empty stomach: twenty minutes before a Carbos meal,

one hour before a Pro/Fats meal, two hours after your last meal.

3. Eat Pro/Fats with Veggies.
4. Eat Carbos with Veggies.
5. Keep Pro/Fats separate from Carbos.
6. Wait three hours between meals if switching from a Pro/Fats meal to a Carbos meal, or vice versa.
7. Do not skip meals. Eat at least three meals a day, and eat until you feel satisfied and comfortably full.

Plus, you need to drink eight 8-ounce glasses of water each day. That's it in a nutshell. It is so easy to follow. Somersize is not a diet, it's a way of eating. It's a lifestyle that you can live with and that you will love. Here are the details of the program.

ELIMINATE

As I have explained, it is essential that we eliminate foods that cause blood sugar to fluctuate too much. In addition to sugar and white flour, there are other Funky Foods that cause similar problems.

There are several types of Funky Foods and I have listed them here. The first group of Funky Foods is made up of sugar sources. Some are natural and some are refined, but natural or not, they're still sugar and we avoid them completely when losing weight in Level One.

SUGARS

White sugar	Corn syrup
Brown sugar	High-fructose
Raw sugar	corn syrup

Sucrose	Maple syrup
Molasses	Beets
Honey	Carrots

Fructose is a low-glycemic sugar that causes low to moderate rises in your blood sugar. SomerSweet, which I have mentioned throughout this book, contains a small amount of fructose that occurs naturally in the sweet chicory fiber. I do not add any fructose to the blend. Plus, SomerSweet is concentrated (it's five times sweeter than sugar), so you get only a very small amount. Each 1-gram serving has so little fructose that by FDA standards, SomerSweet is considered sugar-free, with less than .5 gram of sugar per serving. If you are freely using straight fructose to sweeten your foods, those sugars can add up and upset your balance. Some Somersizers are able to use moderate amounts of fructose without disrupting their weight loss. Others report that when they start to use fructose they gain weight.

The next group of Funky Foods is made up of foods that are high in starch. These foods turn directly to sugar (glucose) upon digestion.

STARCHES

Acorn squash	Potatoes
Bananas	Pumpkin
Butternut squash	Sweet potatoes
Corn	White flour
Hubbard squash	White rice
Parsnips	Yams

Alternatives to white flour include whole wheat, pumpernickel, rye, amaranth, spelt, farro, and kamut, to name a few. White rice can be replaced with brown rice, which has a wonderful earthy flavor, or better yet, wild rice, which has even less starch. Instead of corn and potatoes, you should be eating greater amounts of green vegetables. And bananas are very high in sugar, so we eliminate them while we are losing weight.

The third group of Funky Foods doesn't seem to fit into any of our four Somersize Food Groups because these foods contain protein or fat and carbohydrates, and we don't combine fats wirh carbohydrates on Level One. However, these are the least funky of the Funky Foods. When you graduate to Level Two these are the first foods you may incorporate back into your meals. Some people eat nuts, olives, avocados, and soy products on Level One and still enjoy all the effects of losing weight and feeling great. I regularly eat soy beans (edamame) without any problems.

BAD COMBO FOODS

Avocados	Nuts
Coconuts	Olives
Liver	Soy
Low-fat or whole milk	

The last group of Funky Foods is made up of caffeine and alcohol. Just like other Funky Foods, caffeine can cause highs and lows in your blood sugar, which leads to insulin resistance. You could be Somersizing perfectly and then get out of balance by drinking a cup of coffee. And remember that caffeine is a real no-no for you fellow adrenaline junkies out there! Decaffeinated coffee and herbal teas, especially decaf green tea, are fine. If your body is in balance from Somersizing, you won't need caffeine to perk you up during the day.

Certain types of alcohol, such as beer and white wine, will raise insulin levels. Other types of alcohol are not as bad, since they do not act as carbohydrates. This is new information for Somersizers. I have recently discovered that many types of hard alcohol do not act as carbohydrates. However, when your body needs energy, it will choose to burn hard alcohol first over fat, so I still recommend that you eliminate all alcohol when you are on Level One. During Level Two and occasionally on Almost Level One, you may enjoy a drink. The best choices are red wine and hard alcohols such as vodka, rum, scotch, gin, brandy, bourbon, and whiskey. Red wine has a small amount of carbohydrates and has been found to have beneficial effects for heart health. As for the hard alcohols mentioned, they contain no carbohydrates. I was stunned to hear this! Many tequilas are cut with sugar water and can contain up to 60 grams of carbohydrates per ounce. High-end tequilas, such as 100 percent agave tequila, are pure and not mixed with sugar water. This type of tequila does not contain carbohydrates.

The biggest problem with hard alcohol is the sugary mixers! Avoid tonic water, juice, or sodas, which are all high in carbohydrates. The worst offenders are the "foofy" drinks, like margaritas, piña coladas, and fruit daiquiris. The mixers for these drinks are loaded with sugars and high-fructose corn syrup. Use club soda or diet sodas (if you must), or try Somersize Cocktail Mixers to make a delightful drink with or without alcohol.

Again, steer clear of all alcohol in Level One. I do, however, make an exception with regard to cooking. If you are doing well on Level One you may use wine in some of my recipes because it creates only a slight imbalance and leaves a delicious flavor in your cooking. If you want an occasional drink in Almost Level One or Level Two, choose red wine or hard alcohol with sugar-free mixers.

As for beer, last year I got a call from an angry beer manufacturer who was upset that I had advised Somersizers to stay away from beer. He argued that light beer does not have that many carbs—you've seen the ad campaigns. My response is that you cannot argue with the fact that beer has a higher glycemic index than pure glucose. Your body accepts it as sugar. Now that you understand the connection between insulin and weight gain around the midsection, a "beer belly" makes perfect sense.

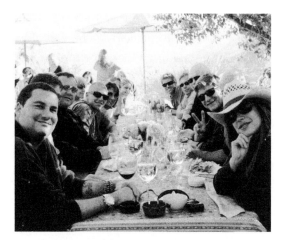

Friends, family, good food. That's Leslie in front.

CAFFEINE AND ALCOHOL

Beer	Coffee
Caffeinated teas	Hard alcohol
Caffeinated sodas	Wine
Cocoa	

Don't worry; you don't have to say good-bye to caffeine and alcohol forever. They'll be back in moderation when we reach our goal weight and advance to Level Two, the maintenance portion of Somersizing.

SEPARATE

To combine our foods in a way that maximizes our digestion, we must first separate foods into our four Somersize categories: Pro/Fats, Carbos, Veggies, and Fruits. I have grouped them by their predominant feature to help simplify the program, though many foods are combinations of proteins, fats, and carbohydrates. For instance, all the foods found in the Carbos, Veggies, and Fruit groups contain carbohydrates, but the carbohydrate levels vary greatly, which is why I have broken them down into different groups. I have briefly described each group here and have included complete lists of these foods in the Reference Guide, which you'll find at the back of the book.

PRO/FATS

The first Somersize group is made up of foods high in protein and/or fat. I put these two food groups together because many of the foods that contain protein also contain fat. Meat, poultry, fish, eggs, cheese, butter, and cream are just a few of the Pro/Fats you'll enjoy.

Proteins are made up of organic compounds called amino acids. These amino acids are the building blocks for the human body. Proteins play a role in virtually every cellular function: they regulate muscle contraction, antibody production, and blood vessel expansion and contraction to maintain normal blood pressure. Eating protein is critically important because it supplies us with new amino acids that are needed to make these different proteins.

Fats provide a major storage form of metabolic fuel. When they break down they provide us with energy. Fats also help to facilitate the use of essential fat-soluble vitamins like A, D, E, and K. Vitamin A is necessary for healthy eyes and skin; vitamin D helps to absorb calcium; vitamin E prevents cholesterol deposits; and vitamin K contributes to healthy blood clotting. Fat also helps to stabilize blood sugar. And fat is the body's fuel source that causes the lowest insulin response. Essential fatty acids cannot be manufactured by our bodies on their own; they, too, must be included in our daily meals. Unsaturated fats, like olive oil, canola oil, and fish oils, help to lower cholesterol levels and should be included in our meals.

Any of the foods in the Pro/Fats group can be eaten together, or in combination with Veggies. (See the complete list of Pro/Fats on pages 287–88.)

CARBOS

Carbohydrates are mostly derived from plant sources, rather than from animal sources. Carbs are the primary metabolic fuel in our Westernized diets. As I explained earlier, carbs break down into glucose, which is one of the body's main sources of energy. Since we have other mechanisms in our bodies to produce glucose, carbs are the one nutrient that is not absolutely essential in our diet. However, completely eliminating carbohydrates from our diet is dangerous. On the Somersize system we eliminate refined carbohydrates like sugar, white flour, and white rice, but we do enjoy complex carbohydrates, like whole-grain pastas and cereals, which still have many essential vitamins and nutrients intact. In addition, complex carbohydrates provide fiber and roughage necessary for the digestive process.

Any of the foods in the Carbos group can be eaten together, or in combination with Veggies. (See the complete list of Carbos on page 288.)

VEGGIES

All vegetables are technically carbohydrates, but those found in this Somersize category have been chosen because they are low in starch and cause only a minute rise in the blood sugar. These include green beans, broccoli, cauliflower, artichokes, tomatoes, peppers, onions, and more. Vegetables are packed with vitamins and minerals and provide essential roughage for proper elimination.

Any of the foods in the Veggies group can be eaten together. And since vegetables can easily be digested with either Pro/Fats or Carbos, you may eat them with either group. (See the complete list of Veggies on page 289.)

FRUITS

Fruits are also technically carbohydrates, but because of their unique sugar content, fruit must always be eaten alone. Fruits are a great source of fiber and help to keep the digestive track moving. They are loaded with antioxidants, but if you mix fruit with other foods, it can lose its nutritional benefits and upset the digestive process. Fruit turns to acid when combined with other food groups and spoils in the stomach, causing gas and that horrible bloated feeling. Fruit as a supposedly "healthy" option for dessert can ruin a perfectly combined meal. Not only will it make you feel uncomfortable, it can trap the energy of other foods and cause unnecessary storage of fat.

I recommend you eat the whole fruit to receive the fiber and drink fruit juice sparingly, as most nutrients are pressed out. You are essentially just drinking fruit sugar. Unfortunately, your body reacts exactly the same to fruit sugar as it does to regular sugar, because it makes your insulin spike. Highly concentrated fruit-juice-sweetened sorbets or ice pops should be eaten infrequently. They sound healthy, but they are not good on Level One. The same goes for dried fruit; the sugar concentration becomes far more intense with dried fruits. I avoid

them on Level One and eat them rarely, if at all, on Almost Level One.

Here are some guidelines on how you can eat delicious and nutritious fresh fruit and gain all the benefits without creating digestion problems.

Eat Fruit on an empty stomach.

Eat Fruit alone, then wait twenty minutes, and you may follow up with a Carbos meal. (The twenty-minute lead time gets the digestion of the fruit going and eliminates problem combinations.)

Eat Fruit alone, then wait one hour, and you may follow up with a Pro/Fats meal.

If you want Fruit for a snack or for dessert, you must wait two hours after your last meal to avoid any problems.

Any of the foods in the Fruit group can be eaten together. (See the complete list of Fruits on page 289.)

FREE FOODS

There are a few items that may be combined with Pro/Fats, Veggies, or Carbos because they do not conflict with any of the food groups. These include soy sauce, vinegar, mustard, herbs, and spices. In addition, lemons and limes, though technically fruits, are very low in sugar and therefore may be used to flavor any of the four food groups. Of course, the most exciting Free Food of all is . . . SomerSweet!

CHAPTER 10

Level One and Almost Level One

I hope you have a basic understanding of the program now. In my previous books I've walked my Somersizers through each meal to show them how to Somersize, and I will do the same here. Every time you sit down for a meal you are in for a treat.

BREAKFAST

Each meal is an opportunity to eat something great, even on Level One when you're trying to lose weight. Let's talk about all the delicious breakfast options. I love breakfast! Cereal, toast, fruit, eggs, bacon, or sausage! As long as you follow the Somersize combinations, you may eat any of those foods for breakfast, just not in the same sitting. Here are your choices.

#1—*Fruit Meal*
#2—*Carbos Meal*
#3—*Fruit, wait twenty minutes, then Carbos Meal*
#4—*Pro/Fats and Veggies Meal*

BREAKFAST #1—FRUIT MEAL

Start your day off with a couple of plums, an orange, or half a cantaloupe. Combine your favorite fruits in a blender with some juice and a few ice cubes for a frosty fruit smoothie. Dice some mangoes, pineapple, papaya, and grapes for a tasty fruit salad. Remember, you may eat any kind of fruit except bananas, which are a Funky Food. Fruit is best in the morning when eaten on an empty stomach. Fruit keeps you regular, is loaded with vitamins and nutrients, and is a natural source of energy.

Examples of Breakfast #1—
Fruit Meal

- Fruit smoothie with peaches, raspberries, strawberries, and fruit juice
- Fruit smoothie with pineapple chunks, papaya, and orange juice
- Fruit salad of melon, grapes, and oranges
- An apple
- A bowl of fresh cherries
- A slice of watermelon

TO DRINK: Decaf coffee or tea, black (or sweetened with SomerSweet)

BREAKFAST #2—CARBOS MEAL

Morning is the best time of the day to eat your carbohydrates so you can use the natural energy they supply throughout the day. There are a number of wonderful options to satisfy your hunger. I like whole-grain toast with nonfat cottage cheese or yogurt. Or I like hot or cold whole-grain cereal with nonfat milk. Since we cannot combine any fat with our Carbos, this is the only time we choose fat-free products, specifically nonfat dairy products. Read your labels and look for brands that are free of starches, fillers, and chemicals.

When checking your labels, focus on the ingredient list, rather than the nutritional panel. If all the ingredients are acceptable Carbos, without any Funky Foods, you may eat the food. Do not look at the number of carbohydrates, proteins, or fats listed in the panel. If there are unpronounceable

ingredients, you are better off avoiding that product.

And remember, you may have Veggies with your Carbos, so feel free to top your toast with tomato and basil or a slice of red onion, if you like.

Examples of Breakfast #2—
Carbos Meal

- Whole-wheat toast with nonfat cottage cheese and tomato
- Rye bagel with nonfat ricotta cheese
- Fat-free wheat tortilla with black beans and salsa
- Somersize Crispy Sweet Whole Wheat Flakes with nonfat milk
- Nonfat yogurt sprinkled with Grape-Nuts
- Shredded wheat with nonfat milk
- Oatmeal with nonfat milk

TO DRINK: Decaf coffee or tea, black or with nonfat milk (and/or sweetened with SomerSweet)

BREAKFAST #3—FRUIT, WAIT TWENTY MINUTES, THEN CARBOS MEAL

Fruit, then Carbos is my favorite choice for breakfast because these foods provide me with necessary fiber and numerous vitamins and nutrients. Morning is the best time to eat your Fruit and Carbos so that you have plenty of time to burn off the natural sources of energy they provide. Here are a few more examples of Fruit and Carbos.

Examples of Breakfast #3—Fruit, then Carbos Meal

- Melon. Wait twenty minutes.
  Oatmeal with nonfat milk
- Fruit smoothie with cantaloupe, raspberries, and grapefruit juice. Wait twenty minutes.
  Whole-grain toast with nonfat cottage cheese and a sprinkle of cinnamon
- A couple of oranges. Wait twenty minutes.
  Puffed wheat cereal with nonfat milk
- Pineapple slices. Wait twenty minutes.
  Toasted rye bagel and a bowl of nonfat yogurt sweetened with vanilla extract and SomerSweet
- Fruit salad. Wait twenty minutes.
  Oatmeal with nonfat milk

TO DRINK: Decaf coffee or tea, black or with nonfat milk (and/or sweetened with SomerSweet)

BREAKFAST #4—PRO/FATS AND VEGGIES MEAL

In a Pro/Fats and Veggies breakfast, you may have anything from the Pro/Fats group with anything from the Veggies group. You have so many choices with this breakfast. Start with eggs, then scramble, fry, boil, poach, or make them into an omelette or a frittata. Don't be afraid of eggs! Have as many as you like. Cook them in butter or oil and serve them with sausage or bacon (I look for brands with no nitrates). For additional flavor, you can even cook your eggs in the bacon fat or sausage fat. And you wonder why I don't call

it a diet! You can have meat, fish, or poultry, including chicken, shrimp, crab, lox, and smoked fish. Feel free to add some cheese to that omelette! And don't forget your vegetables, like onions, tomatoes, zucchini, spinach, mushrooms, asparagus, and more.

Examples of Breakfast #4— Pro/Fats and Veggies Meal

- Omelette with zucchini, Swiss cheese, mushrooms, and sour cream
  Side of turkey sausage
- Fried eggs with bacon
  Side of tomatoes
- Scrambled eggs with smoked salmon, asparagus, and sour cream
- Huevos rancheros—fried eggs with caramelized onions, Cheddar cheese, salsa, and sour cream (hold the tortilla)
- Poached eggs on a bed of spinach with Canadian bacon and hollandaise sauce
  Side of green beans
- Eggs Florentine with ham, cheese, and spinach

TO DRINK: Decaf coffee or tea, black or with cream (and/or sweetened with SomerSweet)

Any of these foods would make up a perfectly combined Somersize breakfast, so you may eat until you are full. This is a great breakfast option when you're eating out because there are so few restrictions. Just stay away from toast, jelly, potatoes, and fruit with your Pro/Fats and Veggies breakfast.

If you want to start this meal with Fruit, you must wait one hour until you have your Pro/Fats and Veggies.

LUNCH AND DINNER

For lunch and dinner you may have salads, soups, sandwiches, chicken, steak, fish, pasta, and more! You just have to decide which food group you feel like eating and then design a meal in the proper Somersize combination. Here are your choices.

#1—Pro/Fats and Veggies Meal
#2—Carbos and Veggies Meal
#3—Single Food Group Meal

LUNCH OR DINNER #1— PRO/FATS AND VEGGIES MEAL

The possibilities are endless with this option. Order from any restaurant menu with the Pro/Fats and Veggies meal: meat, poultry, or fish can be grilled, broiled, baked, roasted, or fried (no flour) and served with plenty of fresh vegetables, raw, steamed, sautéed, or grilled. It is important to balance your meals with vegetables because they give your body the small amount of carbohydrates it needs to stay balanced and to produce serotonin. Enjoy cooking with oil or butter and don't forget to add the cheese! Preparing meals for yourself at home or eating in a restaurant is a pleasure with this option.

Examples of Lunch or Dinner #1—Pro/Fats and Veggies Meal

- Cobb salad with lettuce, chicken, bacon, egg, tomato, blue cheese, and green onions with full-fat sugar-free dressing of your choice (Hold the avocado.)
- Taco salad with lettuce, shredded beef, tomatoes, Cheddar cheese, salsa, onions, and sour cream (Hold the beans and chips.)
- Grilled fish with lemon-butter sauce
  Snow peas tossed in butter
  Green salad with full-fat sugar-free dressing of your choice
- Caesar salad (hold the croutons) with grilled chicken breast
  Grilled red peppers, zucchini, and fennel
- Hamburger patty with melted Jack cheese and a pile of onions
  Green salad with cherry tomatoes and blue cheese dressing.
- Egg salad tossed with celery, green onions, and mayonnaise, served in lettuce cups with tomato slices and alfalfa sprouts
- Rotisserie-style chicken
  Steamed broccoli and cauliflower covered with cheese
- Steamed crab legs and grilled filet mignon
  Steamed artichoke with butter or mayonnaise dip
  Butter lettuce salad with zucchini and Parmesan cheese
- Turkey cutlet served over sautéed Swiss chard with a butter-wine sauce
  Green salad with goat cheese and Somersize Candied Roma Tomatoes
- Grilled lamb chops with lemon and olive oil
- Greek salad with tomatoes, cucumber, red onion, feta cheese, and olive oil
- Stir-fried shrimp with napa cabbage, celery, broccoli, yellow peppers, Italian squash, bamboo shoots

- Chopped salad with salami, roasted peppers, tomatoes, onions, and provolone cheese
- Fresh raw vegetables with dip
- Steak with peppercorn cream sauce and sautéed mushrooms
- Steamed green beans tossed in butter
- Radicchio and endive salad with blue cheese and tomato

TO DRINK: Water, mineral water, Somer-Sweet drinks, decaf coffee or tea with cream (and/or sweetened with SomerSweet)

Your Pro/Fats and Veggies meals will range from the incredibly simple to the luxuriously extravagant. With so much to choose from, you won't ever get bored eating the same old thing. In fact, your food will taste better than ever as you trim your way down to your ideal body weight.

LUNCH OR DINNER #2—CARBOS AND VEGGIES MEAL

I choose this option with very little frequency, because I prefer to eat my carbohydrates only in the morning when I'm trying to lose weight. But every now and then you just need a carbohydrate fix at lunch or dinner, and it really hits the spot. You can have any whole grains or beans with nonfat dairy products and any of the Somersize vegetables on the list. Be careful when you look for whole-wheat products . . . many manufacturers are now listing "wheat-flour" for regular white flour. It must say "whole-wheat flour" to really be a whole grain. In general, if it looks too white to be whole wheat, it probably isn't.

You might have brown rice with peas or black bean chili with fresh tomato salsa and whole-wheat tortillas or whole-grain pasta with tomato basil sauce or whole-wheat pita bread with hummus, baba ghanoush, and fresh vegetables. With any of these meals you could have a green salad. Try my Somersize Pasta, Sauces, and Rice Packets (with no fat) for a perfectly Somersized meal. The key to the Carbos and Veggies meal is to make sure there is absolutely no fat in the ingredients list. (There may be traces of fat on the nutrition panel. Don't worry about these.)

Examples of Lunch or Dinner #2—Carbos and Veggies Meal

- Brown rice with soy sauce and steamed vegetables
  Green salad with a splash of vinegar
- Whole-wheat pita bread with nonfat ricotta cheese, roasted peppers, and eggplant
  Grilled zucchini and yellow squash
- Whole-wheat pasta with tomato, basil, and garlic sauce
  An artichoke with a squeeze of lemon
- A bowl of black beans with whole-wheat tortillas and fresh salsa
- Whole-wheat pita bread with hummus, baba ghanoush, lettuce, and tomato
- Spinach whole-wheat pasta with fresh garden vegetables, peas, and stewed tomatoes
- Whole-wheat cheeseless pizza with marinara sauce, mushrooms, onions, tomatoes, and artichoke hearts
  Green salad with a squeeze of lemon

TO DRINK: Water, mineral water, Somersize drinks, decaf coffee or tea with nonfat milk (and/or sweetened with SomerSweet)

This is a very satisfying and healthy option with all the whole grains and fresh vegetables. It can be a little restrictive, however, because on Level One you can't have any fat with your carbs and you must watch for hidden sugars and Funky Foods. Because this meal is more difficult to obtain in a restaurant, I normally prepare Carbos and Veggies at home.

LUNCH OR DINNER #3— SINGLE FOOD GROUP MEAL

Every now and then you might want to have a meal made up of only one food group, like the all-Fruits meal or the all-Veggies meal. Of course, this is perfectly fine on rare occasions, but I do not recommend it with any frequency.

FINDING A RHYTHM THAT WORKS

When I'm losing weight on Level One, I find that the fewer carbohydrates I eat, the more results I see. As I explained earlier, carbohydrates are an energy source, and if you're not giving your body many sources of energy, it will have to break down your fat reserves and use them as energy. But we don't want to cut out carbohydrates completely, because they are an important source of fiber and help keep your system moving properly. And if you go too low with carbohydrates, your body will break

down its protein, instead of its fat reserves, to be used as energy. Plus, you will become depleted of serotonin.

Here's what works best for me. I like to eat the Fruit, then Carbos breakfast. Because carbs are a good energy source, it's best to eat them in the morning so that you can use that energy throughout the day. For lunch and dinner I find more options with Pro/Fats and plenty of Veggies. Don't forget to add your vegetables! Eating proteins and fats alone, for any length of time, does not promote a healthy balance, so like Mom always says, "Eat your vegetables." Carbohydrate meals for lunch and dinner are a little more restrictive because you can have absolutely no fat.

My recommendation is that for breakfast you frequently choose Breakfast #3—Fruit, then Carbos. For lunch and dinner I recommend Pro/Fats and Veggies as a rule with the Carbos and Veggies meal as the exception. If you eat too many carbohydrates, even the right kind of carbohydrates, they could get stored as fat for later use. (And if you're filling up on carbs, you're probably not giving your body enough protein and fat.) Remember, you're giving your body the small amount of carbohydrates it needs because your Pro/Fats and Veggies meals include some carbohydrates in the form of the many vegetables you'll be enjoying. Once again, make sure to include your vegetables. A meal of meat and cheese alone is not a good idea on a regular basis.

This is only a blueprint of how I divide my Pro/Fats and Carbos meals. For me, too many carbos or too few will cause weight gain, especially at this age, when I am fighting hormonal imbalances. You may find that your body can handle more carbohydrates and that you feel better eating mostly grains and vegetables. On the other hand, if you are eating mostly Pro/Fats, you must balance your meals with plenty of fresh vegetables. I cannot stress this enough. It is unwise to eat only meat and cheese without the fiber and nutrients added from vegetables. Also, this gives your body the essential serotonin it requires for balance.

BALANCE

I have talked throughout this book about balance—how to eat in balance, how to balance our hormones. We have to remember to use our common sense. Even though I stress throughout the books not to overdo it, sometimes we forget and push the envelope too far. Just because your cheesecake is made with SomerSweet, you should not eat the whole thing. One piece of cheesecake is plenty; don't wolf down half a cake or eat it for breakfast just because it's Level One.

If you are on strict Level One, there is no portion control. Hurray! I like to give you the freedom to eat without measuring or weighing your foods because it allows you to live your life and not obsess about every morsel that goes into your mouth. You know that eating a whole wheel of Brie is too much . . . so don't do it. Unlike other programs, you will always have enough to eat when you Somersize. The key is knowing when you are eating just for the sake of eating. So many of us are used to rigid diets that we gorge ourselves when we Somer-

size, just because we can. Once you realize that you will never again go hungry on this program, you will lose the urge to overdo it. Don't forget—*you* are in control.

WATER—THE FLOW OF LIFE

If you have read my other books, you know that I highly recommend drinking eight to ten glasses of water a day. The more water you drink, the faster you will lose weight! (Now you're listening, aren't you?) Water assists your metabolism in running at optimum speed. It is essential to weight loss. But try not to drink with your meals because water can dilute your digestive juices, which slows down the digestive process. Your stomach acids are strongest right before you begin a new meal. When you eat, the acids break down the food quickly and pass it from the stomach. If you drink a big glass of water before your meal, these gastric juices become diluted and are less effective at breaking down the food. Therefore, if you must drink with your meal, eat a portion of your food before you drink anything so as not to dilute the strength of the gastric juices. It's best to drink your eight to ten glasses between meals. Besides water, you can also have decaffeinated coffee, teas, and even diet sodas, if you must. Personally, I stay away from soft drinks; they are loaded with things I don't want to put into my body. You would be doing your body a favor to eliminate them as well.

Many people ask me if the beverages they

drink that are not pure water count toward their eight to ten glasses of water per day. Yes: decaf coffee, iced tea, Somersize Drinks, they all count. So drink up!

NO CHEATING

Cheating is not for Level One. Level One is when we first start the program and we are trying to unload the stored sugar from our cells and heal our metabolism. If you are finding little ways to cheat, you are only cheating yourself. Remember, *any* sugar you eat at this point will throw you out of balance.

Rewarding yourself with a bite of something sweet every now and then will actually inhibit your success. Cheating is a very personal decision. If you want to cheat, there is a sacrifice. You simply will not lose weight as quickly, and may not lose weight at all, if your cheating is throwing off your entire meal. Without the presence of insulin, the amount of calories and fat grams you eat does not matter (but you still should not overdo it). This scenario changes drastically when you add foods that create the presence of insulin, such as sugar and carbohydrates. If you are eating foods that create an insulin response, the entire mass of food has the potential to be stored as fat. Now the calories and fat grams *do* matter because there's simply more energy to be converted to fat. If you are going to cheat, cheat with an isolated food rather than adding it to a large meal.

If you are going to eat a piece of cake, you do not want to eat a high-calorie, high-fat meal right beforehand. You would be better off having a light salad and vegetables if you know you are going to blow it on cake. The fiber in salad helps diminish the effects of the insulin. Plus, salad is low in calories and fat, so at least if you're going to send a meal to the fat reserves, it is only salad and cake. Now if you're *not* going to have the cake, you can eat mozzarella marinara and salad with full-fat dressing. You can eat the chicken with butter sauce, but if you add the cake, you now put a high-fat and high-calorie meal at risk of being converted to fat. Stay on Level One until you feel the fat start melting away. Some drop weight the first week while it takes longer for others. It took me two months for "the melt" to begin! Be patient and stick with it. When your cells are unloaded from the built-up sugar, you can cheat a little in what I call Almost Level One and still maintain your progress.

The moral of the story is . . . if you are not seeing results, you are probably cheating without even knowing it. Reexamine your meals, then reread all the food lists to make sure you are on track. If you are doing everything right and still not seeing results, you may be overeating. Yes, you can eat too much even when you Somersize. Listen to your tummy. Remember, eat until you are full, not stuffed. If you are a compulsive eater, you may be giving your body more food than it needs. Other reasons for slowed weight loss can be eating too much fruit and carbohydrates. My husband, Alan, got fat from eating too much fruit. He was eating fifteen to twenty servings of fruit a day, thinking he was doing his body good! It was too much sugar. It even made his cholesterol increase. Again, here's an example of someone pushing the envelope . . . and he lives with me, Queen Somersizer! If you are eating a lot of Fruit and Carbos meals, you should consider cutting back until your weight loss gets jump-started. That does not mean you should eliminate these foods completely. If you still do not see results, you may have a hormonal imbalance that requires hormone replacement therapy as discussed in the beginning of the book.

A SAMPLE WEEK ON LEVEL ONE

People always ask me, "Well, what do you eat?" I tell them that I may have a Carbos breakfast and then a Pro/Fats and Veggies lunch, but they want to know what I literally eat for every meal and snack.

I don't think about every meal with such detail because this way of eating has become second nature to me, but one week I did keep a food diary and I have included here a whole week's worth of meals on Level One. I have not included portion size because, as you know, you simply eat until you are full. In addition, some people get confused by the timing between eating Pro/Fats and Carbos. You need to wait three hours when switching from one to the other so that your system is cleared and you are not mixing these groups without knowing it. Again, the reason we separate these groups is that when we eat proteins or fats we don't want the presence of insulin. Carbos and Fruit will both cause the release of insulin and that is why we eat them separately from Pro/Fats. This sample week will give you some suggestions on how the timing works. Once you get the hang of it, it becomes second nature. Your own meals can vary from mine tremendously, but perhaps this will give you some additional ideas for meal plans. (For tons of recipe suggestions, check out *Eat Great, Lose Weight*; *Get Skinny on Fabulous Food*; *Eat, Cheat, and Melt the Fat Away*; *Fast and Easy*; *Somersize Desserts*; and *Somersize Chocolate*.

SUNDAY

9:00 BREAKFAST
   Omelette with Fontina, Wild Mushrooms, Pancetta and Sage (page 162)
   Side of turkey sausage
   Decaf coffee

1:00 LUNCH AT HOME
   Summer Tomato Soup with Basil Pistou and Parmesan Crisps (page 168)
   Mixed green salad

4:00 SNACK ON THE BEACH
   Two peaches

7:00 FAMILY DINNER
   Pot roast with onions and tomatoes
   Steamed asparagus
   Green salad with vinaigrette

MONDAY

BREAKFAST
   (7:00) Fruit smoothie (peaches, raspberries, orange juice)
   (7:30) Whole-wheat toast with nonfat cottage cheese
   Decaf coffee

10:00 SNACK
Apple

1:00 LUNCH AT A RESTAURANT
Caesar salad with grilled chicken (no
croutons)

4:00 SNACK
Hard-boiled egg

7:30 DINNER AT HOME
Pan-Roasted Sole with Thyme Butter
Sauce (page 242)
Steamed asparagus

TUESDAY

7:00 BREAKFAST
Fried eggs
Crisp bacon

1:00 LUNCH
Salad of iceberg lettuce with blue cheese
dressing
Grilled chicken breast with assorted
grilled vegetables (zucchini, onions,
peppers)

7:00 DINNER AT HOME
Peppered Pork Chops with Fried Sage
Leaves (page 253)
Braised Red Chard (page 206)
Steamed broccoli and cauliflower with
lemon garlic butter
Butter lettuce salad with garlic vinai-
grette

9:00 SNACK
Plum

WEDNESDAY

BREAKFAST
(6:00) Honeydew melon
(6:45) Decaf cappuccino with nonfat milk

(9:00) Toasted whole-wheat bagel
Nonfat yogurt

2:00 LUNCH
Baby greens with Parmesan cheese, sun-
dried tomatoes, and chicken breast

6:00 DINNER
Chicken Patty Lemon Piccata (page 230)
Steamed broccoli
Radicchio, arugula, and endive salad
with Parmesan cheese

9:00 SNACK
A piece of Cheddar cheese

THURSDAY

7:00 BREAKFAST
Scrambled eggs with turkey sausage links
Decaf coffee

10:00 SNACK
Piece of string cheese

1:00 LUNCH
Taco salad—romaine lettuce, ground
beef, Cheddar cheese, sour cream, and
salsa (no beans, tortillas, or guacamole)

4:00 SNACK
Apple

7:30 DINNER AT HOME
Roast chicken breast with Somersize
Tuscan Sea Salt Rub
Lemony artichokes
Salad with Somersize Green Goddess
dressing

9:30 DESSERT
Somersize Vanilla Ice Cream (made with
cream and sweetened with Somer-
Sweet)

BREAKFAST
(9:00) Papaya
(9:30) Shredded wheat with nonfat milk

12:30 **LUNCH**
Cobb salad (no avocado)

3:00 **SNACK**
Celery sticks with Somersize Ranch
Dressing

7:00 **DINNER**
Zucchini noodles alfredo with grilled
chicken
Green salad

SATURDAY

BREAKFAST
(9:00) Strawberry and peach fruit
smoothie
(9:30) Somersize Crispy Sweet Whole
Wheat Flakes with nonfat milk

12:30 **LUNCH**
Chopped Vegetable Salad with Roasted
Chicken (page 181)

6:30 **DINNER**
Lamburger with Tomato Chutney and
Mint (page 249)
Tomato and basil salad with feta cheese

ALMOST LEVEL ONE

Level One is for weight loss and Level Two is for maintenance—these are very clear guidelines. When you want to lose weight you must stick to Level One, but for many who have a substantial amount of weight to lose, the task seems too daunting to think of giving up ALL the Funky Foods until we reach our goal weight. That is why I created Almost Level One. This category is for when you are achieving steady weight loss and can incorporate the occasional treat on your way to your goal.

This is an important category because it allows us to be human on our journey to our ideal body composition. For example, I tell you not to concentrate on nutrition facts, but rather to focus on ingredient lists to see if a product fits into one of the Somersize food groups. If you are at Level One that would mean absolutely no chocolate until you reach your goal weight. Even chocolate made without sugar! Take my SomerSweet Chocolates, for example. The only ingredient that is forbidden for Somersizers is unsweetened chocolate. Everything else is acceptable. My SomerSweet Chocolates are made with high-quality Belgian chocolate and sweetened with SomerSweet. That means these are not allowed on Level One, but once you are steadily losing you may enjoy them, in moderation, during Almost Level One. There is no reason that you should have to wait until you've lost all your weight to enjoy these divine little treats. In addition, having one of these chocolates every now and then will keep you away from the sugar treats that will seriously disrupt your progress and lead to more sugar cravings.

When you first begin the program, stick to the Level One guidelines . . . all of them. I encourage you not to cheat so that your body will release all the stored sugar from your cells and convert your fat reserves to

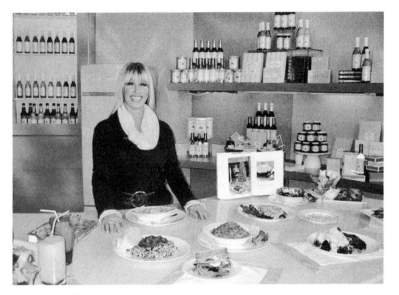

On the set of HSN—my other home in Florida!

fuel. This is how you jump-start your weight loss. Do not halt the process by giving your body sugar or refined carbohydrates for energy. You need to be vigilant so that you train your body to unload your stored sugar and use your fat for energy. As I said, this takes a different amount of time for each person. Some lose ten pounds in the first couple weeks; for me it took much longer to clear out all of my stored sugar. The speed of your weight loss may vary greatly depending upon how much healing your metabolism needs. Be patient. One day it hit me and "the melt" began. It felt as if the pounds were literally melting off my body while I ate fabulous, rich foods.

Once you are steadily losing weight, you may begin to incorporate Almost Level One treats on occasion. How often? As often as your body can handle without disrupting your progress. For example, Somersizers often ask me if they can have berries

with sugar-free whipped cream on Level One. Again, the hard and fast rules say, "Eat fruit alone," but berries are the easiest fruit to combine with other foods because of their high fiber content. This is a perfect Almost Level One treat. Should you start eating berries with whipped cream on Level One? No, wait for your weight loss to kick in. When it is in full swing, add the berries.

Your next question will be, "How many Almost Level One treats can I have in a day?" I don't have a number for you. You will have to figure that out for yourself by using trial and error on your own body. When I am losing weight on Level One, and having little cheats on Almost Level One, a typical day might include a Level One breakfast, a Level One lunch, an Almost Level One treat in the afternoon (such as a couple of my SomerSweet Butter Toffees), and a Level One dinner with an Almost Level One dessert, such as

Somersize Chocolate Mousse or Crème Brûlée.

Do not eat desserts all day! A big part of this program is to help you eat like a normal person. This does not include binge eating. That means that you shouldn't binge on steak—even though you can and still be within the Somersize guidelines. This also means you shouldn't binge on Somersize desserts, even though they have "Somersize" in the name. Please don't overdo it. Eat three meals a day and include healthy snacks. Eat real food. I cannot stress this enough. Real food with treats in moderation is the Somersize way.

I have many Somersizers who push the envelope and try to cram in as many desserts as they can, since technically they are Level One. You must undo this psyche. This is your former dieting self who is looking for ways to beat the system and still get results. There is no beating the system with Somersize. You get wonderful foods and as much as you need to feel full. This is your opportunity to undo the fear of food, the fear of dieting, and the fear of failure. Take this moment to decide to control your food rather than letting it control you. You are given all the tools to do this with Somersize. You will not go hungry. You will not have to go without sweets. You will not have to go without bread. You just need to be moderate and you need to make selections that will help you rather than hinder you. Once you get into this rhythm you will stop trying to push the limits of the program and simply enjoy the freedoms you have within it and the results you will see because of it.

I know you have questions about the guidelines, and my customer service representatives at SuzanneSomers.com are very knowledgeable about the program. Every now and then they will forward me a question in which an issue seems unclear. Can you use fat-free chicken broth in a Carbos and Veggies soup? Or can you use egg whites in a Carbos and Veggies dish? I have seen long threads on the discussion boards or long chats in the chat room. This is when I am asked to settle an "argument" since both sides feel they are right. No, you may not use fat-free chicken broth or egg whites with Carbos and Veggies in Level One. Technically, that is not within the guidelines of the program. However, each of these instances would create a tiny imbalance and I promise you that no one is getting fat off a cup of fat-free chicken broth with some brown rice and broccoli or with an egg white in a whole-grain bread mix. Stop worrying and start enjoying the delicious food you can eat on Level One and Almost Level One. Follow the guidelines as best as you can and you will see results. As you heal your metabolism and begin to lose weight, you will also heal these issues with food.

I hope this explanation of Almost Level One is helpful to you. Follow the rules, but bend them as you see fit. If you notice a slowing in your weight loss, you know you have gone too far and you need to get back to Level One. Don't try to beat the program. Let the program help you to beat your battle with weight. Conquer it once and for all and let this be the last time you get down to your goal weight.

CHAPTER 11

Level Two: Somersize for Life with the All-New Level Two!

The information in this section is new to existing Somersizers. In the past I basically referred to Level Two as Level One with cheating. Now I am a bit more specific about those cheats. With the information I have on the effects of low-carbing for too long, I have modified the way I describe Level Two. Level Two is the maintenance portion of the program, and in order to sustain all your hard work for life you need to rethink your Somersize meals.

Old Level Two thinking was that you continue to eat on Level One, then cheat with wine, desserts, or carbohydrates when you feel like it. If you start to gain weight you have had too many treats and need to cut back to find your balance. Now I realize that I need to be much more specific to make sure you are creating a balance that will last for your whole lifetime. This means getting back to basics and including protein, vegetables, a moderate amount of fats, and

whole-grain carbohydrates at each meal. Now that your body is in balance you can handle the carbohydrates with your proteins and you should include them!

Here's how it works: When you stand naked in front of the mirror and you are thin through the middle, and you are feeling happy with the way you are looking, you can graduate to Level Two, the maintenance portion of Somersizing. Your insulin levels are balanced, which is evident by your beautiful new slim waistline, so you can afford to add the carbohydrates and even indulge every once in a while.

MIXING PRO/FATS AND CARBOS

As I detailed in the carbohydrate section, now that your system is clean, you will find that your body needs a small amount of carbohydrates with your Pro/Fats meal. In fact, your body will welcome it. Eating proteins, fats, and a small portion of carbohydrates at every meal will help keep your entire hormonal system balanced. On Level One, that small portion of carbohydrates comes from the low-starch vegetables we eat. Now that you are on Level Two, you may give your body those carbohydrates in higher-starch forms without upsetting your maintenance. You may add one slice of whole-wheat toast with your eggs. You may add half a cup of brown rice with your turkey soup. You may have about half a cup of whole-wheat pasta with your steak and broccoli. You may add one slice of whole-grain bread with your salad. You may even have formerly forbidden starchy vegetables like a small buttered potato—yes, a potato!—with your chicken and asparagus. Or half of a sweet potato with a pork chop and green beans. I add these carbohydrates to my meals a few times a week. Just make sure that the carbohydrate is not the main portion of the meal. It should be a small side dish within a Pro/Fats and Veggies meal. Your body can now handle the moderate insulin release and will enjoy the benefits of the release of serotonin it gets from ingesting carbohydrates.

Remember, if we deplete our system of carbohydrates for too long, we can lower our serotonin levels. Eating too many carbohydrates, or not eating enough, can throw off our hormonal balance. When our serotonin levels are low, we will crave carbohydrates and sugar. That's when we become prone to cheating and we pig out on a gigantic chocolate bar. Adding these little carbohydrate treats on Level Two keeps our hormones balanced, and therefore keeps those sugar cravings away.

When you combine carbohydrates with Pro/Fats, don't go overboard. For instance, you might have one slice of buttered whole-wheat toast with your eggs in the morning, but a stack of pancakes made from white flour would be overdoing it. Or you could have a tuna melt on one slice of whole-grain bread for lunch, but white bread would not be advised. For dinner you might have a small portion of wild rice with your chicken and vegetables, but a side of white pasta would be a bit much.

Every now and then you may really want those pancakes, white bread, or pasta. Just make sure the imbalance is really worth it to you. Then go back and eat a few strict Level One meals for a while until you get your system back in balance. That's how Level Two works; you eat most meals with protein, vegetables, and moderate amounts of fat and carbohydrates. Plus, every now and then you decide to treat yourself. When I give myself a sugar treat I do not add the carbohydrate. In Level Two I am free to add a little olive oil on my whole-grain pasta or some wild rice in my chicken soup. About once or twice a year I have a big treat, like French fries. (I eat them with a salad. The fiber helps to minimize the effects of the insulin.) We are all human!

I find that on Level Two I can eat a few more Carbos meals, even with a little bit of fat. Sometimes I have whole-grain pasta or brown rice for lunch with vegetables. On Level One I have no oil with this meal, but on Level Two I can sauté the vegetables in some oil and have a more flavorful stir-fry without causing a significant imbalance. But adding protein to a carbohydrate meal is a little tricky. If I want to have meat with my pasta or brown rice, I would make the meal predominantly a Pro/Fats meal with a small portion of pasta or rice (about a half cup or so), rather than have a big bowl of pasta with a few pieces of meat. The protein in combination with a significant amount of carbs is harder on your body than a little fat in combination with the carbs.

If you want to have a sandwich you can stick to lettuce cups in place of bread or you can use one slice of whole-grain bread. You can even add the avocado every now and then. The avocado has fat and carbohydrate, but the new you can handle this imbalance. If avocado isn't your thing, you might add a little mayonnaise or olive oil, depending on the sandwich.

Everyone cheats in different ways. I find I rarely create an imbalance cheating on sugary desserts. Now that I have SomerSweet, I don't miss real sugar. The sugars I miss the most are a glass of wine once or twice a week. When I drink a glass of wine or two, I know I have created a slight imbalance. As a result I will go back to clean eating with protein, vegetables, and moderate amounts of carbohydrates and fat. You have to be the judge of how many times per week you can cheat. When your pants are feeling tight, or your waistband starts cutting into your skin, it is time to go back to Level One. I used to be able to cheat more without having any adverse effects on my body. Now I find that if I keep my cheating to a couple of times a week, I can maintain my figure. If I cheat any more than that, I find I start getting thick through the middle.

It's comforting to know that no foods are forbidden. Somersize simply asks that you first lose the unwanted weight, and when you have reached your goal, you can begin to incorporate previously forbidden foods in moderation. That means adding a small amount of whole-grain carbs or starchy vegetables to your proteins and even occasionally adding back the sugars you miss the most. I encourage you to add the carbohydrates in moderation! Now that your body is in balance you can handle the small amount of insulin because your cells are cleaned out of sugar. This combination of protein, fats, vegetables, and whole grains is the key to sensible eating.

During this time, you are your own policeman. You can't blow it. If you find that you have gotten off the Somersizing track, simply go back to Level One and resume eating delicious, flavorful foods, but be sure to eliminate all sugars, so you can give your body a chance to lower its insulin levels and efficiently metabolize the foods you are ingesting.

In general, I eat moderate portions of all the foods my body needs to thrive—protein, vegetables, and moderate amounts of fat and carbohydrates. I also include plenty of fruit and continue to eat it alone. Level Two involves cheating to some degree or another, so I remain vigilant because I do not want to go back to struggling with my weight. I am in control of my weight by Somersizing. I have been eating this way for more than ten years. The reason I know I will eat this way for the rest of my life is that

Somersize recognizes how human we all are. If you are craving or missing certain foods, have them, and then return to Level One eating.

Be careful not to slip back into bad habits. On Level One, by eliminating Funky Foods, you have trained your pancreas not to oversecrete insulin. And rather than filling up on empty carbohydrates that give your body a quick source of energy, you have trained your body to use your fat reserves as an energy source. You've conditioned your system to digest quickly and efficiently by cutting out bad combinations. You have released the stored sugar from your cells and healed your metabolism. Now your body is in great shape and can handle a few imbalances.

The last thing we want is for all your hard work to be thrown away by resuming old habits. Level Two is about helping you find a balance so you can enjoy previously forbidden foods in moderation, without completely throwing caution to the wind. On Level Two, you are the only person who can determine how much imbalance your body can handle. Some people have to stay very close to Level One guidelines, with the small addition of carbohydrates in order to maintain their weight. Other people find they can create quite a few imbalances and still maintain their weight. By using trial and error, you will soon know how many imbalances your body can handle. Listen to your body. I know I've created too much of an imbalance when I feel bloated after a meal. Another warning sign for me is if I feel tired an hour or two after a meal. These are signs that I have strayed too far from

Level One and need to pull in the reins. Of course, the most obvious sign is if you start to gain weight. Then you know you need to cut back on the treats and eat more moderately!

There are specific guidelines necessary to lose weight on Level One, and if you've gotten down to your goal weight, you have followed them diligently. I wish I could give you specific guidelines for Level Two, but actually that's the beauty of it . . . there are no hard and fast rules for Level Two. You are in control of your body and you need to find a rhythm you can live with for the rest of your life.

The great thing is that no matter how large an imbalance you create, you can always find your equilibrium. Level Two is really an extension of Level One, but there are some serious differences. In Level One there is no portion control as long as you are within the guidelines of the program. In Level Two we are going to add the carbohydrate back to our protein meals and once you do that you must watch your portion size and must be careful not to overdo it with fats. In addition, you must not overindulge in treats. It goes without saying, but moderation is the key to maintaining your weight.

On Level One I would enjoy a piece of chicken or fish with a lovely butter sauce, a vegetable, and a salad. On Level Two I will add a moderate amount of whole-grain carbs (about $1/2$ cup). This way my body is getting protein, fat, vegetables, and carbohydrates. If I wanted to indulge myself, I would hold the carbs and maybe have a piece of flourless chocolate cake (made with SomerSweet, of course). Certainly, I would not have chocolate cake every day or it would catch up with me. And I would not eat the protein with the carbohydrate and the cake because that would be too much insulin present to store the protein and fat as fat. The protein meal with a white-flour roll as well as the cake would be out of the question.

I also find on Level Two that I can handle a few more Carbos and Veggies meals. Whereas on Level One I almost exclusively eat my carbs at breakfast, on Level Two I might incorporate an occasional lunch and dinner revolving around whole-wheat pasta or brown rice. Again, only you can determine how many of these Carbos meals you can eat without upsetting your system.

FRUITS

I still try to eat from the Fruits group completely separately. The only fruit I play around with is berries, because berries are easier to digest than other fruits. They have a very high fiber content and give me little trouble when I combine them with other foods. On Level Two I do not even think twice about eating fresh berries with whipped cream after a Pro/Fats and Veggies meal. Also, when I get tired of toast with nonfat cottage cheese or nonfat yogurt, I use SomerSweet jam on my toast in the morning. And if I just have to have pancakes, there's no need to cheat because I can use my Somersize Pancake and Waffle Mix, which is made with whole grains. Then I top it with Somersize Syrup or Jam. Regular pancakes with butter and maple syrup

would create a huge imbalance, whereas these whole-wheat or multigrain pancakes create less of an imbalance and still satisfy my craving. I also like to use berries in tarts and pies made with whole-wheat crusts; certainly not Level One fare, but easier on your system than an apple tart or a pumpkin pie. And for breakfast or a snack in the afternoon, I like to have fresh berries with nonfat yogurt.

I also may add a few products that are sweetened with fruit juice. At health food stores I've found a few cereals made from spelt and amaranth and kamut flakes that are sweetened with a little fruit juice. Fruit juice, like sugar, creates an insulin response, but your body can handle it now in moderation because your cells are not overloaded with sugar.

ADDING A LITTLE SUGAR AND FUNKY FOODS

As far as sugar goes, I loosen the reins a little. I'm not quite as diligent about hunting for sugar in sauces and salad dressings. If I'm at a restaurant, I don't worry about eating a prepared blue cheese dressing on my salad, even if it has a little sugar in it. It's not enough to cause a problem for me on Level Two. I continue to avoid gravy made with white flour and very sweet sauces, like barbecue sauce. And watch out for those thick Chinese sauces made with sugar and cornstarch. Most restaurants are happy to prepare your food without these ingredients.

I also find I can freely enjoy the foods on the Bad Combo list such as nuts, olives, liver, avocado, and tofu. These are the easiest foods on your system to bring back because they are all real foods and they have incredible health benefits. Now your body can handle the small amount of carbs naturally occurring with the proteins and fats. Nuts are a wonderful Level Two snack.

And how about desserts? With Somer-Sweet, I enjoy Level One desserts a few times a week. Almost Level One desserts can be eaten as frequently as you can handle. It depends on your system. As a rule, I still try to stay away from desserts made with sugar. For me it really isn't worth it and my SomerSweet desserts are so delicious, how could I ever feel deprived?

Check out some of my recipes for desserts made with SomerSweet. Chocolate Espresso Gelato. Wild Berry Crostada. Velvet Chocolate Pudding. Yum! They are delicious Almost Level One treats. For additional dessert recipes, check out my books *Somersize Desserts* and *Somersize Chocolate*. Oh, my. The beauty of this program is that if you want dessert, you can have it!

Another good dessert option after a Pro/Fats meal is Somersize Ice Cream with Somersize Triple Hot Fudge. Even regular ice cream is often lower in sugar than other desserts and is made mostly of Pro/Fats (eggs and cream). If you can't make your own Somersize Ice Cream, make sure to buy the best-quality ice cream, because you want it to have more cream than milk (remember, milk has carbohydrates; cream does not). Pudding, crème brûlée, and chocolate mousse are generally lower in sugar than most other desserts and do not include white flour as many other pastries do. My Somersize versions of these products are made completely with SomerSweet. And as I mentioned, flourless chocolate cake is a great option on Level Two, or chocolate-dipped strawberries with freshly whipped cream!

You really can eat these desserts and maintain your weight if you are Somersizing properly. Check out my recipes in all the books for Level One, Almost Level One, and Level Two desserts. You'll be knocked out by how great they are. They are all made with SomerSweet. The Almost Level One and Level Two desserts contain whole-wheat pastry flour instead of white flour and chocolate with no refined sugars. With SomerSweet, we can enjoy many more desserts the Somersize way.

YOU'RE IN CONTROL

As far as Level Two goes, you are in control. How you choose your imbalances depends on many factors. How many imbalances have you had today and how big were they? How many big imbalances have you had this week? Don't get cocky with your new figure! The pounds can creep back onto your body if you're not careful.

Beware of the slipups. It usually starts with one dessert, which leads to another, and then another. Before you know it, you've started adding bad combinations and a little white flour here and there. Your body will signal you with warning signs. Learn to listen to them! If you start craving sugar and carbohydrates, it means you are eating too much of them. That's what happens; the more sugar you eat, the more you crave. Then come the energy dips, the extra pounds—and don't forget about the damage you're doing on the inside to your healthy cells. And remember, the best way to take away a sugar craving is to eat a Pro/Fat because Pro/Fats help to stabilize blood sugar. So next time you have a craving for sugar or carbohydrates, eat a piece of cheese and it should help. Or try my Somersize Crave Control to naturally take your cravings away. All in all, if you notice signs that your body is starting to crave sugar again, go back to Level One until you get rid of the problem. Stay on top of the new you. Take care of your body.

I also want to mention portion control one more time. On Level One you may eat as much as you want as long as you are following all the Level One guidelines. (That means technically you can eat until you are full and not gain weight. I'm sure you learned not to overeat, because your appetite was fully satisfied with wholesome, nutritious foods.) On Level Two, you must consider limiting your portions when you are creating imbalances. You can't have it both ways—the bonus of Level One is that you can eat as much as you want. The bonus of Level Two is that you have more variety, but you must limit your portions moderately now that you are adding foods that will create moderate amounts of insulin. Your cells are clean . . . let's keep them that way!

Good luck in this new phase. You have such freedom on Level Two; I just know you will love it. Any questions you have will be answered by your own body as you experiment with Level Two. Eating this way is truly a pleasure and I'm sure you will be the envy of all of your friends who can't believe what wonderful foods you eat while still managing to keep your beautiful figure.

A SAMPLE WEEK ON LEVEL TWO

From week to week my meal plans will vary greatly on Level Two. Make sure to balance your Pro/Fats with moderate amounts of Carbohydrates and get plenty of Fruits and Vegetables. Watch the portion size and watch the fats! You will see that there is a combination of Level One meals and Level Two meals. Remember, your body may be able to handle more or less imbalance, depending on your unique metabolism. I can handle about this many imbalances and still maintain my weight. To help you see how I choose my treats, I have put an asterisk next to the items that are Level Two with a brief explanation regarding the imbalance.

SUNDAY

9:00 BREAKFAST
  Spinach and Parmesan frittata
  Decaf coffee

1:00 LUNCH
  Sliced gyros served over lettuce with
    tomato and garlic cucumber sauce
  1 piece of whole-wheat pita bread★
    (★I combined whole-wheat pita with
    a Pro/Fats and Veggies meal.)

4:00 SNACK
  Hard-boiled egg

7:00 DINNER
  Grilled chicken breast
  Steamed broccoli and cauliflower tossed
    in garlic vinaigrette
  Small buttered potato★
  Green salad with garlic vinaigrette
  A glass of red wine★

Somersize Chocolate Mousse★
(★Wine, a Funky potato, and the Almost
Level One Somersize Chocolate
Mousse)

BREAKFAST
(9:00) Mango
(9:30) Rye toast with Somersize Berry
Jam★
Decaf coffee
(★Berry jam creates a slight imbalance
with my toast.)

1:30 LUNCH
Warm goat cheese salad with chicken,
pine nuts, and sun-dried tomatoes★
(★I added pine nuts to my salad.)

4:30 SNACK
SomerSweet Butter Toffee★ (two pieces)
(★An Almost Level One treat.)

7:30 DINNER
Pan-fried pork tenderloin
Celery root purée
Steamed green beans
Butter lettuce salad with balsamic vinai-
grette

TUESDAY

BREAKFAST
7:00 New Mexican Huevos★ (page 163)
(★The whole-wheat tortilla with the
eggs makes this Level Two)

12:30 LUNCH
Roasted Yellow Pepper Soup with
Crostini with Homemade Ricotta
Cheese★ (page 172)
Green salad

(★A small amount of whole-grain bread
with the Pro/Fats and Veggies soup
makes this Level Two)

3:00 SNACK
Somersize Butterscotch Pudding★
(★I use half and half to make this delicious
pudding. It adds only a few carbs to
the fats, making it Almost Level One)

7:30 DINNER
Bruschetta Artichokes (page 205)
Grilled Lamb Chops with Lavender Lamb
Jus (page 247) and Grilled Fennel and
Zucchini (page 213)
1/2 cup Farro Risotto★ (page 227)
(★The whole-grain risotto with the
Pro/Fats makes this Level Two)

WEDNESDAY

BREAKFAST
(6:00) 1/2 melon and decaf coffee
(6:45) Somersize Apple Cinnamon Oatmeal

12:00 LUNCH
Sautéed Cabbage with Pine Nuts★ and
Goat Cheese (page 215)
Crispy-Skinned Salmon with Roasted
Garlic Aïoli and Warm Radicchio–
Shiitake Mushroom Salad (page 238)
and ★French Lentils (page 216)
(★I included nuts and lentils with my
Pro/Fats for a Level Two lunch.)

4:00 SNACK
One SomerSweet Peppermint Cream
Truffle★ (An Almost Level One treat)

7:00 DINNER
Apple Salad with Blue Cheese Vinai-
grette★ (page 184)

Braised Veal Stew with Gremolata (page
250) and celery root potato puree★
(★The apples in the salad and the potatoes
in the puree make this Level Two.)

THURSDAY

6:30 BREAKFAST
Fruit smoothie with mango, papaya,
and pineapple

12:00 LUNCH
Vegetable sandwich (made with Somersize Onion Bread, tomato, cucumber,
lettuce, and Somersize Sun-Dried
Tomato Dip Mix combined with
nonfat cream cheese)

3:00 SNACK
Somersize Chewy Caramel Balls★
(★An Almost Level One treat)

6:00 DINNER
Tuscan White Bean Soup★ (page 171)
Grilled Tuna with Lemon-Thyme Aïoli
and Chilled Asparagus with Lemon-
Thyme Aïoli (pages 241
and 208)
Wild Berry Crostada★ (page 264)
(★Adding the beans to the Pro/Fats, plus
the dessert makes this Level Two.)

FRIDAY

BREAKFAST
(6:30) 2 ripe persimmons
(7:00) Somersize Blueberry Muffin★
(★The muffin mix is Almost Level One
because there is egg white with the
whole-wheat flour)

12:45 LUNCH
Chicken Caesar Salad
Somersize Crème Brûlée

3:30 SNACK
Sliced jicama and celery

7:00 DINNER
Butter lettuce salad with fennel
Lamb chops with steamed green beans
and $1/2$ of a potato★
(★Adding the potato to the Pro/Fats
makes this Level Two)

SATURDAY

8:00 BREAKFAST
Alan's fried eggs in onion nests
One slice of buttered toast★
Decaf coffee
(★I added whole-grain toast to Pro/Fats
for Level Two)

12:00 LUNCH
Cheeseburger (no bun) with lettuce,
tomato, onion, and Somersize Secret
Sauce
Somersize Strawberry Ice Cream with
Triple Hot Fudge Sauce★
(★The ice cream is made with half and
half and the hot fudge is Almost
Level One)

3:00 SNACK
A piece of string cheese

8:00 DINNER
Stir-fried chicken and vegetables with
brown rice★
(★The whole-grain rice with the Pro/
Fats makes this Level Two)

CHAPTER 12

Plateaus

At some point in your life you just get sick of the way you look and you decide to make a change. This time you really mean it. You start a weight-loss program. You commit fully and are thrilled when you see results. The pounds begin to drop. Your clothes fit better. People ask, "What are you doing? You look great!" All is going well, until, after a certain period of time, the magic begins to fade. Suddenly the scale keeps staring back at you with the same number you've seen for the past few weeks. You are still sticking to the plan, but what happened to your results? It's the word no dieter wants to hear . . . yes, you've hit the dreaded plateau. During this phase you are tested to the max. You can either choose to stick with it and ride it out or you can let the frustration get you down. If you choose the latter, you start eating poorly, thinking, "It doesn't matter either way, so I might as well splurge." That's when the pounds

slowly creep back on and you end up as heavy as when you started—or worse, even heavier.

How can we stop the roller-coaster dieting? First of all, we cannot diet. We must change to a new lifestyle that lasts a lifetime. Somersize provides that lifestyle, but even with Somersize some of us still hit plateaus. What to do? I have received many letters and e-mails from Somersizers who have experienced this exact scenario. I have hit plateaus myself. As I have said, when you are Somersizing, the initial period of weight loss will vary from individual to individual. Some drop several pounds in the first week. Others, like me, take longer to clean out the stored sugar in their cells and it takes weeks before they begin to see results. Once "the melt" begins and the weight begins to fall off, it's like a whole new world! You happily greet each day with your Somersize plan because you know it is working and you feel satisfied by the delicious foods you eat. Then the weight loss hits a stall and you wonder what you've done wrong. You can't figure out why your body and your once beloved Somersize program have betrayed you. The answer is not the same for everyone so I will give you several layers of advice to see what piece may fit you.

SCENARIO #1: HOW DARE YOU CALL ME A CHEATER!

Take a good look at your meals and snacks. Are you truly following the Level One guidelines or have you slipped so far into Almost Level One that you are actually eating on Level Two? You could be eating "little treats" here and there that are adding up to more insulin than your body can handle. This happens frequently when you've been on the program for some time and have enjoyed weight loss, even with a slight bending of the rules.

My advice is that you keep a food journal of everything you eat for a full week. Write it down in any format you like; just make sure you document every meal, drink, and snack that goes into your mouth. This will help you to see where you might be straying too far from Level One. I designed a Somersize Journal for this purpose which is available on my Web site. Of course, any journal will do.

If you notice that you are including too many treats, you need to back off. Have you been slipping up with sugary condiments and salad dressings when you're out to eat? Have you been eating cereal, convincing yourself that it is legal even though it is just slightly sweetened? Are you including "just a couple" French fries with your cheeseburger patty and salad? Are you eating chicken that has been coated with flour? All of these slight imbalances add up. Once you begin to lose weight, you may have an imbalance here and there in Almost Level One, but too many at one time can and will throw you off.

My own Somersize products can be the biggest culprit here. Many of my desserts and candies are Almost Level One. That means they need to be eaten in moderation. They are designed to give you a taste here and there to keep you away from sugar and refined carbohydrates. If you are filling up on Almost Level One treats, back off and see if your weight loss resumes. Remember, a couple of squares of a SomerSweet Chocolate Crunch Bar are plenty. You don't need to eat the whole bar! As for SomerSweet Butter Toffee, you may be tempted to open a dozen of those golden foil-wrapped delights, but that is not the idea behind the treats I have provided for you. Enjoy one toffee so that you don't give in to temptation and eat a real piece of candy. Somersize Chewy Caramel Balls are great to bring to the movies to keep your hands out of the popcorn and candy; but don't eat half a bag! I suggest five to six balls at most. As for Somersize Brownies, Devil's Food Cake, Triple Hot Fudge Sauce, and more—think moderation. One piece of brownie is enough! Don't think you can eat the whole pan just because they are Somersized. They are still a treat! My suggestion would be that you stop eating all Almost

Level One Somersize treats and see if you can push past the plateau. If you begin to lose weight you can see that you were indulging too much in these treats and you need to limit your consumption should you choose to include them again.

You also need to watch out for the many "low-carb" products on the market. I have a friend who was Somersizing with great success for over a year. Suddenly she started gaining weight and couldn't figure out why. When I went to her house I saw that she had loaded up on grocery-store "low-carb" products that she assumed fit into Somersizing. It's not that each product was so bad, but a day of eating these foods intermittently rather than real food was adding up and so, too, the pounds.

I myself have also been known to add too many imbalances. I remember at one point I had put on a couple of pounds and I wasn't eating any differently than I had been. I was discussing with my daughter-in-law, Caro-

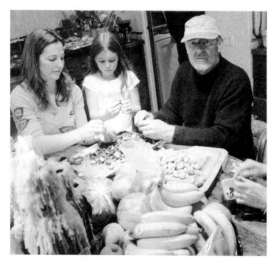

Alan and the girls busy at work peeling roasted chestnuts for Christmas dinner.

line, the fact that I had gone back to Level One and the program didn't seem to be working for me anymore. Caroline and I are always talking about ways to improve Somersizing. I was sharing my frustration with her and she said, "You know you are a little cheater, right?" I must admit I got a tad indignant. Me? A little cheater? Then I thought about it. Yes, I have been known to have a few white-flour noodles with my chicken soup or perhaps a little Dove Miniature for dessert. C'mon, it's not a whole Dove Bar, just a little Dove "bite"! I was eating a whole-grain cereal sweetened with cane juice (this was before I had Somersize cereal). At our favorite Mexican place, I would carefully order pork chili verde and a green salad (no croutons) for lunch. Then I would mindlessly eat a few chips with salsa. And here I was, convinced that I had been Somersizing perfectly! You must realize when you are eating like you're on Level Two, but expecting results like Level One. I know the reason it happens—sometimes you can add those little imbalances and still get results, but eventually it catches up with you, so you need to watch it.

As soon as I cut out the extras and went back to the real Level One, those extra pounds dropped off immediately. I called Caroline and laughed, "Hey, this Somersizing really works when you do it right!" That's when I decided to create the Somersize Journal. It's like truth serum . . . it really helps!

Another thing to look at: portion size. Perhaps you are eating too much or too little. If you are truly eating on Level One I have explained that you may eat until you are full. Are you listening to your body? Or are you eating more because you still fear that you will go hungry? You could simply be eating more food than your body requires. Or are you one of those people who drinks decaf for breakfast, has a few bites of salad for lunch, and eats a small dinner? That is not enough food and your body may be holding on to the food to keep you from starving to death. Be sensible when it comes to portions.

Finally, you must look at your level of exercise. You may be the type of person who does not exercise and has still enjoyed weight loss with this program. If you have now hit a stall you need to jump-start your metabolism with exercise. You must move!!! Remember, lean muscle mass increases your metabolism. Find an activity that you can commit to and stick with it. One of the testimonials I received in the last book, from September, wrote to give me an update. She started exercising and pushed past her plateau. It could work for you, too.

SCENARIO #2: HOW LOW CAN YOU GO? WITH CARBS, THE ANSWER IS "TOO LOW"

If you truly are eating on Level One, without cheating, and you have still hit a plateau, you need to look at what else could be creating the stall. After keeping a journal and checking all your ingredients on the reference guide, if you are staying true to the program and still not getting through you need to move to the next step. This is new information to Somersizers.

When I started the program more than a decade ago, I was not aware of the syndrome of going too low in carbohydrates. I have always recommended including whole-grain carbohydrates, but warned about overdoing it. Too many carbs, even the right kind, can lead to weight gain if your body has more than it needs to supply immediate energy. Most people figure out that the lower you go on the carbs, the faster you lose weight. However (and this is a big "however"), IF YOU GO TOO LOW IN CARBOHYDRATES FOR TOO LONG, YOU CAN ALSO CREATE HORMONAL IMBALANCE! As we know, hormonal imbalance leads to weight gain. I'm sure this is confusing to you. I have explained that if you are not eating carbs or sugar, your body will not produce insulin, and insulin is responsible for deciding if food gets stored as fat or burned as fuel. How can food be stored as fat if you're not eating any foods that cause an insulin response?

After trial and error on my own body, learning from other Somersizers, and studying this phenomenon with endocrinologists, I have determined that over long periods of time, some people will actually adjust to not eating carbs and their bodies will rebel against it. In much the same way that your metabolism will slow to protect you against starvation when you are on a low-calorie diet, your body may also adjust to the lack of carbs and stop burning your fat as fuel. This can be especially true for people who have lost a significant amount of weight. Our bodies are programmed to protect us from drastic weight loss. Sadly, the reverse is not true and our bodies don't

LEPTIN — THE SABOTAGER!

When it comes to obesity, many people blame individuals for being weak. Only recently are scientists discovering how our hormones may be sabotaging our weight-loss efforts. Our bodies don't seem to have any problem letting us put on an amount of weight that could kill us, but there is mounting evidence to show that our hormonal system works on overload to keep us from losing a significant amount of weight.

Our bodies are wired to want food—more and more food. Our hormones are finely tuned to regulate both what we eat, when we eat, and how that food will be processed. All of the body's major organs are working together with hormones to regulate these systems. Here are a few of the signals that control our eating habits.

The short-term signals are related to feeling hunger and feeling full. Ghrelin is a hormone that tells us when we are hungry. It's the metaphoric grumble in the tummy. When enough food reaches the small intestine, another hormone, called cholecystokinin, signals that we are full and triggers the release of enzymes in the gallbladder and the pancreas. That is why you hear people say, "Wait a few minutes and see if you're still hungry before you have another helping." You are waiting for the cholecystokinin to kick in and signal your body that you are full.

The hormones leptin and insulin are longer-term signals. Leptin is produced by the fat cells and helps you manage the amount of fat you store around your organs and under your skin. When you are losing weight, your fat stores are being depleted. When this happens, the amount of leptin also decreases. At this point, your body may view this as starvation. This is when your body kicks into gear in an effort to hold on to the food, make you burn fewer calories, and slow down the metabolism to help you regain the weight. The tricky part is that the greater the weight loss, the stronger the signals to eat more and replenish the fat stores.

With this information, you can see that the more weight you have to lose, the harder it may become. Scientists hope to be able to uncover more about this phenomenon. In the meantime, don't give up hope! Resist the temptation to go off track during a plateau. Try going to all new Level Two and see if that helps you break through.

seem to protect us from deadly weight gain! In this way evolution has not caught up to societal norms that now make obesity the common course. Our bodies are programmed to keep us alive—not to let us starve to death. You have to be able to trick your system into allowing a steady weight loss. Don't despair. I have finally figured out this passage and I will explain how to conquer this plateau and continue with your weight loss so that you can reach your goal weight and live there forever.

When you go too low in carbohydrates for too long, it is not insulin that creates the problem; it is a different type of imbalance that has to do with the hormone serotonin. As I explained in the Carbohydrates section, serotonin is the "feel-good hormone" and is produced by the foods we eat. If you are low in serotonin, you will crave carbohydrates, sugar, and caffeine. These are the very foods that will destroy your progress. You must heal your serotonin if you are to have success.

First of all, make sure you are having a Carbos breakfast at least four times a week. This is the best way to have your carbohydrates, since you burn off the energy they supply throughout the day. If you are eating your carbohydrates in the morning and still are stuck at your plateau, you must go the next phase of healing your serotonin, which is a move to Level Two. Level Two? I know this is confusing, since Level Two is for maintenance, but if your serotonin levels are low, a move to Level Two will help repair the damage so that you can resume your weight loss. It must be noted, however, that

this is a modified version of Level Two and does not include the occasional sugar or refined carbohydrate treats. These types of treats add up to maintenance and you do not want maintenance since you are still trying to lose weight.

To break your plateau, this modified version of Level Two simply means at each meal you must add a small helping of whole grains or complex carbohydrates to your Pro/Fats. Have one slice of whole-wheat toast with your eggs. Add about a half cup of whole-grain pasta or brown rice, or even half of a potato with your chicken or steak. If gluten is a problem as it is for me, try quinoa. The recipes in this book offer a variety of ways to prepare this delicious grain. Quinoa is now my favorite grain. This addition of carbohydrates with your protein and fats will balance your hormones and get you back on track. Yes, you are introducing insulin into your protein meals, but you need to do this to create serotonin to keep your system balanced.

Most important, during this phase, you must watch your portions! Once you start adding the carbs back to your meals, you are introducing insulin and you must watch your portions since proteins and fats will be in the presence of insulin. Also, you must watch the saturated fats! Too much fat in the presence of insulin will lead to weight gain. The fun part is that you get to add the carbs, but you must watch the portions and fats. When you are eating these foods without the presence of insulin, there are no portion restrictions, but now you are at the point where you need a balance of protein, fats, and carbohydrates at every meal to place your body back into balance. The good news is that you get that serving of wild rice or a couple of new potatoes, but you cannot eat a block of cheese as an appetizer!

How much is too much? You know I am going to tell you to use your common sense, but if I had to give you amounts, I would say to eat about six to eight ounces of protein, plenty of vegetables, a moderate amount of healthy fats, and about a half cup of complex carbohydrates.

SCENARIO #3:
NOT CHEATING, EATING ENOUGH CARBS, AND STILL NO RESULTS

What if you are Somersizing perfectly, including enough carbs, and *still* seeing no results? Well, if you are at an age where you could be experiencing hormonal loss, you need to see an endocrinologist and have a hormone panel run, as I have described in depth. Other symptoms that may (or may not) accompany weight gain are difficulty sleeping, hot flashes, memory loss, mood swings, depression, and lack of sex drive. How can you be sure? This type of hormonal imbalance can only be detected through a blood test, as I have explained at great length in previous chapters. If you are low in estrogen and progesterone you must replace these lost hormones to achieve balance. This balance will not only make you feel better, but if you Somersize, you will also find your ideal body composition once again.

SCENARIO #4:
NOT CHEATING, EATING ENOUGH CARBS, ON BHRT, AND STILL NO RESULTS

What if you have gone down the complete checklist above and still cannot identify with any of these scenarios? You are not cheating. You eat a good balance of whole-grain carbohydrates. You are eating sensible portions. You exercise. You have had your hormone panel checked. And still you are not losing weight. What now? You could be experiencing adrenal burnout. The serious type A person who is the super-over-achiever and fills every minute of each day with activity and stress will at some point fall off the cliff and have nothing left to give anyone. As you have read earlier, with this type of burnout comes hormonal imbalance, which always leads to weight gain. It can take months to repair the damage. The solution is the same as that for Scenario #2. Go to the modified version of Level Two. Include a half cup of whole grains with your Pro/Fats meals; eat moderate portions and don't overdo it on the saturated fats. Do not include sugar or refined carbohydrate treats. It can take some time to heal from adrenal burnout. Make sure to reread the section on adrenals to get the full advice on how to recover from this scenario.

I hope this helps you to identify why you may be stuck at a plateau. The most important thing to remember is that throwing caution to the wind and returning to old eating habits will only make the situation worse. Stick with it and modify the program as I have suggested above and I'm sure you will find a way to resume your weight loss. Best of luck, and please send me your stories about beating plateaus so that I can continue learning what works for my fellow Somersizers.

WILLPOWER IS NOT ENOUGH: HELPFUL HINTS TO STAY ON YOUR PROGRAM

Do you realize that in the last two decades, the average American diet has expanded by hundreds of calories per day and nearly two-thirds of the population is now overweight? If current trends continue, virtually ALL Americans will be dangerously overweight within a few decades. As a society we must become aware of this vicious cycle of over-supply and overdemand.

Somersizing is a beautiful and easy method of keeping those unwanted pounds at bay, but it is important to understand that willpower alone is not going to do it for us. With Somersizing there is no portion control in Level One; we simply eat until we are full and satisfied . . . not stuffed. Haven't you ever reached a point at which you are full but you keep eating because it tastes so good? This is where we must have internal controls in place to decide "I have had enough." Easier said than done . . . it is practically impossible to discipline yourself out of your desire for food.

Hunger is such a basic biological urge that very few of us can use willpower alone to resist it. Because of that, I have come up with some simple steps to make your Somersize weight-loss program more effective.

First of all, don't keep offending foods in the house. When you are at the store and you pick up that bag of cookies, ask yourself, "Who is this for?" Most of the time on some subliminal level we are buying those cookies for ourselves, tricking our brain into thinking we are buying them "in case company comes over" or to have something around for the kids. Keep all bad foods out of the house. Then when you feel out of control and might go on a binge, there will be no bad foods to indulge in and you will be more likely to satisfy your cravings with a celery stick, a nice piece of Cheddar, or maybe a Somersize chocolate.

Watch your stress level. Stress makes us overeat. The fight-or-flight reaction to stress is hardwired into our brains. Also take your time eating. Chew, taste, enjoy. Pay attention to the sensory qualities of the food you're eating, the taste, texture, aroma. Give your body time to know when you've had enough. For so many of us, eating becomes a way to ease anxiety. If this is the case, make a list of what's bothering you and take action to eliminate unnecessary stresses. Carry a small notebook with you and write down how you're feeling each time you eat. If you are under pressure, take a short walk around the block or up and down the stairs at work. You might try calling a friend or taking a great luxurious warm bath, or putting on some music and dancing. These are enjoyable distractions that will take the desire for food off your mind. If you have to eat, then go for something sensible.

Don't shop when you are hungry . . . go to the grocery store after you have had a meal. The tendency to buy offending foods is greater when you are starving. Also, shop the periphery of the supermarket. The major offending foods that are loaded with chemicals and trans fats are most often found in bags and containers that are located in the center aisles.

Slow down. It takes ten to fifteen minutes for your hormones to signal that you are full. If you eat on the run and wolf down your meal in minutes, your body doesn't have enough time to tell you that you are satisfied. If you eat too quickly, you are almost guaranteed to overeat. Enjoy your food, but stop before you are stuffed.

Take time to plan and prepare food to eat during the week. Jot down some meal ideas and make a grocery list. Then do a big shop and steal an hour on Sunday to make a large batch of soup or stock, or cut up vegetables to nibble on during the week. I often eat the same meal several times in one week. If I make a great pot of soup on Sunday, Alan and I may eat if for three nights before we get bored and want something new. This sure makes mealtime quick and easy when you take a day to prepare something.

Avoid fast foods and treats that are full of chemicals and refined sugar. These foods are digested so quickly that they send blood sugar levels on a roller-coaster ride, causing hunger pangs soon after you eat them. Consequently you can consume a lot of these foods before your body signals your brain that you are satisfied.

Look for foods that are fiber-rich: whole grains, vegetables, and a moderate amount of fruits. These foods keep hunger at bay and they are nutritious.

Add water to your daily intake. We need eight eight-ounce glasses of water every day. You also get water from food you eat. Foods high in water content also control cravings. Celery, peppers, berries, apples, and oranges are all great foods to nibble on.

Studies have shown that people tend to overeat by as much as 40 percent when they're tired. The body's wiring interprets exhaustion as a trigger to fuel up for more energy; also, fatigue makes it harder to be disciplined about the size and quality of meals. Scientists have even identified "night-eating syndrome," which is associated with depression and low self-esteem. Enjoy small meals throughout the day to keep your body energized. If you still find yourself overeating before you go to bed, allow yourself a snack but keep the portion small and choose something healthy to take the craving away. Also, make sure to get your rest. If you're dragging during the day, take a twenty-minute nap. Make a habit of going to bed early enough to get a full eight hours of sleep. If you have trouble sleeping, try an herbal formula that contains valerian and lemon balm. Bigelow Sweet Dreams tea is a nice one.

Don't feed your moods. Eating is inherently pleasurable and some foods also chemically affect your mood. Carbohydrates, for example, boost levels of the feel-good hormone serotonin. That is why we turn to food when we're feeling bored or upset. If you suffer from clinical depression, feelings of worthlessness, or a lack of pleasure in things you normally enjoy, consult a therapist or qualified doctor. This was one of the best things I ever did for myself. Feelings of irritability and low energy or an inability to concentrate are also important signs. Depression should be taken seriously. In mild cases, Saint-John's-wort is helpful, and it can be bought over the counter. If you are of menopausal age, find a qualified endocrinologist to help you determine your hormone levels and put back the hormones you have lost. The depression you are feeling might have a lot to do with chemical (hormonal) imbalance and, if so, can be rectified. Exercise is a good antidote for garden-variety blues. Numerous studies have shown that physical activity can improve self-esteem and ease mild forms of depression. It's also essential for maintaining weight loss.

Boredom is most often a problem for people who don't have a highly structured schedule, such as people who are out of work. Distract yourself by organizing the house, writing letters, tending to the garden, or doing volunteer work.

Watch for hunger cues. You may think you are hungry, but most Americans don't know what genuine hunger is. The real problem is that most of us eat so often, and in so many different locations, that we experience hunger cues almost everywhere we go, so our appetites can be whetted even when we've just had a big meal.

Limit the places you eat. Stop mindless snacking in front of the TV or in bed. Eat exclusively in one room, preferably sitting at a table. It makes a big difference. You tend to eat more slowly and less frantically if you are seated at a table. If you need a snack at work, get up from your desk and go to the employee cafeteria or break room. This is where a Somersize Protein Bar or a Somersize Protein Shake would help. Make a rule not to eat in the car or while you're walking. (I am a big offender of eating in the car.)

Do a hunger check. It's important to eat something before you are so hungry that you won't "counter surf" (eating anything on the counter). Become more aware of your feelings of satiety. When you've had enough to be comfortable but not completely stuffed, you'll be at the right place for you.

You can do it! Make the change today, right now, and start experiencing a new lifestyle that will keep you healthy and slim.

And, finally, if you are experiencing any of the seven dwarfs of menopause—Itchy, Bitchy, Sweaty, Sleepy, Bloated, Forgetful, and All Dried Up—please, please get yourself to a qualified endocrinologist. All the willpower in the world will not help you. By now you must understand that eating properly, the Somersize way, will help you to maintain your beautiful slim body, but not if your hormones are not balanced. You must put back the hormones you have lost in the aging process or that extra weight will not go away.

This is an essential step to achieve your goal of being slim and sexy forever.

Once you find your balance, you may need to adjust things from time to time. Don't decide "it doesn't work" if your results are not immediate. If you feel things are off, go in for another blood test and have your levels adjusted. It takes some tweaking, but it's worth the effort!!

CHAPTER 13

Exercise

You didn't think I would skip this one, did you? I have said this to you many times: You don't have to be a fanatic about exercise, you just have to get over being lazy. One in four Americans gets no exercise at all. Fewer than one-third get the recommended thirty minutes per day to reduce the risk of chronic disease.

Create even small ways to get exercise. They add up and make a difference. It's so easy to drive everywhere, but what about walking whenever it makes sense instead of driving the car? What about buying yourself a nice new shiny bike? My husband and I have a tandem bike (bicycle built for two) and we love it. We are able to talk and look at the sights while we are getting effortless exercise. I have a lot of stairs on my property so I try to take two stairs at a time to get the best stretch and cardio benefit.

Weight-bearing exercise is essential in the second half of life. After the age of thirty-

five our muscles begin to deteriorate. *We must include weight training to keep our muscles intact.* Start with simple moves using five-pound weights. As you gain strength, increase to ten pounds. If you are able, keep on increasing the poundage as you progress. Every time you do weight-bearing exercise the muscle you are using stimulates bone growth. Loss of bone is a huge factor in aging. Weight-bearing exercise plus hormone replacement is your greatest defense against bone loss.

Also, building lean muscle mass increases your metabolism to help you burn more calories every day. This can really give you a boost and is another great suggestion for pushing through plateaus. Plus, you have the added benefit of beautifully defined muscles to make you look and feel better.

Take a brisk walk every day. The fresh air and benefits to your heart are immeasurable. Remember my analogy of the brand-new car. If it just sits in the garage it is going to sputter and choke when you go to start it. The same goes for your body. If you don't use it, how can you expect it to work at maximum? Don't allow your body to sputter and choke. If you want to get motivated, take a look at someone in a wheelchair. Don't you think they would do ANYTHING to be able to move their body?

Diet, exercise, balanced hormones, and a good mental attitude all add up to optimum living. It's a choice . . . you choose—life or a slow death of disease and poor mental attitude. Exercise is an integral part of maximum health, and let me tell you, at my age you can really see a difference between those who exercise and those who don't. I want to look and feel and be healthy so I drag my sorry ass out of bed each day and I start by doing something. Every day that you exercise is a day you feel better and happier. And on the days you exercise you tend to feel better about yourself so you are more inclined to stay on course with your eating. Positive mental energy affects every part of your day and exercise releases endorphins that make you feel great.

Exercise is also your greatest asset in keeping your system working well. Constipation is a huge problem in the second half of life. Exercise helps to ensure regularity. When your body is all clogged up you feel sluggish and without energy. Don't lie there all cozy in the morning. Get up! Move! Save your quality of life! Exercise is a gift.

So what are some of the ways you can get on the road to a normal exercise routine?

Make an investment in a piece of home exercise equipment. I live in California, so I

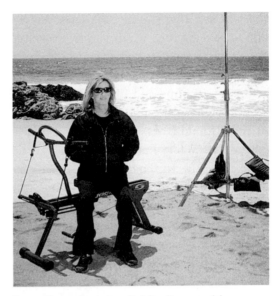

My son, Bruce, directed my BodyRow™ commercial.

have several machines that I leave outside because I don't have room for a home gym. It's actually much nicer to exercise outside in the warmer months. Machines are great because they force you to do each exercise correctly. Doing an exercise incorrectly greatly diminishes the effects of your efforts. Of course, I use the machines that I have developed over the years: the ThighMaster, the BodyRow™, the Ultra Track, and the Torso Track. These machines have been targeted for most of our problem areas. There are many wonderful machines out there, so choose one that appeals the most to you. If it looks like something you will actually use, then go for it.

Remember, these machines only work if you do! So many of us buy these great machines, use them fanatically for the first couple of weeks, then retire them to the workout cemetery in the back of the house or the garage. Keep your machine where you will use it. If you like to watch television to pass the time when you are working out, then put your machine right in front of the TV, or put it in the backyard, or in your bedroom. My husband plunked his Body-Row™ right in the middle of the kitchen. At first I found it very annoying and then I got over it. While I am cooking he can sit there endlessly working his body, talking to me. I have grown to love it for all those reasons. It makes me happy to have him be in good shape—mainly for health reasons, but he also looks incredible and quite easy on the eyes, if I do say so myself.

I think the worst place to put workout equipment is in your home gym. That's the loneliest room in the house. These machines are usually put in the basement or some other dark, unattractive, out-of-the-way place, which gives you a constant reason not to go there. Exercise is a joy if you choose to look at it that way. Try this: Instead of saying to yourself, "I have to work out," change the *have* to *get*. Now say the sentence again: "I *get* to work out." See how it changes everything? Again, think of how many people would love to be able to walk, ride a bike, or climb stairs, but cannot due to physical limitation. I *get* to work out.

My friend Barry taught me this simple adjustment in thinking. I use it every day with everything I do. I *get* to write these books, I *get* to travel to Milwaukee, I *get* to organize my closets. See the difference a word makes? It's an attitude adjustment. Simply changing the word *have* to *get* alleviates stress and changes your entire view of the work at hand.

So try it: I *get* to work out every day to keep myself healthy. I *get* to work out while I am watching television . . . while my butt is lifting. See how it changes things? It will change your body shape and your health as well.

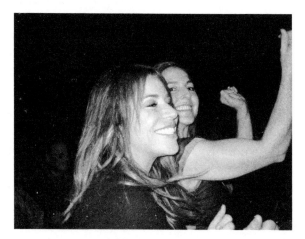

Leslie and Caroline sing at the Copacabana.

CHAPTER 14

Sticking with It

This is time for a little tough talk. I have people who come up to me and want me to explain everything to them . . . how to balance the hormones, how to lose the weight. I always tell them to read the book or books because it's all in there, but when they keep on calling asking how it works, I know that this is a person who is going to fail at her attempt to get her weight and/or hormones balanced.

If you don't have enough interest to read the books (over and over, if necessary), then you will never find success in this program. This is about your health, your weight, and your hormonal balance. This is about your quality of life. It's available to you, but at some point you have to take responsibility for the life you are living. So many people blame genetics: "Well, my mother was fat, my whole family was fat," or "My mother and grandmother had type 2 diabetes and were tired all the time; I'm sure I will be the

same way when I get older." That is not your sentence. In most cases the problem is not genetics but entrenched dietary and lifestyle habits. Your mother probably ate the same food as your grandmother. Your family probably did not make it a priority to stay healthy.

Many people will say, "Well. It's easy for you. You are able to hire a private trainer and to buy great equipment. You can even hire a private chef if you want to keep yourself on the program. You can afford expensive foods. Some of these jabs are true, but they do not have to do with commitment.

We are bombarded with stories and pictures of celebrities who lose and gain and lose and gain. I myself have been the subject of the tabloids, since there's nothing better for magazine sales than watching a woman who writes diet books gain weight. Mary-Kate Olsen is too thin; Kirstie Alley is too fat; and how many times do we need to see

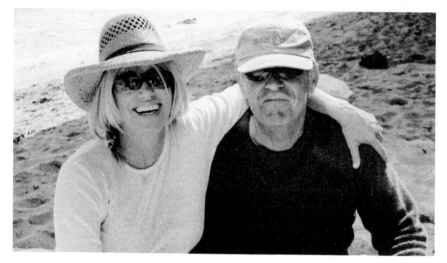

My pal, Al.

actresses pose nude or nearly nude after having a baby to prove that the baby fat is gone? We are obsessed with weight in this country and most of us are losing the battle. We hold ourselves up to unrealistic expectations based on comparing ourselves to the über-trained bodies of models and celebrities who grace the covers of magazines, yet many people cannot afford trainers, gym memberships, exercise equipment, diet counselors, and expensive weight-loss foods. Part of that argument is true: It is easier to lose weight if you can afford to buy the things you need to assist in the matter. HOWEVER, a walk around the neighborhood works as well as any treadmill, running stairs at the local school works as well as any expensive stairclimber, jumping jacks work your body as hard as any trainer would, and buying real, fresh food at any local grocery store and preparing a salad with a chicken breast may not be as convenient as having specialty food delivered to your door . . . but they are all

ways that you can get serious about your health without spending too much money. I work hard to stay in shape. Alan and I work out almost every single day and we eat well.

You probably think I'm being hypocritical by saying that you don't need to buy all that stuff, since I sell a huge variety of exercise equipment and food products to go with my Somersize weight-loss plan. It is no secret that people love convenience. You don't *need* any of those things to be successful on my program, but I offer them because so many of you have asked me to develop convenience items for you that are better than the ones on the market. I do my best to bring you high-quality, affordable goods that help you to achieve your goals. I know not all of you can afford them, but I just cannot compromise quality. I do my best to keep the cost low, but when it comes to quality I will not budge.

So here's your chance. You can accept who you are and stop using the excuse that you don't have money or that you are destined to be fat since your family is overweight. Instead, in one fell swoop, you can be the person who turns the family around.

I come from a long line of alcoholics. My father was an alcoholic, my grandfather was an alcoholic, and there were many other people on that side of the family who also struggled with alcoholism. Just because I come from alcoholics does not mean I am sentenced to be one as well. Life is about choices. The information I give in my books is for people like you and me . . . people who desire a better life in every way and are willing to do the work to get it. Life is what you put into it. The easy way is to sit on the couch and eat pizza and complain. The only person who gets hurt in this situation is you. Is this the example you want to set for your children? Is this the "genetic" lifestyle and dietary example you want them to inherit? If you change, by example they will follow suit.

Start today. Embrace this way of life. You have read the testimonial letters in this book; you see the progress of these fine people. They are talking to you. These are people who have shared their stories so that you can be inspired. Making the choice to get your weight in check, and to eat delicious food beautifully prepared without chemicals and preservatives, will have an incredibly positive effect on your health and that of your family. Commit to eating real food. Shop the periphery of the supermarket, and leave the packaged goods in the center for others. Commit to some form of exercise each day. Take a walk or go up and down the stairs until you hear your heart beating. Get your hormones balanced.

Remember that technology is going to keep us alive until we are ninety to one hundred years old. The changes you make today are going to improve these extra years we all get to live. It's a choice . . . do you want to be in a wheelchair with tubes up your nose because you made the choice to smoke and eat sugary foods all your life? We now have the advantage to restore health through good dietary habits and exercise and by avoiding chemicals and harmful additives like tobacco.

Choose health. Choose to grow and learn and not be "stuck" in the same old patterns of negative behavior. In therapy, I learned many years ago that insanity can be defined as "repeated patterns of negative behavior." For instance, if someone were to keep on banging her head against the wall, even though she was bruised and bleeding, you would call her insane, wouldn't you? Well, look at a person who keeps on eating and not exercising and not trying to balance her hormones, even though she has type 2 diabetes, or heart problems, or high blood pressure, or knees too weak to walk. To keep on doing the same thing to exacerbate this condition even though there is another way is insanity.

STOP THE INSANITY!

Please remember that you can choose to be slim and sexy forever. You are in control; you can do it. All you have to do is commit. Deciding to lose weight and balance your hormones will change your life for the better. Then, by your example, others around you will want what you have. In doing so, you will have changed the family "genetics"; you will have turned not only your own life around, but your family will also be on a new path.

This book makes it easy and fun to get on track. The recipes show you the possibilities of the beautiful food you can have. You've read about hormones and the positive effect they can have on your weight and health. Take advantage of all the research and work I have done. I did this initially for myself, and it has worked. Now I want you to have it also. It gives me great joy to bring you this fabulous information. It is a privilege to be of service. The joy I receive every time one of you stops me on the street to show me your new body, or to tell me how hormone replacement has turned your life around, is indescribable. We are all in this together. We have to help one another. The only thing I need from you is your commitment to change your life.

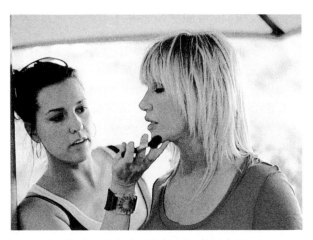

Getting touched up during the photo shoot
for this book.

Part Four

THE RECIPES

CHAPTER 15

Somersize Menus for Every Occasion

Since this is my seventh book in the Somersize series, you may be wondering what I have in store for you in the kitchen. This is always my favorite part of these books, since my true love is cooking. In fact, I only developed the Somersize program so that I could continue to eat my favorite foods and stay in good health!

My love affair with food began early—at age five. I was given a little Golden Book called *Susie's Cookbook*. I loved that book and thought it was written about me. The little girl had blonde hair and I identified.

My mother always prepared real food for us, not because she was a health freak; it's what was available. Preservatives and chemicals had not yet been introduced into our diets, so food was eaten in season. On Saturday mornings, the vegetable man would honk his distinctive horn, we would run outside, and he would sell us fruits and vegetables straight from the farm: artichokes,

tomatoes, potatoes, strawberries, peaches, watermelons. Fresh milk was delivered to our front door three times a week and every once in a while my mom would let me put out the little tag that instructed the milkman to also leave a bottle of fresh chocolate milk. Each summer we waited for Mrs. Best's plum tree to ripen. My mother would spend a week making jars of delicious plum jam.

It never entered my mind that food was anything other than real. On Sunday nights my mom would prepare yummy pot roast with creamy mashed potatoes and her wonderful gravy (something Irish women do really well). When we could get them we would have freshly shucked peas and I would swirl them around in my mashed potatoes and gravy. For dessert, a delicious spice cake with mocha frosting. It was, and still is, one of my favorite all-time meals.

Somewhere along the line, things changed. I distinctly remember when it happened, although at the time it rolled into our lives so easily and smoothly that none of us ever noticed. TV dinners! The beginning of fast food! This was the answer to the new phenomenon of having our mothers go to work for the first time. It was so easy. I used to beg my mother to let us have frozen TV dinners, sometimes a turkey dinner, sometimes (yum) a frozen chicken pot pie. I loved them. How exciting when these things showed up at the corner market. They were in the freezer right next to the ice cream! My favorites were turkey or meatloaf with the cranberry sauce and the apple crisp in its own little separate compartment in the aluminum tray. It seemed as though it took forever to heat up for those 25 minutes in the oven (we didn't have microwaves yet). When the timer finally went off I was always first to get mine out of the oven, ripping the aluminum covering off and taking a bite when it was still too hot. Even though I repeatedly burned my tongue it was worth it to feel the excitement of this first taste. For the life of me I can't imagine why I was so excited to eat what tasted like the worst airplane food ever—cardboard turkey and slimy apple crisp. But I was sold. I bought into it hook, line, and sinker.

I remember when the first Jack in the Box rolled into town. What fun! What a great hangout for us teenagers! As long as we kept on ordering Cherry Cokes and French fries, they let us stay. This is where the bad habits started. Who wants a roast beef dinner when you are all filled up on potatoes and sugar? And so the struggle began. Fast foods, chemicals, preservatives, frozen foods, canned foods, food in bags, trans fats, hydrogenated oils.

Soon we were eating our TV dinners on TV trays in front of the newest fad, television! All family conversation stopped while we numbly stared at the TV set and ate our frozen dinners. Not only did TV and TV dinners change family dynamics, but it forged a blueprint for unhealthy eating. By the next generation (mine) we had stopped learning at our mother's knee how to make the special dishes that women passed down in families for generations. Food was now something that you bought preprepared as much as possible and grabbing a quick meal in a bag at McDonald's became a standard part of our culture.

My hope is that this book will help you return to real food. I know we are all busy, but eating real food around a family table is so important for our health and well-being.

If you are like me and you love great food, you are in for a treat with these recipes. I pride myself on these meals. This is the food that I cook for people at my home and that makes them say "Wow!" for many days to follow (she says humbly!). These are meals loaded with taste sensations in every bite. Whether you're cooking dinner for the family on a Tuesday night or entertaining a crowd on the weekend, you will impress yourself and your friends with these fabulous tastes.

As always, I select very high-quality ingredients for my recipes. I do not skimp on quality, because quality makes the difference between mediocre food and great food. I understand that the costs are simply too high for many people, so I suggest that you buy the best ingredients you can afford. Additionally, I use some exotic ingredients that may be hard to find at your local grocery store. I try to give you options so that you can substitute more readily available and more affordable ingredients. I also provide an Ingredients Source Guide (page 294) so that you can order many of these ingredients for yourself.

Please do not be intimidated by the food! Some of these recipes sound more difficult than they are. You can create simple, elegant meals in a snap—or you can spend all day making culinary creations that the finest restaurants would be proud to serve. The choice is yours and I give you a spectrum of recipes from which to choose.

You will find the very easiest recipes in a section called Convenience Cooking (page 271). These recipes are for those who don't like to (or don't have the time to) cook from scratch, but want the satisfaction of a home-cooked meal. All you need are some small kitchen appliances and some of my Somersize food products and you can make meals in minutes. Can you imagine, Beef Bourguignonne with a two-minute prep time? All it takes is a slow cooker and a splash of my Traditional Burgundy Simmer Sauce. You supply the chuck roast, some pearl onions, and some celery. Set it to Low and you'll return eight hours later to a fabulous meal with a beautiful sauce made with the natural juices from the meat. You'll find a whole section of wonderful meals like this that you can make in a snap.

For those of you who are more advanced in the kitchen, wait until you try Braised Veal Stew with Gremolata or Crab Bisque with Sweet Corn and Crab Relish or Bittersweet Chocolate Citrus Tart. Divine! Since I am focusing more closely on Level Two and the importance of balancing your Level Two meals with a small amount of carbohydrates, you will find more ways to create Level Two foods in these recipes. Whenever possible I give you the adjustments to make them Level One, but I wanted to give you ideas for Level Two to teach you how to incorporate the carbs without upsetting your progress. It also adds wonderful variety to these meals.

In addition to the recipes, I have also included several entertaining menus so that you can see how I put all these delicious foods together for my family and friends. I certainly don't expect that any of us are eating four-course meals during the week, but it's nice to see how you can put these recipes together if you so desire. I entertain frequently and I pull out all the stops. I love to create a fantasy evening around the most delicious soup, a unique salad, a memorable entrée with vegetable and side dish and, of course, a dazzling dessert. That being said, on most nights Alan and I are very happy with a pot of soup and a salad.

At the end of the recipe section you will find a chapter called "Convenience Cooking." You know I love to cook from scratch, but sometimes I need a little help in the kitchen—that's when my Somersize products come to the rescue. You'll find prepackaged foods and quick and easy appliances can be a real help when you are short on time. I have also included some recipes that are delicious and easily made with my Somersize products.

Enjoy these recipes. I hope you will try something new and experience the wonderful flavor sensations in this book.

SOMERSIZE MENUS

◇

LEVEL ONE

Summer Tomato Soup with Basil Pistou and Parmesan Crisps (page 168)

Grilled Halibut with Spicy Rock Shrimp Salsa and Grilled Asparagus (pages 236 and 207)

Level Two: Add ¹/₂ cup Red Rice (page 226)

◇

ALMOST LEVEL ONE

Crab Bisque with Sweet Corn and Crab Relish (page 170)

Pan-Roasted Rib-Eye Steak with Slow-Roasted Sweet Onion and Sautéed Spinach (page 244)

Level One: Omit corn in soup

◇

LEVEL ONE

Baby Greens with Sherry Shallot Vinaigrette (page 180)

Roast Chicken Breast Stuffed with Herbed Goat Cheese with Wild Mushroom Sauce (page 231)

Steamed green beans

Level Two: Add ¹/₂ cup Sautéed Herb Quinoa (page 222)

◇

LEVEL ONE

Grilled Tomatillo and Red Onion Soup with Fresh Mint (page 167)

Achiote Chicken with Radish and Cucumber Salad (page 232)

Almost Level One: Add Chocolate Espresso Gelato (page 257)

◇

LEVEL ONE

Caramelized Roasted Fennel Soup

Baby Greens with Sherry Shallot Vinaigrette (page 180)

Pan-Roasted Sole with Thyme Butter Sauce (page 242)

Steamed asparagus

Level Two: Add ¹/₂ cup Forbidden Rice (page 220)

◇

LEVEL ONE

Asparagus Soup (page 174)

Warm Frisée Salad with Poached Egg and Pancetta (page 182)

Veal Patties with Lemon-Caper Sauce and Caramelized Root Vegetables (pages 251 and 212)

Almost Level One: Add Chocolate Marquise (page 263)

◇

ALMOST LEVEL ONE

Roasted Yellow Pepper Soup with Crostini with Homemade Ricotta Cheese (page 172)

Whole-Wheat Linguine with Candied Roma Tomatoes (page 221)

◇

LEVEL TWO

Sautéed Cabbage with Pine Nuts and Goat Cheese (page 215)

Crispy-Skinned Salmon with Roasted Garlic Aïoli and Warm Radicchio–Shiitake Mushroom Salad (pages 238 and 194)

Level One: Omit pine nuts in salad and lentils in salmon

◇

LEVEL TWO

Apple Salad with Blue Cheese Vinaigrette (page 184)

Braised Veal Stew with Gremolata (page 250)

Level One: Omit apples in salad

◇

LEVEL TWO

Peppered Pork Chops with Smashed Tuscan Potatoes and Braised Red Chard (pages 253, 217, and 206)

Level One: Omit potatoes

◇

LEVEL TWO

Bouillabaisse with Red Pepper Rouille and Whole-Wheat Crostini (pages 240 and 198)

Wild Berry Crostada (page 264)

Level One: Omit crostini and dessert

◇

LEVEL ONE

Bruschetta Artichokes (page 205)

Grilled Lamb Chops with Lavender Lamb Jus (page 247)

Grilled Fennel and Zucchini (page 213)

Level Two: Add $1/2$ cup Farro Risotto (page 227)

◇

LEVEL TWO

Chopped Vegetable Salad with Champagne Mustard Vinaigrette (omit chicken) (page 181)

Chipotle-Glazed Pork with Candied Tomato Salsa (page 254)

Level One: Omit Mango Salsa and Tomatillo Salsa on the pork

◇

LEVEL TWO

Thai Beef with Cucumber Salad with Soba Noodles and Asian Greens (pages 178, 225, and 179)

Level One: Omit Soba Noodles

◇

LEVEL TWO

Baby Black Lentil Salad (page 185)

Lamburger with Tomato Chutney and Mint (page 249)

Grilled Asparagus (page 207)

Level One: Omit Lentil Salad

◇

LEVEL TWO

Thai Butternut Squash Soup (page 175)

Curry Chicken Skewers with Roasted Eggplant Relish (pages 233 and 192)

$^1/_2$ cup Forbidden Rice (page 220)

Level Two: Omit soup and rice

◇

LEVEL ONE

Grilled Tuna with Lemon-Thyme Aïoli and Chilled Asparagus (pages 241 and 208)

Level Two: Start with Tuscan White Bean Soup (page 171)

◇

LEVEL ONE

Caesar Salad with Black Pepper Parmesan Crisps (pages 183 and 169)

Pan-Roasted Halibut with Zucchini Ribbons, Candied Roma Tomatoes, and Parsley Pesto (page 237)

Level Two: Replace Zucchini Ribbons with Potato Ribbons. Add Wild Berry Crostada (page 264)

◇

LEVEL ONE BRUNCH BUFFET

Leg of Lamb with Porcini Mushroom Rub (page 248)

Herb and Leek Frittata (page 164)

Chilled Asparagus with Lemon-Thyme Aïoli (page 208)

Caesar Salad (page 183)

Level Two: Add Strawberry Rhubarb Cobbler (page 267)

◇

LEVEL TWO HOLIDAY MEAL

Roasted Tomato Soup (page 166)

Christmas Roast (page 246)

Sautéed Brussels Sprouts with Pancetta (page 211)

Deadly Scalloped Potatoes (page 218)

Warm Chocolate Soufflé Cakes with Chocolate Espresso Gelato (pages 266 and 257)

Level One: Omit potatoes and dessert

◇

LEVEL TWO

Apple Salad with Blue Cheese Vinaigrette (page 184)

Herb-Roasted Loin of Pork with Pan Drippings (page 252)

Caramelized Root Vegetables (page 212)

Warm Cranberry Relish (page 193)

Bittersweet Chocolate Citrus Tart (page 269)

Level One: Omit apples in salad, cranberry relish, and dessert

CHAPTER 16

Egg Dishes

Omelette with Fontina, Wild Mushrooms, Pancetta, and Sage

PRO/FATS AND VEGGIES—LEVEL ONE

SERVES 1

I am nuts for pancetta. Pancetta is a cured Italian bacon that is salty and meaty and absolutely wonderful, especially when sautéed and added to just about anything. This omelette will knock your socks off. If you can't find pancetta at your deli, you may substitute regular bacon.

1 tablespoon olive oil, plus more if needed
$^1/_2$ cup wild mushrooms, sliced (or regular mushrooms)
2 ounces pancetta (or bacon), diced well
3 eggs
$^1/_4$ cup heavy cream

Sea salt and freshly ground black pepper
1 tablespoon unsalted butter
$^1/_2$ cup grated Fontina cheese (or Monterey Jack or mozzarella)
1 tablespoon finely chopped fresh sage (or $^1/_2$ teaspoon dried)

Place a medium sauté pan on high. Add the olive oil and mushrooms and sauté until the mushrooms are golden brown and crusty, about 10 minutes. Remove the mushrooms from the pan and set aside.

Return the pan to medium heat. Add more oil if needed and add the pancetta; sauté until crisp. Remove the pancetta from the pan and set aside.

In a medium bowl, whisk the eggs, cream, and salt and pepper to taste.

Melt the butter in a small nonstick sauté pan (with an ovenproof handle) and add the egg mixture. Cook over medium heat, gently stirring, just until the eggs begin to set. Add the mushrooms, pancetta, cheese, and sage on half of the omelette. Place the omelette pan under the broiler for 1 to 2 minutes. Remove from the oven and fold in half. Serve immediately.

New Mexican Huevos

L E V E L   T W O

S E R V E S   1

Here's a delicious Level Two breakfast that is just incredible. It's similar to huevos rancheros, but it's a Santa Fe version with a whole-wheat tortilla, sautéed chard, black beans, and a fresh chipotle salsa rather than a ranchero sauce. Wow.

1 tablespoon olive oil
$^1/_2$ red onion, sliced
$^1/_2$ cup stemmed and chopped red chard
2 tablespoons plus 1 teaspoon unsalted
    butter
1 whole-wheat tortilla

$^1/_2$ cup black beans
Juice from $^1/_4$ lime
Sea salt and freshly ground black pepper
2 eggs
Chipotle and Tomato Salsa (page 199)

In a medium nonstick sauté pan over medium heat, add the olive oil and onion and sauté until soft and caramelized, about 5 minutes. Add the chard and sauté until wilted. Add 1 tablespoon of the butter. Remove from pan and set aside.

In the same pan, warm the tortilla over medium heat, 2 minutes on each side. Remove the tortilla and set it onto a plate.

In a medium saucepan, heat the beans over medium until warm. Add the lime juice and season to taste with salt and pepper. Add 1 teaspoon of the butter. Place the beans in the center of the tortilla and surround with the chard.

Return the pan to medium; add the remaining 1 tablespoon butter and melt. Crack in the eggs and cook until the whites are set (the yolks can remain runny if you prefer); do not flip the eggs. Slide the eggs out of the pan and place on top of the beans. Garnish with 2 heaping spoonfuls of salsa.

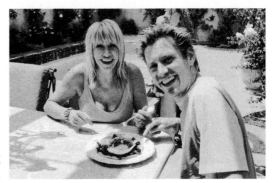

Bruce loves the days when we test recipes at his house. We are eating New Mexican Huevos.

Herb and Leek Frittata

PRO/FATS AND VEGGIES — LEVEL ONE

SERVES 6 TO 8

I love frittatas because they are so versatile. They can take on whatever flavor profile you wish and they are great for entertaining, since they taste equally good hot or cold. I served this at an Easter brunch. I kept it warm in my Somersize Slow Cooker. Or you can simply bake it in an ovenproof sauté pan, slice it into wedges, and serve warm or at room temperature.

3 leeks, thinly sliced (white parts only)
1 tablespoon olive oil
unsalted butter
18 eggs
1 cup heavy cream

Sea salt and freshly ground black pepper
$^1/_2$ cup chopped fresh flat-leaf parsley
1 tablespoon chopped fresh thyme leaves
   (or 2 teaspoons dried)
1 cup grated Parmesan cheese

Preheat the oven to 350 degrees.

In a large sauté pan over medium heat, sauté the leeks in the olive oil and butter until crisp and golden brown, about 4 minutes.

In a large mixing bowl, add the eggs and cream and whisk until frothy. Season with salt and pepper. Add the parsley, thyme, and Parmesan cheese, reserving a bit of cheese for the top of the frittata. Whisk gently to combine.

FOR THE SAUTÉ PAN METHOD

Pour the egg mixture over the leeks in the sauté pan. Sprinkle the remaining Parmesan over the top. Cook over medium heat until the eggs begin to set, about 3 minutes. Do not stir. Place the sauté pan into the oven and bake for 10 to 12 minutes, or until the center is just set.

FOR THE SLOW COOKER METHOD

Place the sautéed leeks into the porcelain pot of the slow cooker. Add the egg mixture and sprinkle the top with the remaining Parmesan cheese. Cook on High for $2^1/_2$ to 3 hours. To cook faster, place the porcelain pot into the preheated oven and bake for about 15 minutes, or until the center is set. Either way, when cooked to desired liking, place the slow cooker on Keep Warm setting and serve.

CHAPTER 17

Soups

Roasted Tomato Soup

PRO/FATS AND VEGGIES—LEVEL ONE

SERVES 4 TO 6

This is a great soup to make when tomatoes are in abundance. If you grow your own tomatoes, even better. When I want to WOW my guests, this is my starter. You can make this in one day or over a couple of days. Here's how you do it. Remember, your food is as good as your ingredients. Use ripe, delicious tomatoes; heirloom or vine-ripened have the best flavor. The secret to this soup is the SomerSweet to balance the acid in the tomatoes. All good Italian cooks know to add a spoonful of sugar when cooking with tomatoes. I don't know why, but to me, SomerSweet tastes better than sugar. You may want a little more or a little less. This soup tastes great hot, room temperature, or cold . . . whatever your pleasure.

10 ripe delicious tomatoes
$^1/_4$ cup olive oil
Sea salt and freshly ground black pepper
1 bunch fresh thyme, leaves only (or
    1 tablespoon Somersize Tuscan Sea
    Salt Rub)
1 bunch fresh basil, coarsely chopped, plus
    10 extra leaves, julienned, for garnish

2 cups chicken stock (homemade, if
    possible)
2 teaspoons SomerSweet (or more to taste)
$^1/_8$ teaspoon crushed red pepper flakes
    (optional)
$^1/_4$ cup heavy cream
Sour cream (or crème fraîche), for garnish

Preheat the oven to 350 degrees.

Cut the tomatoes in half through the middle and lay them cut side up on a baking sheet or roasting pan. Drizzle olive oil on top of the tomatoes. Sprinkle the tomatoes liberally with sea salt. Top with the thyme leaves. Place the tomatoes into the oven for about 2 hours or until slightly darkened on top.

When done, remove from the oven and scrape into a medium saucepan, including drippings from the bottom of the baking sheet. Add the chopped basil. Bring to a boil over medium heat for 10 minutes. Then add the chicken stock, reduce the heat, and simmer for 45 minutes. Add the SomerSweet and red pepper flakes, if using. Remove from the heat and purée the soup with a hand blender or transfer to a blender and purée until smooth. Add the heavy cream and ladle into serving bowls. Garnish with a dollop of sour cream and sprinkle with julienned basil.

Grilled Tomatillo and Red Onion Soup with Fresh Mint

PRO/FATS AND VEGGIES—LEVEL ONE

SERVES 8

This soup is for tomatillo lovers. If you've never had them, they are like small green tomatoes with the taste of lemon, apples, and herbs. In this recipe they are grilled, then finished with a little kick of jalapeño, then smoothed out with cream and SomerSweet for balance. This is perfect to serve in small portions in your favorite demitasse cups as a first course. If you are not familiar with this new and unusual flavor, I urge you to try this one. It might end up being your favorite.

1 pound tomatillos, husked and washed
1 red onion, sliced into thick rings
$^1/_2$ bunch fresh cilantro leaves, roughly chopped
$^1/_2$ bunch fresh mint leaves, roughly chopped, plus $^1/_2$ bunch julienned, for garnish

1 tablespoon balsamic vinegar
Sea salt and freshly ground black pepper
$^1/_4$ cup heavy cream
$^1/_4$ cup chicken broth
1 jalapeño chili, seeded and diced
$^1/_2$ teaspoon SomerSweet
2 tablespoons unsalted butter

Place the tomatillos, onion slices, cilantro, chopped mint, balsamic vinegar, salt, and pepper into a bowl. Toss gently to combine. Let sit for about 10 minutes to let the flavors combine.

Preheat the grill to high. Add the tomatillos and onions, reserving the marinade for later. Grill for 10 to 15 minutes, or until the tomatillos are slightly charred and the skin is bubbling. Return the tomatillos and onions to the bowl. Transfer to a blender with all the juices and purée until smooth. Strain into a saucepan and heat over medium. Add the cream, broth, jalapeño, and SomerSweet. Cook until just boiling, then reduce the heat to a simmer and add the butter. Ladle into demitasse cups and garnish with the julienned mint.

Summer Tomato Soup with Basil Pistou and Parmesan Crisps

PRO/FATS AND VEGGIES—LEVEL ONE

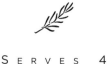

SERVES 4

There are so many ways to prepare tomato soup. This version is fresh and light, a perfect starter for a summer evening meal. Alan sneaks it right out of the pot.

6 to 8 ripe tomatoes (preferably heirloom or vine-ripened)
2 tablespoons olive oil
1 yellow onion, thinly sliced
2 cloves garlic, smashed
Sea salt and freshly ground black pepper

1 whole sprig fresh basil with stem (optional)
1 recipe Basil Pistou (page 188)
4 Black Pepper Parmesan Crisps (page 169)

Coarsely chop the tomatoes and set aside. Heat a small stockpot on medium and add the olive oil and onion. Cook the onion until translucent, about 10 minutes, then add the garlic cloves and continue caramelizing the onion for another 10 minutes. Add the tomatoes and bring just to a boil. Season with salt and pepper. Reduce the heat and add the basil, if using; simmer for about 2 minutes. Remove the pot from the heat. Take the basil out, remove the stem and discard, then return the leaves to the pot and purée with a hand blender (or transfer to a blender and purée). Adjust the seasoning.

Garnish with a dollop of Basil Pistou and a Parmesan crisp. Serve immediately.

Black Pepper Parmesan Crisps

PRO/FATS — LEVEL ONE

MAKES 4 CRISPS

I first introduced you to Parmesan crisps in *Eat, Cheat, and Melt the Fat Away.* In this version I have added cracked black pepper, and I cook them in the oven rather than on the stovetop. You can leave these flat or cool them over an inverted glass or bowl to create different shapes. Whatever the case, you'll love these delicious, cheesy chips to garnish soups or salads or just to snack on. For variety add any of your favorite herbs, or a sprinkle of one of my Somersize Sea Salt Rubs. You can even make "barbecue chips" by using my Memphis Sea Salt Rub!

Black peppercorns
$^1/_2$ cup freshly shredded Parmesan cheese

Preheat the oven to 350 degrees.

Place a handful of peppercorns onto a cutting board. Using the bottom of a heavy skillet, press onto the peppercorns until they crack. You do not want any whole peppercorns.

Line a baking sheet with parchment paper (or a Silpat). Sprinkle the cheese into 3-inch circles, making several mini "pancakes." Season each with cracked black pepper. Place into the oven for about 5 minutes, until just golden.

Remove from the oven and place each crisp over an inverted small glass or bowl. When cool enough to touch, form into different shapes as desired.

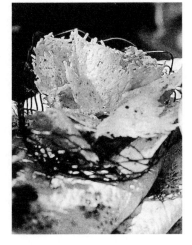

Crab Bisque with Sweet Corn and Crab Relish

LEVEL TWO

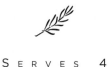

SERVES 4

The key to making this soup is to have your fishmonger steam the crab, then clean it for you, reserving the meat AND the shells, which are essential to making the base of the bisque. Alan loves corn more than anyone I know. He taught me to use the cob to make the most flavorful soups. Obviously, this becomes Level Two for that reason, but, oh my, is it worth it. If you only make one thing out of this book, this is the one. If you make this without the ear of corn and without the corn relish, it is a Level One soup and still worthy of my highest recommendation.

1 tablespoon butter
1 onion, sliced
1 celery stalk, sliced
1 red bell pepper, seeded and sliced
1 whole Dungeness crab, steamed whole
2 tablespoons tomato paste
2 cups white wine

4 cups chicken broth
2 cups heavy cream
1 ear fresh corn, corn shaved off and
  reserved for garnish
1 recipe Sweet Corn and Crab Relish
  (page 191)

Heat a large stockpot on medium. Add the butter, onion, celery, and bell pepper. Cook for about 10 minutes to let the vegetables slowly sweat. Add the crab shells and meat to the pot, mashing with a wooden spoon to break up the shells and release the flavor. Add the tomato paste, stirring with the shells until it begins to caramelize.

Add the white wine to deglaze the pan. Bring to a boil, then lower the heat to a simmer and let reduce by half. Add the chicken broth and let cook over medium heat until it boils. Then lower the heat to a simmer for 10 minutes. Add the cream and reduce the entire soup again by half.

Strain through a medium sieve, pressing the shells and vegetables to extract all the flavor. Pour the strained bisque into a clean pot and add the corn cob. Cook on low for 5 to 8 minutes, until the bisque is thickened. Ladle into soup bowls and garnish with a generous spoonful of the Sweet Corn and Crab Relish.

Tuscan White Bean Soup

S E R V E S   4

I've always had an affection for cannellini beans, which are Italian white kidney beans. In this tomato-based soup I add kale, which tastes delicious and is so darn good for you. The addition of fresh rosemary and a sprinkle of Parmesan cheese balances the flavors of this divine Level Two soup. I usually cook a whole bag of beans, use what I need for this soup, and use the leftovers for my Cannellini Bean Dip (*Eat Great, Lose Weight,* page 74).

1 16-ounce bag dried cannellini beans
6 cups chicken broth
Extra-virgin olive oil
1 tablespoon unsalted butter
$^1/_2$ yellow onion, diced
1 clove garlic, minced
$^1/_2$ celery root, peeled and diced
1 stalk celery, diced

1 bunch kale, roughly chopped
1 tablespoon tomato paste
Sea salt and freshly ground black pepper
1 sprig fresh rosemary, chopped (or 1
   teaspoon dried)
1 sprig fresh thyme (or $^1/_2$ teaspoon dried)
Freshly grated Parmesan cheese, for
   garnish

Place the dried beans into a large mixing bowl and cover by 3 inches with cold water. Allow to soak overnight at room temperature.

Drain the beans and place into a stockpot. Cover with the chicken broth and bring to a boil. Reduce heat to low and simmer until the beans are tender, about 1 hour.

Place another stockpot on medium heat and add the olive oil, butter, onion, garlic, celery root, and celery. Sauté until the vegetables are soft, about 20 minutes. Add the kale and cook for 2 to 3 minutes, until just wilted. Add the tomato paste and stir to combine. Add the cooked beans, including the broth if the soup has become too thick. Season with salt and pepper. Add more broth if the soup has become too thick. Add the rosemary and thyme. Ladle into soup bowls and garnish with a generous sprinkle of Parmesan cheese.

Roasted Yellow Pepper Soup with Crostini with Homemade Ricotta Cheese

L E V E L   T W O

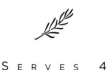

S E R V E S   4

There is a distinct difference in taste between red, yellow, and green bell peppers. Red peppers are sweet, yellow peppers are smooth and subtle, green peppers are spicy and tart. This soup is made with yellow peppers: smooth and dreamy. The color is beautiful and the basil garnish provides just the right accent. Made in this manner it would be Level One Pro/Fats and Veggies, but what really makes it special is the Crostini with Homemade Ricotta Cheese.

2 yellow bell peppers, cut in half and
    seeded (or red peppers)
4 yellow tomatoes, cut across the width (or
    red tomatoes)
3 cloves garlic
$^1/_2$ yellow onion, cut into 2 quarters

2 sprigs fresh basil (or $^1/_2$ teaspoon dried)
Extra-virgin olive oil
Sea salt and freshly ground black pepper
1 cup chicken broth (or more)
1 recipe Crostini with Homemade Ricotta
    Cheese (page 224)

Preheat the oven to 350 degrees.

Place the peppers, tomatoes, garlic, onion, and 1 sprig of the basil (reserving the other for garnish) onto a baking sheet. Drizzle with olive oil and season with salt and pepper. Roast in the oven for 45 minutes, or until the vegetables are soft.

Transfer to a blender or food processor. Add the broth and purée until smooth. Adjust the consistency with more broth, if necessary. (This will depend upon the amount of juice in the tomatoes.) Season with salt and pepper, then strain into a soup pot. Heat over medium until hot. Remove the basil leaves from the remaining sprig and julienne.

Ladle the soup into bowls, then garnish with the basil and a slice of Homemade Ricotta Crostini.

Caramelized Roasted Fennel Soup

PRO/FATS AND VEGGIES—LEVEL ONE

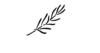

SERVES 4

This recipe serves four . . . or just me! I love it.

3 bulbs fennel, sliced $^1/_4$ inch thick
1 medium yellow onion, sliced $^1/_4$ inch
  thick
3 cloves garlic
Extra-virgin olive oil

Sea salt and freshly ground black pepper
3 cups chicken broth
$^1/_2$ cup heavy cream
Crème fraîche, for garnish
Chopped fresh chives, for garnish

Preheat the oven to 375 degrees.

Place the fennel, onion, and garlic on a baking sheet. Drizzle with olive oil and season with salt and pepper. Roast in the oven for 45 minutes, or until the vegetables are caramelized and soft. Scrape all of the vegetables into a blender or food processor. Add the chicken broth and purée until smooth. Adjust with more broth if necessary.

Strain into a soup pot and add the cream. Heat over medium until hot. Adjust for seasoning with additional salt and pepper. Ladle into soup bowls and garnish with crème fraîche and a sprinkle of chives.

Asparagus Soup

SERVES 4

This soup is yummy hot or cold. As always, fresh stock is best, but canned will be fine. The garnish is not necessary, but the addition of the lightly whipped unsweetened cream and the slight flavoring of fresh tarragon really puts the finishing touch on. Asparagus is a great vegetable to keep your system alkaline and it's always best to get your nutrients from fresh food. I love this soup. It's easy to prepare for an everyday dinner, yet spectacular enough to serve at the fanciest dinner party.

2 tablespoons unsalted butter
1 yellow onion, finely diced
$^{1}/_{2}$ cup heavy cream plus 2 tablespoons for garnish
3 cups chicken broth

2 bunches asparagus, cut into $^{1}/_{8}$-inch pieces
Sea salt and freshly ground black pepper
Fresh tarragon, for garnish

In a medium saucepan over medium heat, melt the butter. Add the onion and cook until very soft. Add the $^{1}/_{2}$ cup cream and $1^{1}/_{2}$ cups of the broth and bring to a boil. Add the asparagus and bring back to a boil, adding the remaining broth if necessary. Lower the heat to a simmer and cook until the asparagus is just cooked through, 3 or 4 minutes. Remove from the heat and purée immediately in a food processor or blender. Strain through a fine strainer into another pan. Season with salt and pepper.

For the garnish, whip the 2 tablespoons of heavy cream in a stainless steel bowl.

When the cream forms soft peaks, add the chopped fresh tarragon.

Serve soup immediately with a dollop of the tarragon cream or chill in an ice bath.

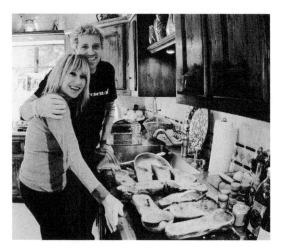

My darling Bruce is helping me turn the roasted squash into delicious soup

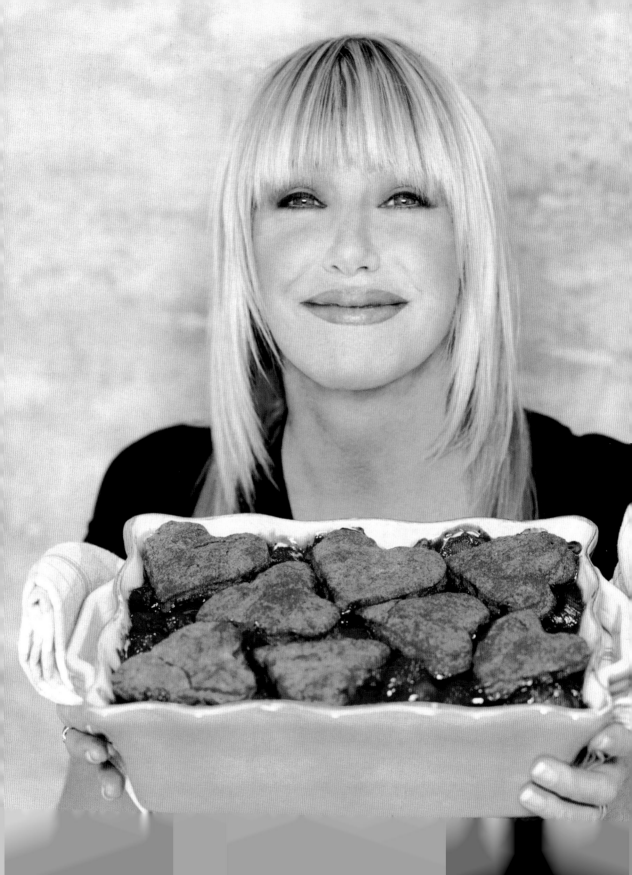

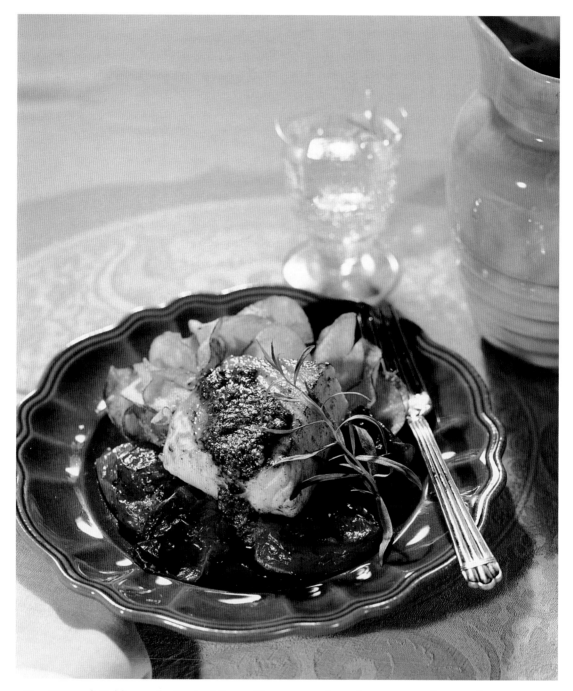

Pan-Roasted Halibut with Candied Roma Tomatoes and Parsley Pesto. In this Level Two version I served it with fried potato ribbons (gasp! so good). For Level One, try delicious Zucchini Ribbons.

PRECEDING PAGE: I'm in love with my Strawberry Rhubarb Cobbler with heart-shaped whole-wheat biscuits.

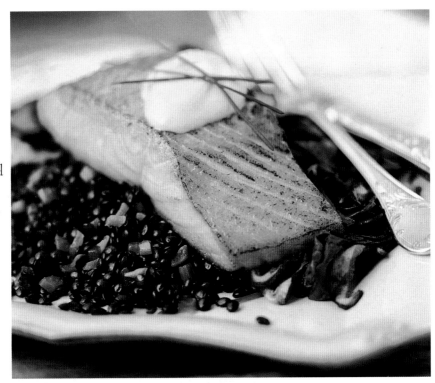

An elegant dish of
Crispy-Skinned
Salmon with Roasted
Garlic Aïoli, Warm
Radicchio–Shiitake
Mushroom Salad,
and French Lentils

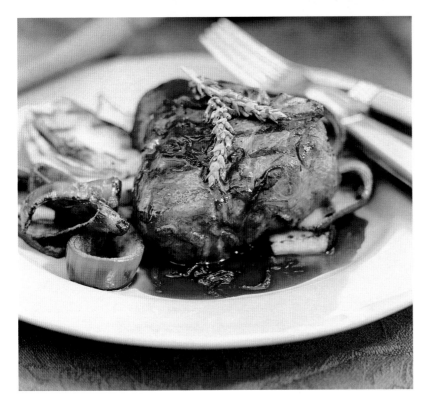

A gorgeous dish of
Grilled Lamb Chops
with Lavender Lamb Jus
served with Grilled
Fennel and Zucchini.

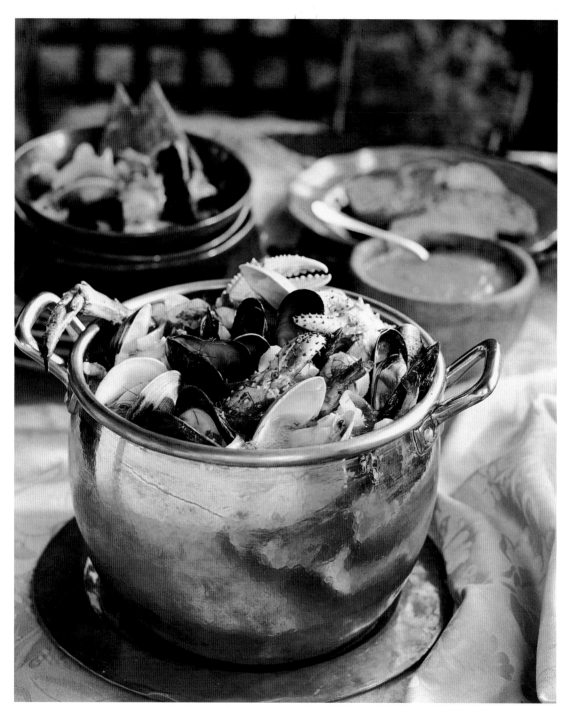

A family-size pot of Bouillabaisse with Whole-Wheat Crostini and Red Pepper Rouille.

OPPOSITE: The family gathers around on the kitchen patio for Bouillabaisse, a delicious seafood stew.

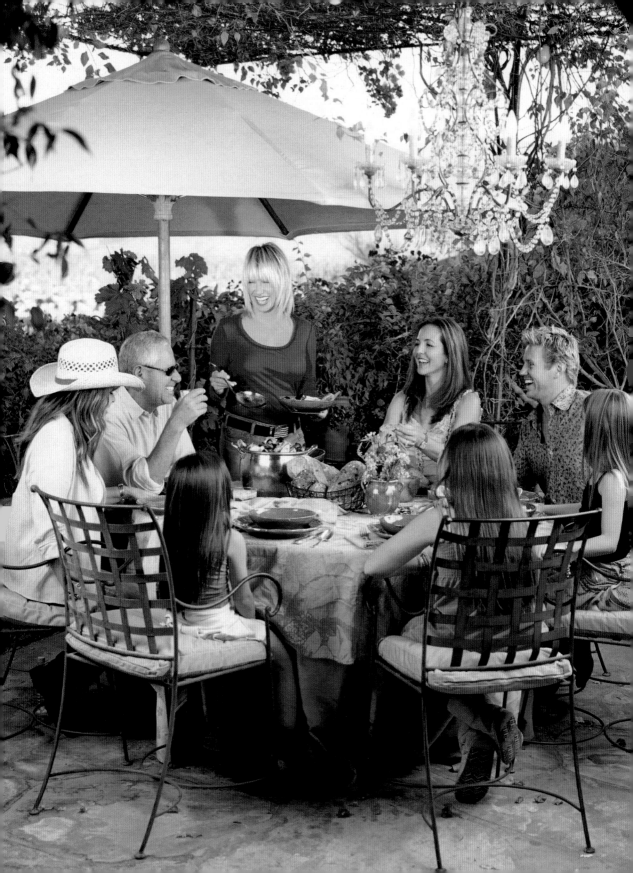

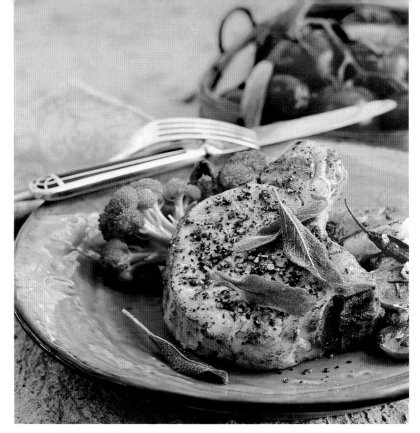

One of my favorite meals—Peppered Pork Chops with Fried Sage Leaves served with Smashed Tuscan Potatoes and broccoli.

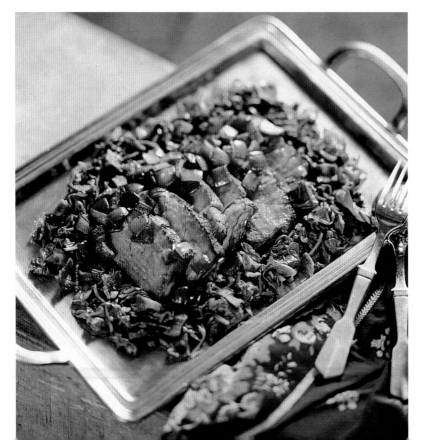

A beautiful tray of sliced Pan-Roasted Rib-Eye Steak with Slow-Roasted Sweet Onion and Sautéed Spinach.

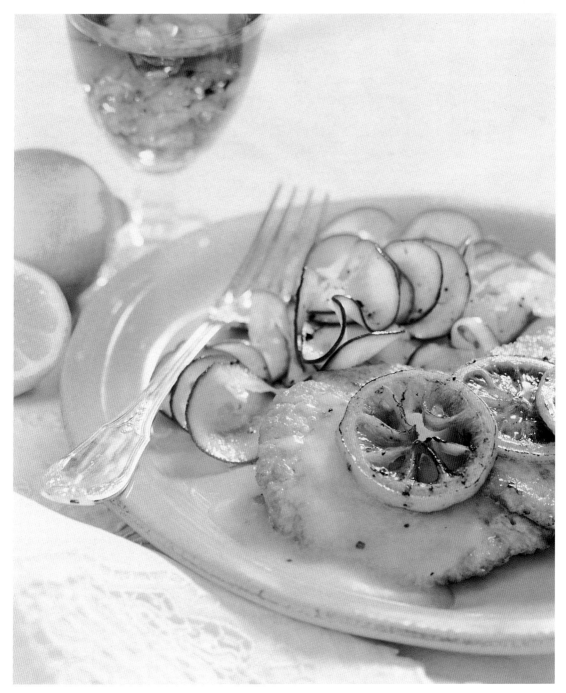

For a simple lunch or dinner, try this fabulous Chicken Patty Lemon Piccata with Zucchini Ribbons.

FOLLOWING PAGE: Sneaking away in the afternoon for some downtime with a magazine and a spoonful of Velvet Chocolate Pudding.

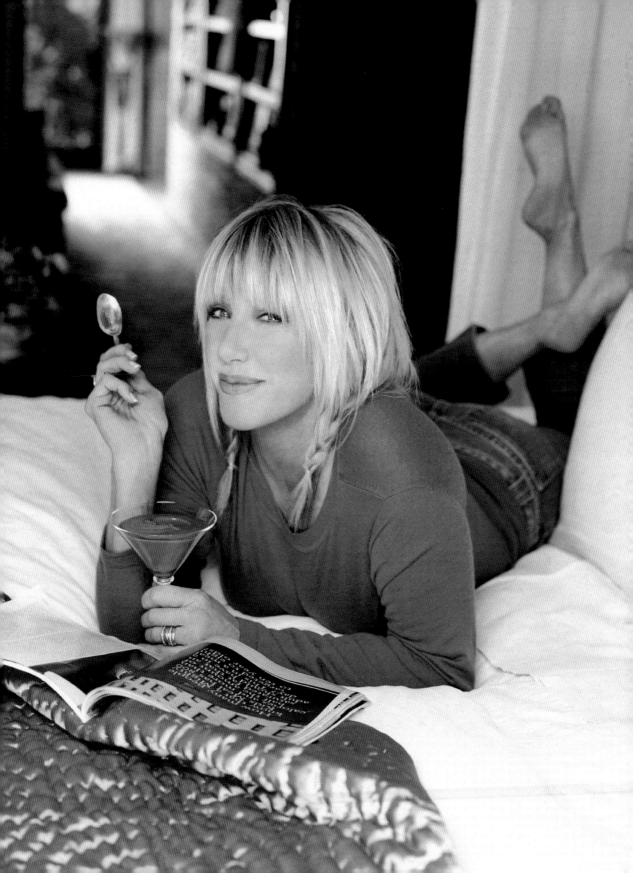

Thai Butternut Squash Soup

PRO/FATS AND VEGGIES — LEVEL TWO

SERVES 4

I often make this soup for my Thanksgiving dinner. I serve it in small demitasse cups so as not to ruin everyone's appetite for the turkey dinner to follow. What makes this soup so spectacular tasting is the roasting of the butternut squash. It gives the soup a deep, rich flavor. The garnish is optional, but the flavors of the mint, red chili, and lightly whipped cream puts the wow into the squash flavor. Adults love the zing of the thin red chili slice, but I leave it off for the grandchildren, 'cause I'm a nice Zannie.

1 butternut squash
Extra-virgin olive oil
Sea salt and freshly ground black pepper
1 tablespoon unsalted butter
1 teaspoon red curry paste or 1 tablespoon
    Somersize Thai Red Curry Sea Salt
    Rub, to taste
2 cups chicken broth, plus more if needed
1 cup coconut milk

$^1/_2$ cup heavy cream
1 stalk lemongrass, split in half

GARNISH

Juice of $^1/_2$ lime
2 tablespoons heavy cream, lightly
    whipped
1 tablespoon fresh mint, finely julienned
1 red chili pepper, thinly sliced

Preheat the oven to 350 degrees.

Cut the squash in half and remove the seeds and pulp. Drizzle with olive oil and sprinkle with salt and pepper. Place the squash halves on a baking sheet with edges. Pour $^1/_4$ cup water onto the baking sheet. Gently cover the entire baking sheet with foil and bake until the squash is soft, about 45 minutes. When cool enough to handle, scoop out the flesh of the squash and set aside.

In a medium saucepan over medium heat, add the butter and curry paste. Start with 1 teaspoon of the curry paste and add more, depending on how hot you like it. Allow the paste to melt and add the squash, stock, coconut milk, and cream. Season with salt and pepper. Add the lemongrass halves to steep. Allow to come up to a simmer and cook for 10 minutes, stirring occasionally. Remove from the heat, remove the lemongrass stalks, and purée in the blender. Add more stock if needed for consistency.

Garnish with a squeeze of lime, a dollop of lightly whipped cream, a sprinkle of mint, and a slice of chili.

Fast and Easy Chicken Soup

PRO/FATS AND VEGGIES — LEVEL ONE

SERVES 8

Chicken soup is my all-time favorite food. If I were stuck on an island with only one food, I would choose chicken soup. I have always made my own broth by letting a carcass cook overnight with vegetables. Now it's easier than ever with my Somersize Fast and Easy Cooker. With a pressure cooker, you can make fabulous chicken soup in just 30 minutes! And it's the best broth you've ever tasted. It's rich and golden and perfect. You can even start your chicken frozen! It doesn't change your cooking time since you don't begin timing until the Fast and Easy Cooker comes up to pressure. By that time your bird will be thawed. Imagine, from freezer to soup bowl in 30 minutes!

1 whole chicken, cleaned
2 leeks, cleaned thoroughly and chopped
1 onion, sliced
3 stalks celery, chopped
$^1/_4$ cup chopped fresh flat-leaf parsley
2 tablespoons Somersize Tuscan Sea Salt Rub

Freshly grated Parmesan cheese, for garnish (optional)
Basil Pistou (page 188) or Parsley Pesto (page 189), for garnish (optional)

Place all the soup ingredients into the large pressure pot of the Somersize Fast and Easy Cooker. Fill with water two-thirds of the way up the pot. Place the pressure lid onto the pot and lock into place. Place on high heat. When the pressure builds, the pressure indicator will pop up. When you hear the hissing of releasing steam, set the timer for 30 minutes.

After 30 minutes, release the steam and open the lid. Check chicken for doneness. If cooked through, remove the chicken from the broth and set aside until cool enough to handle. (If not cooked through, return to pot and bring back to pressure for 5 minutes more.) Remove the meat from the bones and tear into strips; place into serving bowls. Spoon the broth and vegetables over the chicken. Garnish with Parmesan cheese or a spoonful of pesto, if desired.

CHAPTER 18

Salads

Thai Beef with Cucumber Salad

PRO/FATS AND VEGGIES—LEVEL ONE

SERVES 2

This exotic combination of flavors combines sweet, spicy, and tangy. I like to serve this over Asian Greens with Soy Vinaigrette (page 179). For Level Two, I add Soba Noodles (page 225) for a beautifully balanced salad of taste, texture, and pure delight.

CUCUMBER SALAD

1 cucumber, peeled
1 tablespoon freshly grated ginger
1 tablespoon finely chopped fresh mint
$^1/_2$ red onion, thinly sliced
$^1/_4$ cup rice wine vinegar
1 teaspoon SomerSweet
Sea salt and freshly ground black pepper

THAI BEEF

1 8-ounce filet mignon (or rib-eye steak)
2 tablespoons extra-virgin olive oil
1 Thai chili, thinly sliced (or serrano or jalapeño)
$^1/_2$ bunch fresh mint leaves, chopped
1 tablespoon finely chopped fresh cilantro
4 fresh basil leaves, julienned
Juice and zest of $^1/_4$ lime

To make the cucumber salad, slice the cucumber in half lengthwise, scrape out the seeds, then cut into half-moon pieces. Toss in a bowl with the ginger, mint, onion, rice wine vinegar, and SomerSweet. Season with salt and pepper. Set aside to let the flavors combine.

To make the Thai beef, marinate the beef in a resealable plastic bag in 1 tablespoon olive oil, the chili, mint, cilantro, basil, lime juice, and lime zest for 30 minutes.

In a medium sauté pan, heat the remaining tablespoon of olive oil over high heat, then sear the beef for 2 minutes on each side for medium rare. Remove from the heat and let rest for 2 minutes. Thinly slice against the grain. Top with a mound of cucumber salad.

FOR LEVEL TWO

Serve over a bed of Asian Greens with Soy Vinaigrette and a mound of Soba Noodles.

Asian Greens with Soy Vinaigrette

VEGGIES — LEVEL ONE

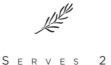

SERVES 2

This is a nice, light salad to accompany Asian foods. It works great as a base for my Thai Beef with Cucumber Salad (page 178).

$^1/_2$ pound mixed greens (preferably baby Asian)
1 tablespoon soy sauce
$^1/_4$ cup rice wine vinegar

$^3/_4$ cup olive oil
Sea salt and freshly ground black pepper
Juice from $^1/_4$ lime

Wash the greens and set aside.

Combine the remaining ingredients in a bowl. Add the greens and toss to coat. Serve immediately.

Baby Greens with Sherry Shallot Vinaigrette

PRO/FATS AND VEGGIES—LEVEL ONE

SERVES 2

This is a basic green salad that is a staple for French housewives. You'll see it in this book in the first photo insert paired with my Grilled Scallops Wrapped in Pancetta (page 239).

$^1/_2$ pound mixed baby greens
2 tablespoons finely minced shallots
$^1/_4$ cup sherry vinegar

$^3/_4$ cup extra-virgin olive oil
Sea salt and freshly ground black pepper

    Wash the greens and set aside.
    In a mixing bowl, combine the remaining ingredients. Toss the greens in dressing until coated. Serve immediately.

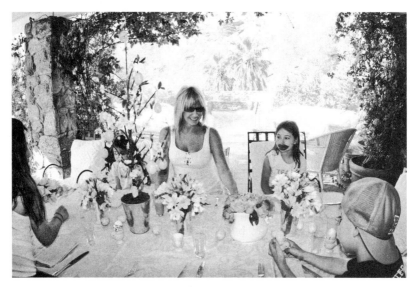

Our beautiful pink Easter table. The kids helped dye the eggs.

Chopped Vegetable Salad with Roasted Chicken

PRO/FATS AND VEGGIES—LEVEL ONE

SERVES 4

How many salads have you had in your life with dry, tough pieces of chicken? No more! In this recipe the chicken is seared and roasted, then coated with vinaigrette and cooled before slicing. Cooling before you slice is the key to keeping the chicken moist so that all the juices do not run out of the poultry. You'll love the combination of crisp vegetables with tender chunks of flavorful chicken in a delicious Champagne Mustard Vinaigrette.

4 small boneless, skinless chicken breasts
Sea salt and freshly ground black pepper
2 tablespoons olive oil
1 recipe Champagne Mustard Vinaigrette
  (page 190)
1 bag baby mixed greens
1 red bell pepper, seeded and medium
  diced

1 yellow bell pepper, seeded and medium
  diced
1 cucumber, peeled, seeded, and medium
  diced
2 stalks celery, medium diced
$1/2$ red onion, medium diced
2 whole scallions, medium diced

Preheat the oven to 450 degrees.

Season the chicken breasts liberally with sea salt and pepper. Heat a large ovenproof sauté pan over medium high. Add the olive oil and the chicken breasts and sear for 3 minutes per side. Place the sauté pan into the oven and roast for 5 to 6 minutes. When done, brush the chicken breasts with vinaigrette. Remove the chicken from the pan and set aside to cool. When cool, dice the chicken into $1/2$-inch chunks.

In a mixing bowl, toss the mixed greens with 2 tablespoons of the vinaigrette until well coated. Divide the greens among 4 salad plates.

Add all the chopped vegetables and chicken to the bowl. Season with salt and pepper. Add $1/4$ cup of the dressing and toss until well coated.

Place the chicken and vegetable mixture on top of the greens and serve immediately.

Warm Frisée Salad with Poached Egg and Pancetta

PRO/FATS AND VEGGIES—LEVEL ONE

SERVES 2

The most difficult part of this recipe is making sure you get the frisée really clean. Cut the top and the bottom off and reserve the middle. Float the bottom and the tops in a bowl of water to let the dirt fall off. The middle part gets cleaned as usual. I first had this dish at Brasserie Lipp on the Left Bank in Paris. It's a classic French staple loved by all. The combination of warm, lightly sautéed frisée, fried pancetta, and a poached egg is heavenly. No wonder the French have been preparing this for so many years.

2 tablespoons extra-virgin olive oil
$^1/_4$ cup pancetta, diced
1 head frisée (or other hearty lettuce), cut
    into 1-inch pieces

$^1/_2$ tablespoon sherry vinegar
Sea salt and freshly ground black pepper
2 eggs

In a large sauté pan over medium heat, add 1 tablespoon of the oil and the pancetta. Cook slowly until rendered and crispy. Add the frisée and toss with the remaining tablespoon of oil. Allow the frisée to wilt slightly. Add the vinegar, salt, and pepper. Remove from the heat and set aside.

In a small saucepan over high, boil 3 cups of water. Reduce the heat to a simmer and crack the eggs into the water. Cook for 3 to 4 minutes or until desired doneness.

Put the salad on 2 plates and place an egg atop each portion. Serve immediately.

Caesar Salad

SERVES 6

I like Caesar salad separated into spears so I can pick them up and enjoy sumptuous mouthfuls of dressing and crunchy lettuce. I don't know why, but eating them like this enhances the taste for me. The presentation of spears dripping with sauce is beautiful; however, you may break the lettuce into bite-size pieces if you find it easier to serve. This dressing is my all-time favorite—a really traditional tableside Caesar. Also, for you anchovy haters, just eliminate those little guys and add some sea salt.

4 anchovies
1 teaspoon cracked black peppercorns
$^1/_3$ cup extra-virgin olive oil
$^1/_2$ cup freshly grated Parmesan cheese,
   plus shavings for garnish
1 refrigerated egg
3 tablespoons red wine vinegar
2 tablespoons fresh lemon juice

1 tablespoon puréed garlic
2 teaspoons dry mustard
1 teaspoon celery salt
3 dashes Tabasco sauce
3 dashes Worcestershire sauce
2 medium heads romaine lettuce or
   4 hearts of romaine

Combine the anchovies, black pepper, and olive oil in a blender. Purée until very smooth, 1 to 2 minutes or until well combined. Add the grated Parmesan and blend briefly to combine.

Bring a small saucepan of water to a boil. Place the egg on a slotted spoon and lower it into the boiling water. Cook for $1^1/_2$ minutes, remove, and reserve.

Place the remaining dressing ingredients into a large bowl and whisk in the anchovy mixture. Crack open the egg and spoon its contents (including the parts that are uncooked) into the mixture. Whisk until well combined. The dressing may be refrigerated at this stage.

Wash and dry the lettuce. Arrange the lettuce spears onto serving plates and drizzle dressing over the top. Garnish with shaved Parmesan, and serve.

Apple Salad with Blue Cheese Vinaigrette

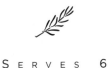

S E R V E S   6

Apples and blue cheese are a fabulous combination. It's sweet and crunchy and tangy and strong at the same time. I love this salad. It is impressive enough to serve to company but easy enough to put together for a simple family dinner. You may omit the apples to make it Level One. Honey Crisp apples are only available for two months of the year, in October and November. They are crisp and sweet and tart. Try them!

$^1/_4$ cup crumbled blue cheese
$^1/_4$ cup sherry vinegar
$^3/_4$ cup extra-virgin olive oil
Sea salt and freshly ground black pepper

1 head butter lettuce
1 bag radicchio
1 large (or 2 small) Honey Crisp, Gala, or
   Fuji apples, thinly sliced

In a small bowl, mix together the blue cheese, vinegar, and olive oil. Season to taste with salt and pepper.

In a salad bowl, combine the lettuce and radicchio with the apples. Toss with the dressing and serve immediately.

Baby Black Lentil Salad

S E R V E S   8

I just love baby lentils. These black lentils are called Beluga lentils and they are one of my favorites because they hold their texture and don't get mushy. If you cannot find this type, check my Ingredients Source Guide (page 294), or substitute any lentils. In this recipe I combine them with the fresh crunch of cucumber, along with tomatoes, scallions, mint, and a squeeze of lime. This makes a great lunch with some grilled whole-grain bread or as a Level Two side dish with a grilled chicken breast.

4 cups cooked baby black lentils (or any lentils), cooled
2 shallots, finely diced
1 cucumber, peeled, seeded, and diced
1 tomato, seeded and diced
2 whole scallions, diced

1 tablespoon julienned fresh mint leaves, plus extra for garnish
Juice from $^{1}/_{2}$ lime
2 tablespoons extra-virgin olive oil
Sea salt and freshly ground black pepper

Combine all the ingredients in a mixing bowl. Gently toss until the lentils are well coated. Garnish with mint and serve.

CHAPTER 19

Sauces, Salsas, Relishes, and Dressings

Basil Pistou

MAKES ABOUT 1 CUP

Pistou rhymes with *ah-choo!* I first encountered pistou during one of my summers in the South of France. The French use it as a flavoring in soups and on top of meat, chicken, or fish. The Italians call it *pesto* and use it on pasta and also as a flavoring for main dishes, salads, and soups. Whatever you call it, it's fantastic. This recipe is particularly unique because the basil is blanched, which helps to keep its bright green color. I like to keep this on hand at all times. It is especially great on my Summer Tomato Soup (page 168).

2 cups basil leaves, loosely packed
$^{1}/_{2}$ cup spinach leaves, loosely packed
$^{1}/_{2}$ cup freshly grated Parmesan cheese

$^{3}/_{4}$ cup olive oil
1 clove garlic, minced
Sea salt and freshly ground black pepper

Set aside a small bowl filled with ice and water. Bring a small pot of water to a boil and add the basil leaves for 30 seconds to soften. Remove immediately and put the leaves into the ice water. Then remove the leaves, squeeze out excess water, and place in a blender. Add the remaining ingredients and purée until smooth.

Parsley Pesto

MAKES ABOUT 1 CUP

They say it's not easy being green, but the color is one of the most beautiful things about this pesto. *Pesto* literally means "pounded" in Italian. When most people think of pesto, they think of basil, which is the traditional ingredient, along with Parmesan, garlic, and olive oil. This twist on the classic is made with parsley for an incredible taste. This is great on fish like my Pan-Roasted Halibut (page 237) or on any of your favorite vegetables, soups, chicken, meats and, of course, pasta!

$^1/_2$ bunch flat-leaf parsley, leaves only
1 bunch tarragon, leaves only
$^1/_4$ cup freshly grated Parmesan cheese

1 clove garlic, minced
$1^1/_2$ cups extra-virgin olive oil
Juice of 1 lemon

Place all the ingredients except the lemon juice into a blender or food processor and blend until smooth. Add the lemon juice at the very end to prevent discoloration of the herbs. Store in an airtight container with a piece of plastic wrap directly on the surface to preserve color. The pesto will keep in the refrigerator for about 2 weeks.

Champagne Mustard Vinaigrette

PRO/FATS—LEVEL ONE

MAKES ABOUT 1 CUP

Champagne vinegar, Dijon mustard, and shallots combine forces to create this sublime dressing. Takes me right back to my summers spent in France.

2 shallots, finely minced
2 tablespoons Dijon mustard
4 tablespoons Champagne vinegar

1 cup extra-virgin olive oil
Juice from $1/4$ lemon
Sea salt and freshly ground black pepper

In a medium-size bowl, combine the shallots, mustard, and vinegar. Whisk in the olive oil until completely smooth. Add the lemon juice and season to taste with salt and pepper.

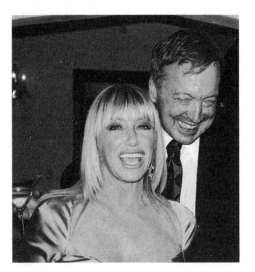

My agent, Al Lowman . . . always laughing.

Sweet Corn and Crab Relish

MAKES 2 CUPS

Welcome to Level Two! How great to be balanced enough that we can indulge in a little fresh corn. This relish is the topping for my incredible Crab Bisque (page 170). When you shave off the corn, be sure to save the cob for the soup. This relish is also fabulous served atop a butter-lettuce salad or right out of the container! Of course, you may delete the corn and have this on Level One. Yum.

2 ears corn on the cob (or $1^1/_2$ cups corn)
$^1/_2$ cup lump crabmeat
1 jalapeño, seeded and finely diced
1 tablespoon freshly chopped flat-leaf
   parsley

Juice from $^1/_2$ lemon
1 shallot, finely diced (or $^1/_4$ red onion,
   finely diced)
Sea salt and freshly ground black pepper

   Slice the corn off the cobs. Reserve the cobs to flavor the Crab Bisque. Toss all the ingredients in a bowl. Serve immediately or store in an airtight container in the refrigerator.

Roasted Eggplant Relish

PRO/FATS AND VEGGIES—LEVEL ONE

MAKES 1 CUP

A lot of people think they don't like eggplant, but eggplant takes on whatever flavors you cook with it. The combination of cumin and fresh mint makes this delicious. Even eggplant haters will be tricked!

4 Japanese eggplant, cut in half lengthwise
1 tablespoon extra-virgin olive oil
Sea salt and freshly ground black pepper

$^{1}/_{2}$ teaspoon ground cumin
1 teaspoon freshly chopped mint
Juice from $^{1}/_{4}$ lemon

Preheat the oven to 350 degrees.

Place the eggplant on a baking sheet and sprinkle with the olive oil, salt, and pepper. Bake until soft and cooked through, about 30 minutes. Remove from the oven and allow to cool. Then dice the eggplant into 1-inch pieces. Mix in a bowl with the cumin, a drizzle of olive oil, the mint, and the lemon juice. Serve immediately.

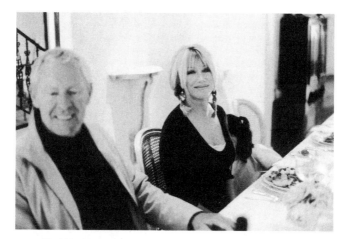

The kids threw me a Mother's Day lunch—I'm one happy mom.

Warm Cranberry Relish

SERVES 6

Everyone thinks of cranberries as something you spoon on your plate on Thanksgiving along with your turkey. Cranberries are loaded with great nutrients and they are remarkably versatile. My husband loves this recipe with roast pork. Cranberry relish is a simple chutney. It is made in a saucepan and not only does it taste great, but it's very beautiful. It takes only 15 minutes to prepare and puts a lot of excitement onto the plate. Try it with my Herb-Roasted Loin of Pork (page 252).

2 tablespoons extra-virgin olive oil
$^1/_2$ onion, finely diced
2 tablespoons fresh ginger, finely minced
2 cups whole fresh cranberries

1 tablespoon sherry vinegar
1 tablespoon SomerSweet
Sea salt and freshly ground black pepper

In a medium saucepan over medium heat, add the olive oil, onion, and ginger. Cook until the onion softens, 4 or 5 minutes. Add the cranberries, vinegar, Somer-Sweet, and $^1/_2$ cup water. Cook until the berries pop and become soft, 10 to 15 minutes. Stir occasionally. Season to taste with salt and pepper. Serve immediately.

Roasted Garlic Aïoli

PRO/FATS AND VEGGIES—LEVEL ONE

MAKES 1 CUP

Aïoli is a garlic-flavored mayonnaise that originated in the South of France. In this version I roast the garlic first for a smooth, mellow flavor. Use this as a topping for chicken, seafood, and vegetables. Try it on my Crispy-Skinned Salmon (page 238) or as a sauce on steamed asparagus.

1 head garlic
1 egg
1 egg yolk

1 tablespoon Dijon mustard
Juice from $^{1}/_{2}$ lemon
1 cup light olive oil

Preheat the oven to 350 degrees.

Wrap the garlic in aluminum foil and roast for about 45 minutes. Squeeze the garlic cloves from their skin and place into a blender or food processor with the egg, egg yolk, mustard, and lemon juice. Purée until smooth. Add the oil in a slow drizzle until the aïoli emulsifies. Store in an airtight container and refrigerate until ready to use.

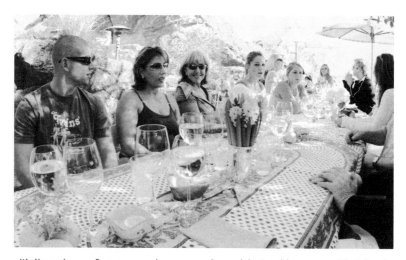

It's November . . . Dungeness crab season, and we celebrate with our annual Crab Lunch at the back of the property. That's my sister Maureen who comes every year.

Lemon-Thyme Aïoli

PRO/FATS AND VEGGIES — LEVEL ONE

MAKES 1 1/2 CUP

This fresh, lemony sauce is perfect on seafood, especially my Grilled Tuna (page 241). It also livens a piece of steamed broccoli.

1 egg
1 egg yolk
1 tablespoon Dijon mustard
1 clove garlic, minced
Juice and zest from $^1/_2$ lemon

1 tablespoon chopped fresh thyme
 (or 1 teaspoon dried)
Sea salt and freshly ground black pepper
$1^1/_2$ cups light olive oil

Place all the ingredients, except the oil, into a blender or food processor. Blend until smooth. With the machine running, add the oil in a slow stream until the aïoli becomes emulsified. Serve immediately or store in an airtight container for 2 to 3 days.

Gremolata

MAKES $^1/_2$ CUP

This is a classic garnish to serve over osso bucco or any dish you want to give a fresh, sprightly flavor. Unlike pestos, which are puréed, this is finely minced so that it retains more texture. It is divine over Braised Veal Stew (page 250).

$^1/_2$ bunch flat-leaf parsley leaves, finely
   minced
Zest from 1 lemon
1 clove garlic, pressed

$^1/_4$ cup olive oil
Sea salt and freshly ground black pepper

Place all the ingredients into a bowl and toss to combine. Let the flavors meld for 30 minutes before serving. Store in an airtight container in the refrigerator for up to 1 week.

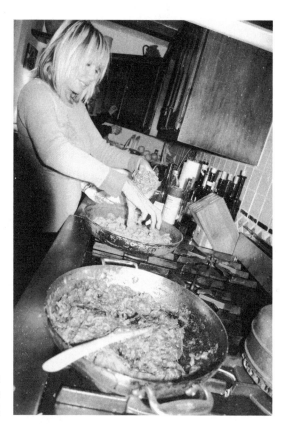

My caramelized onions are done and I am sautéing my turkey sausage for the Thanksgiving stuffing. I love tradition!

Wild Mushroom Sauce

PRO/FATS AND VEGGIES — LEVEL ONE

SERVES 2

This mushroom sauce is a knockout on a simply roasted steak, pork chop, or chicken breast. Try it with Roast Chicken Breast Stuffed with Herbed Goat Cheese (page 231)—heavenly! If you can get wild mushrooms they are a real treat. I like to use a combination of morels and chanterelles, but shiitake or even regular button mushrooms will do the trick. The addition of the veal demi-glace adds an extra wallop of flavor, but it's still delicious without it.

1 tablespoon extra-virgin olive oil
1 clove garlic
1 cup wild mushrooms
2 sprigs fresh thyme, leaves only
  (or $^1/_4$ teaspoon dried)
$^1/_4$ cup white wine

$^1/_2$ cup chicken broth
1 tablespoon veal or chicken demi-glace
  (optional)
1 tablespoon unsalted butter
Sea salt and freshly ground black pepper

Place a sauté pan on medium heat. Add the olive oil and the whole clove of garlic to infuse the flavor into the oil. Sauté the garlic for about 1 minute, and then add the mushrooms and thyme. Sauté until the mushrooms are crusty and golden brown, about 10 minutes. Add the wine to deglaze the pan, scraping the bits on the bottom of the pan to release the flavor. Continue cooking until the wine reduces by half. Add the chicken broth and demi-glace and reduce again by half. Whisk in the butter and remove from the heat. Season with salt and pepper and serve as desired.

Whole-Wheat Crostini with Red Pepper Rouille

LEVEL TWO

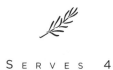

SERVES 4

Rouille in French means "rust." This fiery red sauce is made with peppers, garlic, and olive oil. It's most commonly used to garnish Bouillabaisse (page 240), but it will light up a simple turkey burger like you can't believe! The rouille is Level One, but when you add it to the toast it becomes Level Two.

1 head garlic
1 red bell pepper (or 1 cup drained jarred red peppers)
$1/2$ teaspoon cayenne pepper
Juice from $1/2$ lemon

Sea salt and freshly ground black pepper
1 cup extra-virgin olive oil, plus more for drizzling
4 slices crusty hard, whole-wheat bread

Preheat the oven to 350 degrees.

Slice the head of garlic in half through the middle, so that you have cut off the tops of the cloves. Cover the garlic with aluminum foil and roast for about 1 hour. Squeeze the garlic pulp out of the skins and set aside.

To roast the bell pepper, place the whole pepper on a hot grill or an open flame and char on all sides until the skin is black and bubbling. Immediately put the roasted pepper into a sealed paper or plastic bag and let steam for about 15 minutes. Remove the pepper from the bag and pull off the stem. Break the pepper apart and discard the seeds. Scrape the charred skin off gently with a knife.

Place the roasted garlic, roasted pepper, cayenne, lemon juice, salt, and pepper into a blender or food processor and blend until smooth. Add the 1 cup of olive oil in a slow stream until the rouille becomes emulsified. Serve immediately or store in an airtight container in the refrigerator for about a week.

To make whole-wheat crostini, drizzle olive oil onto the bread and toast or grill until golden. Cut each slice on the diagonal and drizzle the toast with rouille.

Chipotle and Tomato Salsa

PRO/FATS AND VEGGIES — LEVEL ONE

MAKES 2 CUPS

Use this delicious salsa on New Mexican Huevos (page 163) or a grilled chicken breast or steak, or as a dip with Black Pepper Parmesan Crisps (page 169). Chipotles are dried, smoked jalapeños. They have a wrinkly skin and a smoky, almost chocolaty, flavor. They are usually canned in adobo sauce, which is what I use to flavor this salsa.

2 tomatoes (red or yellow), medium diced
2 teaspoons adobo sauce (from canned chipotles)
$^1/_2$ red onion, finely diced
$^1/_2$ chipotle, seeds removed and finely diced

2 tablespoons olive oil
Juice from $^1/_2$ lime
1 tablespoon chopped fresh cilantro (or $1^1/_2$ teaspoons dried)
Sea salt and freshly ground black pepper

In a medium bowl, gently combine all the ingredients and season with salt and pepper. Serve immediately and store leftovers in an airtight container in the refrigerator for up to 3 days.

Mango Salsa

L E V E L   T W O

M A K E S   1   C U P

This fabulous salsa is sweet and spicy all at the same time. It goes with my Chipotle-Glazed Pork (page 254), and it's great with chicken breasts or a piece of Chilean sea bass. It's also a delicious treat with tortilla chips. Try this one. It's a winner.

1 ripe mango, peeled, fruit carved away
   from the seed and diced
$^1/_2$ red onion, finely diced
1 red jalapeño, seeds removed
Juice from $^1/_4$ lime

1 tablespoon chopped fresh cilantro
1 tablespoon chopped fresh mint
1 tablespoon extra-virgin olive oil
Sea salt and freshly ground black pepper

   Mix together all the ingredients. Season with salt and pepper.

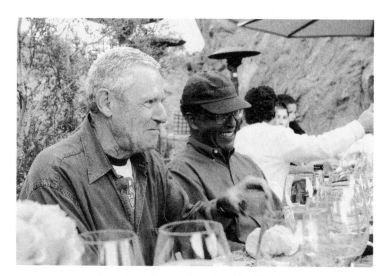

My husband, Alan, and our dear friend Nelson.

Tomatillo Salsa

LEVEL TWO

MAKES 1 CUP

When you live in Southern California or any of the southwestern states, tomatillos are abundant; but most people don't know what to do with them. Tomatillos have a lemony, pungent flavor and look kind of like green tomatoes wrapped in papery husks. They are good roasted, and they also are great in soups; but I especially like them for salsa. This salsa is great with my Chipotle-Glazed Pork (page 254); it's also good on fish or chicken or you can warm it up and use it as a sauce.

Extra-virgin olive oil
1 yellow onion, finely diced
1 cup diced tomatillo, husks removed

$^1/_2$ avocado, chopped
Sea salt and freshly ground black pepper
1 tablespoon chopped fresh mint

In a medium sauté pan over high, add the olive oil and onion. Sauté until caramelized. Add the tomatillo. Cook until soft, 5 or 6 minutes. Remove from the heat and put into a blender. Add the avocado and blend until smooth. Season with salt and pepper. Remove from the blender and fold in the mint.

Candied Tomato Salsa

PRO/FATS AND VEGGIES — LEVEL ONE

MAKES 1 CUP

For those of you who have been following the recipes in my books so far, you know how I feel about candied tomatoes. I love them. My kitchen is never without a container. Use them in a variety of ways: soups, sauces, or salads. My Chipotle-Glazed Pork with Candied Tomato Salsa (page 254) is an awesome combination.

1 recipe Candied Roma Tomatoes (page 204), coarsely chopped
1¹/₂ tablespoons extra–virgin olive oil
1 tablespoon chopped fresh cilantro

1 red jalapeño or Fresno chili, finely chopped
Sea salt and freshly ground black pepper

In a medium-size bowl, mix together all the ingredients. Season with salt and pepper.

CHAPTER 20

Vegetables

Candied Roma Tomatoes

PRO/FATS AND VEGGIES—LEVEL ONE

MAKES 12

As you may know by now, I am a freak for slow-roasted tomatoes. I first brought you candied tomatoes in *Eat Great, Lose Weight*; and in this version I bring them to you with the Roma tomato. Roma tomatoes are readily available; and even on the occasion when they don't taste their best raw, they roast beautifully and the flavor intensifies. The touch of SomerSweet helps the caramelization. Feel free to add your herb of choice and double or triple the recipe as needed. I love to serve these on just about anything. Try them with my Pan-Roasted Halibut (page 237). By the way, tomatoes are an excellent source of lycopene, which significantly reduces the risk of getting prostate cancer.

6 Roma tomatoes
$^{1}/_{4}$ cup olive oil

$^{1}/_{4}$ teaspoon SomerSweet
Sea salt

Preheat the oven to 350 degrees.

Halve the tomatoes lengthwise and squeeze out most of the seeds. Coat in olive oil, sprinkle in the SomerSweet, and season liberally with salt. Place tomatoes cut side down on a baking sheet or roasting pan.

Roast for about 1 hour, or until the skin becomes crinkly and slightly browned. Remove from the oven and peel off skin (optional). Serve warm or store in an airtight container until ready to use.

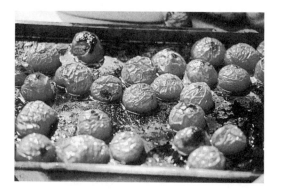

Bruschetta Artichokes

PRO/FATS AND VEGGIES—LEVEL ONE

S ERVES 4

Most people don't realize artichokes are male and female. Males are pointy; females are round. Needless to say, the females taste the best. The most amazing thing about a pressure cooker is that you can cook these in 15 minutes; otherwise, you can steam them for 45 minutes. This is a beautiful first course and a real crowd-pleaser.

Juice of one lemon
4 artichokes
3 tomatoes, chopped

1 bunch fresh basil, chopped
$^1/_4$ cup olive oil
Sea salt and freshly ground black pepper

Place the lemon juice in a bowl of water. Trim the artichokes by cutting off the inedible, prickly outer leaves and barely exposing the purple center off the choke. Trim the tips from the remaining leaves using scissors. Place each prepared artichoke in the bowl of lemon water to prevent discoloration.

Fill the bottom of a steamer with 4 inches of water. Place the artichokes in the steamer basket and steam until tender, 40 to 60 minutes. (Cooking time will vary depending on the size of the artichoke.) If using a pressure cooker, cook according to the manufacturer's instructions. When cool, scoop out the hairy chokes, being careful to keep the heart intact.

In a separate bowl, place the tomatoes, basil, olive oil, salt, and pepper and toss. Spoon the tomato mixture into the center of the artichokes and serve.

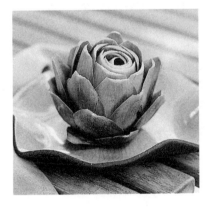

Vegetables *205*

Braised Red Chard

SERVES 4

Swiss chard is loaded with vitamins and nutrients. You'll love the way this tastes sautéed with butter and olive oil.

2 tablespoons olive oil
1 yellow onion, finely diced
2 tablespoons unsalted butter
$1/4$ cup chicken broth

2 bunches red Swiss chard, coarsely chopped
Sea salt and freshly ground black pepper

Place a wok or large skillet over high heat. Add the olive oil and onion and sauté for 2 to 3 minutes. Turn down the heat to medium and cook for another 7 minutes, or until lightly browned. Add the butter, broth, chard, salt, and pepper and let braise for about 15 minutes.

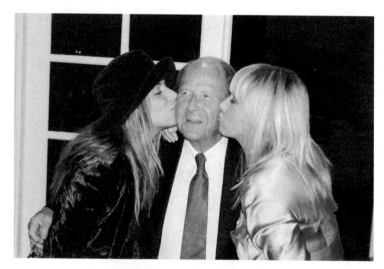

The French father-in-law . . . ooh, la, la!

Grilled Asparagus

S E R V E S 4

I love the taste of freshly grilled vegetables. This asparagus is especially good with the added zing of lemon zest and a squeeze of lemon juice.

1 bunch fresh medium-thick asparagus
Extra-virgin olive oil

Sea salt and freshly ground black pepper
Zest and juice from $^1/_2$ lemon

Preheat grill to medium.

Wash and trim off the tough ends of the asparagus. Drizzle with olive oil, then season with salt, pepper, and lemon zest.

Place the asparagus onto the grill, turning frequently for about 3 minutes. Remove from the heat and sprinkle with fresh lemon juice just before serving.

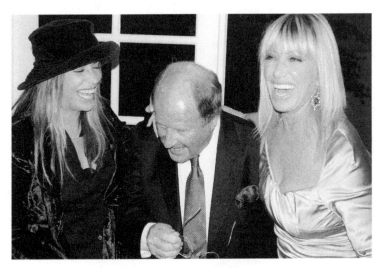

Having a great time with Leslie and Jean-Pierre.

Chilled Asparagus with Lemon-Thyme Aïoli

PRO/FATS AND VEGGIES—LEVEL ONE

S E R V E S   6   T O   8

The key to keeping vegetables bright green and crisp is blanching. This process is very simple. Boil a pot of salted water and have an ice bath standing by. The vegetables cook for just a few minutes, then they are plunged into the ice bath to stop the cooking process. This preserves the color and keeps vegetables from getting soggy. You may use this technique for any of your favorite vegetables to create wonderful crudité platters. In this recipe I like to chill the asparagus, then top it with Lemon-Thyme Aïoli (page 195). Perfect for a buffet.

2 bunches fresh medium-thick asparagus
Olive oil

Sea salt and freshly ground black pepper
1 recipe Lemon-Thyme Aïoli (page 195)

Bring a large pot of salted water to a boil. Prepare an ice bath with water and ice in a large mixing bowl.

Trim the tough ends from the asparagus. Place into boiling water for about 4 minutes (cooking time will vary depending upon the thickness of the asparagus). Check for doneness. The asparagus should be just al dente.

Strain immediately into a colander and plunge into an ice bath to halt the cooking process. Keep in the bath until just cooled through and remove to avoid the asparagus getting soggy. Dry on a kitchen towel and chill.

Arrange on a platter and drizzle with olive oil, then season with salt and pepper. Serve with the aïoli.

Zucchini Ribbons

S E R V E S   4

These zucchini ribbons are the perfect replacement for pasta. Plus, what a great way to get kids to eat vegetables! I use these in so many different ways. I cover them with pesto or alfredo sauce and they are a wonderful side dish with meat, seafood, or poultry. The easiest way to make these is with my amazing kitchen prep tool called the Somersize Su-Chef. With the press of a button, you get a looooooooong, curly, perfectly thin ribbon of zucchini. Look for the Su-Chef on my Web site. If you don't have one, you can use a vegetable peeler to make long, thin ribbons.

4 large zucchini
1 tablespoon olive oil
Sea salt and freshly ground black pepper

Attach the Fancy Food Cutter to the Somersize Su-Chef with the ribbon cutter disk. Follow the directions according to the Su-Chef manual. Or, using a vegetable peeler, make long, thin ribbons by peeling the zucchini lengthwise, turning as you go so you are left only with the center core.

Heat a large sauté pan on medium. Add the olive oil and zucchini. Season with salt and pepper. Sauté for 30 seconds, until just warmed through. Serve immediately.

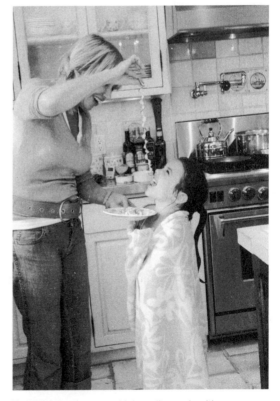

The kids loooooooove zucchini noodles made with my Somersize Su-Chef.

Black Kale (Cavello Nero)

PRO/FATS AND VEGGIES—LEVEL ONE

SERVES 2

This is one of the more unusual greens. If it is not available, ask your produce manager to order it for you. This kale sautés beautifully and has a better flavor for pan-frying than the standard kale available at most grocery stores. That kale is better left for soups, whereas this version cooks more easily in a frying pan. This recipe is garlicky and has a great kick from the pepper. I love this flavor. It's also great with Parmesan cheese.

2 tablespoons extra-virgin olive oil
2 cloves garlic, finely minced
1 bunch black kale, cleaned very well
    (triple wash)

Juice from $^1/_2$ lemon
Sea salt and freshly ground black pepper

In a large sauté pan over medium heat, add the olive oil and garlic. Cook until the garlic is golden brown. Add the kale and toss to wilt. Cook until soft, about 5 minutes. Sprinkle with lemon juice and season to taste with salt and pepper. Serve immediately.

Sautéed Brussels Sprouts with Pancetta

PRO/FATS AND VEGGIES—LEVEL ONE

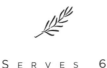

SERVES 6

Brussels sprouts can be the most delicious vegetable if prepared properly. I love experimenting with them. These have a crispy texture and salty taste because of the fried pancetta. Also, cutting them into quarters enhances the flavor and makes them more exciting to taste. Even the Brussels-sprouts hater will be turned around by this recipe. It is truly delicious, and you will find yourself making these on days other than holidays. Try them; you'll like them.

¹/₄ cup diced pancetta (or bacon)
1 tablespoon extra-virgin olive oil
2 shallots, finely diced

1 pound fresh Brussels sprouts, cleaned and cut into quarters
2 tablespoons unsalted butter
Sea salt and freshly ground black pepper

In a sauté pan over medium heat, cook the pancetta in the oil until rendered and slightly crispy, 3 or 4 minutes. Add the shallots and cook until soft and light caramel in color, 2 or 3 minutes. Add the Brussels sprouts and butter and sauté until they are soft and golden, 4 or 5 minutes. Season with salt and pepper to taste. Serve immediately.

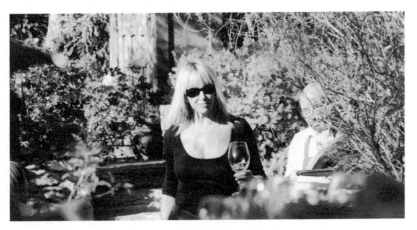

Overseeing the details at our crab luncheon.

Caramelized Root Vegetables

PRO/FATS AND VEGGIES — LEVEL ONE

SERVES 6

It's important that you cut these root vegetables into bite-size pieces. That way each delicious piece gets coated with flavor and buttery, salty sauce. These are pan-fried and make a great accompaniment to your autumn meals.

1 tablespoon olive oil
1 celery root, peeled and cut into small
    pieces
1 turnip, peeled and cut into small pieces

1 rutabaga, peeled and cut into small
    pieces
2 tablespoons unsalted butter
Sea salt and freshly ground black pepper

In a medium sauté pan over medium heat, add the olive oil and vegetables. Cook slowly. As the vegetables begin to caramelize, add 1 tablespoon of the butter.

Continue to cook for 10 minutes. Add the remaining butter. Season with salt and pepper and serve immediately.

Grilled Fennel and Zucchini

PRO/FATS AND VEGGIES—LEVEL ONE

SERVES 2

These grilled vegetables are the perfect complement to my Grilled Lamb Chops with Lavender Lamb Jus (page 247). They bring life to any simple piece of grilled or roasted chicken, fish, or meat.

2 zucchini
1 red onion
2 fennel bulbs

Extra-virgin olive oil
Sea salt and freshly ground black pepper

Preheat grill to high.

Slice the zucchini very thin lengthwise. Slice the onion into thick rings, then separate. Slice the fennel into thick slices. Drizzle the vegetables with olive oil, then season with salt and pepper. Grill the zucchini for about 1 minute per side. The fennel and onion will take slightly longer. Serve immediately.

Warm Spinach with Prosciutto Crisps

PRO/FATS AND VEGGIES—LEVEL ONE

S E R V E S   2

What a great way to enjoy spinach. Yum! It is packed with flavor. Lightly sautéed spinach with crispy fried prosciutto, sprinkled with grated Romano, salt, and freshly ground pepper: a simple and simply delicious way to eat your vegetables.

3 tablespoons extra-virgin olive oil
6 thin slices prosciutto
1 whole clove garlic, minced
1 bag spinach

Juice from $^1/_2$ lemon
2 tablespoons grated Romano cheese
Sea salt and freshly ground black pepper

In a nonstick pan over medium, add 1 tablespoon of the olive oil. Gently lay the prosciutto into the pan and cook until crispy and transparent, about 1 minute on each side. Drain on paper towels and set aside.

In a large sauté pan over high, add the remaining olive oil and the garlic. Allow the garlic to lightly brown. Add the spinach and toss in the oil to coat and wilt gently, but not overcook, about 2 minutes. Squeeze in the lemon juice. Remove from the heat immediately and toss with the cheese, salt, and pepper. Place onto plates, garnish with crispy prosciutto, and serve immediately.

Sautéed Cabbage with Pine Nuts and Goat Cheese

ALMOST LEVEL ONE

SERVES 2

This combination is a real pleaser. Sautéed, toasty pine nuts and warm goat cheese make purple cabbage like you've never tasted before. You'll love it. Omit the pine nuts and it's Level One.

3 tablespoons extra-virgin olive oil
2 tablespoons pine nuts
$^{1}/_{2}$ head purple cabbage, thinly sliced
Sea salt and freshly ground black pepper

2 teaspoons sherry vinegar
2 ounces fresh goat cheese, shaped into
　2 disks

In a large sauté pan over high, add the olive oil and pine nuts. Toast the nuts until light golden brown. Add the cabbage. Cook until wilted, about 3 to 5 minutes. Season with salt and pepper. Add the vinegar.

In a separate nonstick sauté pan over medium, add a drop of oil and warm the goat cheese on each side until soft. Remove from the heat.

Place the cabbage onto plates and add the cheese on top. Garnish with freshly ground black pepper. Serve immediately.

French Lentils

LEVEL TWO

MAKES 2 CUPS

I love, love, love these tiny lentils from France. They hold their shape after cooking and are like piles of little jewels on the plates. They taste even better the next day. They have a wonderful flavor and make a great carb addition to a Pro/Fats meal for Level Two. Have about $1/2$ cup along with the Crispy-Skinned Salmon with Roasted Garlic Aïoli (page 238) and you've got a perfectly balanced and delightfully delicious Level Two meal.

1 tablespoon extra-virgin olive oil
1 stalk celery, very finely diced
$1/2$ yellow onion, very finely diced
2 cloves garlic
1 cup French de Puy lentils (or any dried lentils)

$1/2$ cup white wine
3 to 4 cups chicken broth
Sea salt and freshly ground black pepper
1 tablespoon finely chopped flat-leaf parsley, for garnish
Juice from $1/2$ lemon, for garnish

Place a large saucepan on low heat. Add the oil, celery, onion, and garlic. Sauté the vegetables for about 10 minutes, until they become soft. Add the dried lentils and stir to coat with the oil. Turn the heat up to medium and add the wine to deglaze the pan. Continue cooking until the wine reduces by half. Add 3 cups of the broth and bring to a boil, then reduce the heat and let simmer for 20 to 30 minutes, checking frequently to make sure the liquid does not completely evaporate. (Add more broth as needed.) Season with salt and pepper. Garnish with parsley and a squeeze of lemon juice. Serve warm or cold.

Smashed Tuscan Potatoes

L E V E L   T W O

S E R V E S   2   T O   3

Yum! Smashed potatoes! An Irish girl's dream! This is your treat for progressing to Level Two. Little red potatoes flattened and sautéed in olive oil, infused with rosemary . . . simply delicious. What a treat after all these years of leaving the potato behind. I love these almost as much as cake!

8 new potatoes (small red potatoes)
Sea salt
3 sprigs fresh rosemary (or 3 teaspoons
    dried)

$^{1}/_{4}$ cup extra-virgin olive oil
3 cloves garlic
1 dried red chili (chile de arbol)
Freshly ground black pepper

Place the potatoes into a saucepan and cover with cold water by 1 inch. Add about 2 teaspoons salt and 1 sprig of the rosemary (or 1 teaspoon of the dried). Place over high heat just until it comes to a boil, then simmer for about 20 minutes. The potatoes are done when pierced easily with a fork.

Drain the water then set the potatoes aside to cool. When cool to the touch, smash each with the heel of your hand.

Place a large sauté pan on medium-high heat. Add the olive oil and the whole garlic cloves. Let the garlic get nice and crusty on one side, then turn to cook the other side. Add half the potatoes at a time (this keeps the temperature of the oil nice and hot so that the potatoes don't stick). Shake the pan to loosen the potatoes. Cook for about 2 minutes, then add the remaining potatoes and the remaining 2 sprigs of fresh rosemary (or 2 teaspoons dried). Once the potatoes get crusty on one side (about 4 minutes), turn them with a spatula and cook the other side. Season with salt and pepper and serve immediately.

Deadly Scalloped Potatoes

LEVEL TWO

SERVES 6

Okay, these should be Level Ten! There is nothing Somersized about these potatoes, but I think Christmas is the one day of the year to go for it. These potatoes are in a category all their own. Thinly sliced potatoes (if you have a mandoline, please use it for this), dripping in a sour cream–mascarpone sauce with herbs and seasonings: The result is sumptuous and sinful. *One day only*, then back to your program. Enjoy and indulge, but try to have some restraint.

1 cup sour cream
$^1/_2$ cup mascarpone cheese (or cream cheese)
$2^1/_2$ cups heavy cream
$^1/_2$ cup chicken broth
$^1/_2$ tablespoon freshly chopped thyme

Sea salt and freshly ground black pepper
5 medium-size Yukon Gold potatoes, unpeeled, sliced thin in rounds on a mandoline
$^1/_4$ cup Fontina cheese, grated

Preheat the oven to 400 degrees.

In a medium-size mixing bowl, combine all the ingredients except the potatoes and Fontina cheese. Season to taste with salt and pepper.

Ladle one fourth of the cream mixture into the bottom of a Pyrex or other heavy baking dish. The baking dish can be 9 × 9 inch or 9 × 13 inch, depending on how thick you want the finished dish to be. Place potato slices overlapping one another by one fourth. After finishing each layer, sprin-

kle with salt and pepper. When finished layering all the potatoes, pour the remaining cream mixture over the top. Sprinkle with the Fontina cheese and cover the dish with foil. Bake for 1 hour. Lift the foil and press the potatoes with a spatula to make sure they are evenly covered. Return to the oven until cooked completely through, about another 15 minutes. Remove the foil and cook until the potatoes are golden brown, about 15 more minutes. Serve immediately.

CHAPTER 21

Rice, Pasta, and Grains

Forbidden Rice

LEVEL TWO

MAKES 3 CUPS

Forbidden rice is a black rice from China . . . the emperors' exclusive grain. It is a specialty item that can be ordered; see my Ingredients Source Guide (page 296) for information. It is simply a delicious new grain to add to your pantry. Try it. This goes well with the Curry Chicken Skewers (page 233).

1 cup uncooked Forbidden Rice
$^1/_2$ red onion, finely diced
1 bunch flat-leaf parsley, finely chopped
Zest and juice from 1 lemon

$^1/_4$ cup extra-virgin olive oil
1 tablespoon freshly chopped mint
Sea salt and freshly ground black pepper

Prepare the rice according to the package directions. Place into a mixing bowl and add the other ingredients. Mix well. Season with salt and pepper. Serve at room temperature.

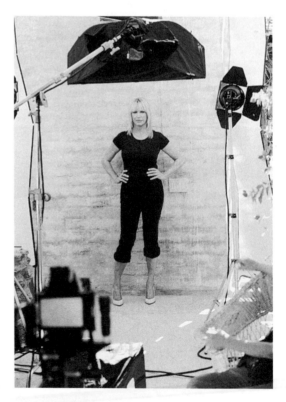

Posing for our *Slim and Sexy* photo shoot.

Whole-Wheat Linguine with Candied Roma Tomatoes

LEVEL TWO

SERVES 2

There are many different types of whole-grain pastas: whole wheat, spelt, amaranth, and my new favorite, farro. When I began Somersizing, I missed my white-flour pasta. Over the years I have grown to prefer the earthy, nutty, fresh flavors of whole-grain pasta. This recipe explodes with flavor. It is fresh and has a great kick depending upon how much red pepper you like to add.

$^1/_2$ pound whole-wheat linguine
$^1/_4$ cup extra-virgin olive oil
1 red onion, thinly sliced
2 cloves garlic, finely chopped
1 recipe Candied Roma Tomatoes

(page 204)
Zest of 1 lemon
1 bunch fresh basil, stemmed
Crushed red pepper flakes
Sea salt and freshly ground black pepper

Cook the pasta according to the package directions.

In a sauté pan over high, add 2 tablespoons of the olive oil and the onion and cook until caramelized and soft. Add the garlic, tomatoes, lemon zest, and basil. Cook until the tomatoes soften, about 10 minutes.

Drain the pasta and add 2 cups of the cooked linguine to the sauté pan. Toss together and add the remaining 2 tablespoons of olive oil, the red pepper flakes, and salt and pepper to taste. Serve immediately.

Sautéed Herb Quinoa

MAKES 3 CUPS

Quinoa (pronounced "keen-wah") was a staple of the ancient Incas, who called it the mother grain. It's considered a complete protein with eight essential amino acids and a rich source of vital nutrients, plus it's lower in carbohydrates than most grains. Did I mention that it's incredibly delicious? It is my favorite new whole grain. I like it even better than brown or wild rice. You simply boil it in water as you would rice, but it takes a fraction of the time to cook. Prepared in this way, with a sprinkle of salt, it's a Carbo dish. In this recipe I add olive oil and herbs and it becomes a perfect Level Two side dish to balance your Pro/Fat meal.

1 cup dry quinoa
2 tablespoons extra-virgin olive oil
2 shallots, finely diced
1 clove garlic, minced

2 teaspoons finely chopped fresh flat-leaf
  parsley
Sea salt and freshly ground black pepper

Prepare the quinoa according to package instructions.

While the quinoa is cooking, place a sauté pan over medium heat. Add the olive oil and shallots; sauté for 2 minutes. Add the garlic and cook for 1 minute longer. Add the cooked quinoa and the parsley and stir to combine. Season with salt and pepper and serve immediately.

Quinoa Tabbouleh

M A K E S   2   C U P S

You know by now that I've fallen in love with quinoa. It's the "super grain" that has so many wonderful vitamins and nutrients (see box, page 76). In this recipe, I use it to create a twist on classic tabbouleh. Speaking of incredibly nutritious foods, I also use about 1 cup of parsley, which is one of the healthiest dark green, leafy vegetables and gives you a huge boost of vitamins A and C. For Level One, omit the olive oil and enjoy this as a Level One Carbos and Veggies dish.

1 cup cooked quinoa, cooled
3 tablespoons olive oil
1 cup freshly chopped flat-leaf parsley
$^{1}/_{4}$ cup finely chopped shallots
   (or $^{1}/_{4}$ red onion)
1 tablespoon freshly chopped dill
   (or $^{1}/_{2}$ tablespoon dried)

1 cup diced tomato
$^{1}/_{2}$ cucumber, peeled, seeded, and diced
1 tablespoon freshly chopped mint
Zest and juice from 1 lemon
Sea salt and freshly ground black pepper

In a medium bowl, combine the quinoa with all the other ingredients and season with salt and pepper. Serve immediately or store in an airtight container in the refrigerator for up to a week.

Crostini with Homemade Ricotta Cheese

LEVEL TWO

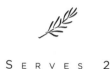

SERVES 2

Imagine . . . homemade ricotta! It's so easy, and it's much fresher and creamier than store-bought. I like to drizzle this over thinly sliced whole-grain bread and use it as a garnish for Roasted Yellow Pepper Soup (page 172). Homemade ricotta is also great served over tomatoes, or you could layer it in your Somersize Slow Cooker Lasagna (page 282) or dollop it into one of your favorite puréed soups. If you don't have time to make your own, buy store-bought ricotta and add a little bit of cream and whip it with a whisk to make it less gritty and give it a creamier texture.

1 cup heavy cream
1 cup whole milk
$^1/_4$ cup whole fat, plain yogurt

Sea salt
2 thin slices hard-crusted, whole-grain
    bread

Place the cream, milk, and yogurt into a saucepan and heat over medium. Stir frequently until small bubbles form around the edge. Lower the heat and simmer for 20 minutes. Turn off the heat and allow to cool so that the whey (the watery liquid) and the curd separate. Turn off the heat. Line a strainer with cheesecloth and ladle the ricotta into it. Allow the liquid to strain out of the cheese for a few minutes; then draw up the sides of the cheesecloth and scrape the ricotta into a bowl. Season with a little salt.

Toast the bread until golden brown. Spread ricotta on the toast and serve. Place any remaining ricotta in an airtight container and store in the refrigerator.

Soba Noodles

S E R V E S   4

Soba noodles are delicious. They are made from pure buckwheat, so they are a great Somer-size choice for soups and salads. Try them in unusual ways, even tossed with pesto for an easy treat. I add these to my Thai Beef with Cucumber Salad (page 178) for Level Two.

$^1/_2$ cup uncooked soba noodles
2 teaspoons soy sauce
1 teaspoon rice wine vinegar

1 tablespoon olive oil
1 tablespoon freshly chopped chives
Sea salt and freshly ground black pepper

Cook the soba noodles according to the package instructions. After the noodles are cooked, run them under cold water to stop them from further cooking. Place the noo-dles into a medium-size bowl. Add the soy sauce, vinegar, oil, chives, and salt and pepper to taste.

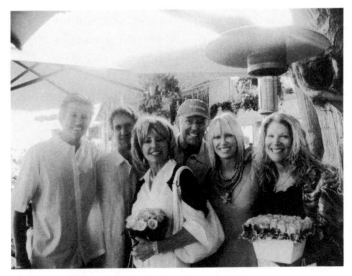

Alan's birthday lunch with our wonderful friends.

Red Rice

LEVEL TWO

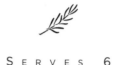

SERVES 6

Here's another wonderful grain: red rice. My friend Shirani, from Sri Lanka, introduced me to this and now it's a staple in my home. In this recipe it's cooked with zucchini and squash with herbs and a squeeze of lemon. Perfect.

2 tablespoons extra-virgin olive oil
2 cloves garlic, finely chopped
2 shallots, finely chopped
1 zucchini, diced
1 yellow squash, diced
3 cups cooked red rice (or any whole-grain rice)

1 tomato, seeded and diced
1 tablespoon finely chopped fresh chives (or 1 teaspoon dried)
1 tablespoon julienned fresh basil
1 scallion, finely minced
Sea salt and freshly ground black pepper
Juice from $1/2$ lemon

Heat a sauté pan over medium. Add 1 tablespoon of the olive oil, the garlic, and the shallots. Sauté until soft, about 4 minutes. Add the zucchini and squash. Sauté until just cooked through, about 2 minutes.

Add the cooked red rice, tomato, chives, basil, and scallion. Season with salt and pepper, the lemon juice and the remaining tablespoon of olive oil. Serve hot or cold.

Farro Risotto

SERVES 6

Farro is an Italian grain that I was first introduced to on a trip to Tuscany. It has a nutty flavor and earthy texture. Most people come home from Italy with fabulous shoes and handbags...my suitcase was filled with bags of farro! It's great in soups or as a side dish. In this recipe I have made it into risotto by adding broth, butter, and Parmesan. It becomes this creamy, wonderful sensation! It's Level Two because of the whole grains combined with the fats. For less of an imbalance, you may use vegetable broth in place of the chicken broth and omit the butter and cheese (of course, it's not as big of a wow, but it's still great). To find farro, see my Ingredients Source Guide (page 295).

4 cups chicken broth
1 tablespoon extra-virgin olive oil
$^1/_2$ onion, medium diced
1 cup raw farro

2 tablespoons unsalted butter
$^1/_4$ cup freshly grated Parmesan cheese
Sea salt and freshly ground black pepper

In a medium-size saucepan, bring the chicken broth to a boil and reduce to a simmer.

In a separate saucepan over medium heat, add the oil and onion and sauté until translucent. Add the farro and stir until coated, then slowly add warm broth 1 cup at a time, constantly stirring until the liquid is absorbed. Continue to add broth until the farro is cooked, about 15 minutes. Add the butter and Parmesan cheese. Season with salt and pepper. Serve immediately.

CHAPTER 22

Poultry

Chicken Patty Lemon Piccata

PRO/FATS — LEVEL ONE

S E R V E S 4

Everybody loves chicken piccata. I particularly love this version made with ground chicken. It's light, yummy, and lemony.

2 pounds ground chicken
4 tablespoons olive oil
$^1/_2$ cup chicken broth
Sea salt and freshly ground black pepper

Juice from 1 lemon
4 tablespoons ($^1/_2$ stick) unsalted butter
1 lemon, sliced

Separate the ground chicken into patties and flatten them. In a heated skillet, add the olive oil and fry the patties until cooked and crusty, about $1^1/_2$ minutes on each side. Remove the patties when cooked. Add the chicken broth to the skillet and scrape up all the bits from the bottom for about 3 minutes, or until the broth is reduced by half. Season with salt and pepper and the lemon juice. Turn off the heat and add the butter, stirring until the sauce is smooth. Pour over the chicken patties. Garnish with the lemon slices and serve immediately.

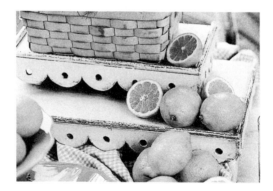

Roast Chicken Breast Stuffed with Herbed Goat Cheese with Wild Mushroom Sauce

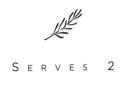

SERVES 2

Ask your butcher if he can cut the chicken into what we call an "airline" breast. In this cut the wing bone is attached, but the breastbone is removed. It is important that the skin stay on. If you can't get this cut, just get a boneless chicken breast with the skin attached.

3 ounces fresh goat cheese
2 teaspoons chopped fresh thyme
  (or $^1/_2$ teaspoon dried)
2 teaspoons chopped fresh flat-leaf parsley
  (or $^1/_2$ teaspoon dried)
2 teaspoons chopped fresh marjoram (or
  $^1/_2$ teaspoon dried)

2 chicken breasts (preferably airline cut)
Sea salt and freshly ground black pepper
1 recipe Wild Mushroom Sauce (page 197)
Extra-virgin olive oil

In a bowl, mix the goat cheese with the herbs. Making sure to keep the skin attached on one side, separate the skin from the chicken breasts to create a pocket. Fill each cavity with half the cheese mixture and press down on the skin to evenly distribute. Season the outside of both chicken breasts with salt and pepper.

Prepare the Wild Mushroom Sauce.

Preheat the oven to 450 degrees.

Heat a large sauté pan (with an ovenproof handle) on medium high. When the pan is nice and hot, add 2 to 3 tablespoons of olive oil, and then add the chicken, skin side down. Sear the chicken for 3 minutes to get a nice brown, crispy skin. Using a wide spatula, gently turn the chicken (so as not to tear the skin) and continue cooking for another 3 minutes.

To finish the chicken, place the sauté pan into the oven and roast for 10 to 12 minutes. (If your sauté pan does not have an ovenproof handle, transfer to a casserole dish or roasting pan.) When the chicken is done, remove from the oven and place each breast onto a serving plate. Spoon the Wild Mushroom Sauce over each chicken breast and serve immediately.

Achiote Chicken with Radish and Cucumber Salad

PRO/FATS AND VEGGIES — LEVEL ONE

SERVES 2

Achiote is ground annato seed from the annato tree. You may think you have not heard of it, but annato is commonly used as a natural coloring. Next time you buy some Cheddar cheese, look at the label and you'll probably see annato. This seasoning is not particularly spicy, but is has an interesting bold flavor. I love it in combination with the crunchy radishes and cucumber of the salad.

CHICKEN

2 tablespoons ground achiote
2 tablespoons extra-virgin olive oil
Juice from 1 lime
Sea salt and freshly ground black pepper
2 boneless, skinless chicken breasts

SALAD

1 bunch radishes, sliced into quarters
1 cucumber, peeled, seeded, and cut into
  half-moons
1 bunch arugula (or spinach)
Extra-virgin olive oil
Sherry vinegar
Sea salt and freshly ground black pepper

TO MAKE THE CHICKEN

Preheat the oven to 400 degrees.

In a mixing bowl, combine all the ingredients except the chicken. Mix until smooth. Place the chicken into a sealable plastic bag. Add the marinade, seal the bag, and let sit for 15 minutes (or up to 24 hours in the refrigerator).

Remove the chicken from the marinade and place into a baking pan. Roast until thoroughly cooked, about 20 minutes. Remove from the oven and allow to cool completely. When cooled, slice on the diagonal.

TO MAKE THE SALAD

In a mixing bowl, combine the radishes, cucumber, and arugula. Drizzle lightly with olive oil and a splash of vinegar. Season with salt and pepper and toss until well coated.

Place the salad greens onto plates and top with sliced chicken. Serve immediately.

Curry Chicken Skewers

SERVES 2

Curry is confounding to most Americans. Unless we have grown up with someone adept at cooking curries, we really don't know how to use these fabulous spices. Curry Chicken Skewers are delicious and easily made with a jar of simple curry paste from the grocery store. They taste best when cooked on a grill; and be sure to reserve a little extra marinade. Bring it to a boil, then cool slightly and blend in a couple of tablespoons of crunchy peanut butter. Makes a great dipping sauce. This creates more of an imbalance because of the carbohydrates in peanut butter, but it's fine if you're doing well on your maintenance.

3 tablespoons red curry paste
$^1/_2$ cup coconut milk
Juice from 1 lime
1 tablespoon extra-virgin olive oil
Sea salt and freshly ground black pepper

2 boneless, skinless chicken breasts, cut
   lengthwise into 4 pieces
1 recipe Roasted Eggplant Relish (page
   192)

In a medium bowl, mix together the curry paste, coconut milk, lime juice, and olive oil. Season with salt and pepper. Add the chicken and coat well. Cover and refrigerate for at least 1 hour or overnight.

Heat the grill.

Remove the chicken from the marinade and skewer with either presoaked wooden skewers or metal skewers. On the hot grill, cook until done, about 3 minutes on each side. Serve immediately with Roasted Eggplant Relish.

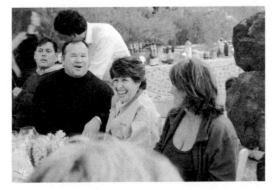

My darling friend Andrea at our outdoor annual lunch.

Roast Turkey Breast Stuffed with Prosciutto, Fontina Cheese, and Sage

PRO/FATS AND VEGGIES—LEVEL ONE

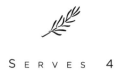

SERVES 4

Turkey gets relegated to Thanksgiving, which is a shame because it is delicious and versatile. A turkey breast cooks in no time, and this version with a classic saltimbocca stuffing is a real crowd-pleaser. Pan juices are an optional pleasure.

$^{1}/_{2}$ cup grated Fontina cheese
$^{1}/_{2}$ cup julienned prosciutto
2 tablespoons julienned fresh sage
Sea salt and freshly ground black pepper
1 2-pound boneless turkey breast

Olive oil
1 cup white wine
$^{1}/_{2}$ cup chicken broth
2 tablespoons unsalted butter

Preheat the oven to 425 degrees.

In a small bowl, combine the cheese, prosciutto, and sage. Sprinkle with salt and pepper.

Create a pocket to hold the stuffing by inserting a carving knife into the middle of the turkey breast almost to the other side of the breast. Twist and turn until you create a cavity. Using your hand, insert the stuffing into the cavity. Season the turkey well with salt and pepper and drizzle with olive oil. Place in a roasting pan and into the oven for 20 minutes. Lower the heat to 350 degrees and roast until done, approximately 45 minutes to an hour or until the temperature

reaches 165 degrees on a meat thermometer. Remove from the oven and allow to cool slightly.

Remove the turkey from the pan and place the pan on top of the stove. Over medium heat deglaze the pan by adding the wine. Allow to reduce by half, scraping the sides and bottom of the roasting pan in order to get all the brown bits into the sauce. Add the chicken broth and bring up to a simmer, then add the butter. Adjust seasoning to taste.

Slice the turkey breast and place it onto plates. Spoon the sauce over the turkey and serve immediately.

CHAPTER 23

Fish and Seafood

Grilled Halibut with Spicy Rock Shrimp Salsa

PRO/FATS AND VEGGIES—LEVEL ONE

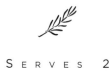

SERVES 2

Rock shrimp are small and buttery with a lobsterlike texture. Mint, cilantro, jalapeños, and lime juice create an awesome shrimp salsa to top this halibut. Of course, you may substitute any small shrimp, but this variety is particularly tasty. Be careful when handling jalapeños not to rub your eyes; or better yet, do what I do and wear rubber gloves. This salsa can be made up to 6 hours in advance.

12 ounces fresh halibut fillet (or other white flaky fish)
Extra-virgin olive oil
Sea salt and freshly ground black pepper
Zest and juice from 1 lemon
4 fresh basil leaves (or 1 teaspoon dried)
1 jalapeño, seeded and finely diced

$^1/_2$ red onion, finely diced
$^1/_2$ pound rock shrimp
2 tablespoons finely chopped fresh cilantro
Zest and juice from 1 lime
1 tablespoon julienned mint leaves
1 tomato, seeded and finely diced

Drizzle the halibut with olive oil, then season with salt, pepper, lemon zest, and basil leaves. Set aside to let the flavors infuse.

Place a medium sauté pan on high heat. Add 2 tablespoons olive oil, the jalapeño, and the red onion. Sauté for about 2 minutes, then add the rock shrimp and cook until they turn white, about 2 minutes more. Pour the ingredients into a mixing bowl and add the cilantro, lime zest and juice, mint, and tomato. Gently toss to combine with a pinch of sea salt.

Preheat the grill to high. When hot, add the fish and cook for about 2 minutes per side. Place onto a serving dish and squeeze fresh lemon juice over the top. Add a little more salt and pepper, then top with a generous portion of rock shrimp salsa. Serve immediately.

Pan-Roasted Halibut with Zucchini Ribbons, Candied Roma Tomatoes, and Parsley Pesto

PRO/FATS AND VEGGIES—LEVEL ONE

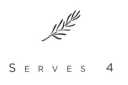

SERVES 4

What I love about this dish is the combination of the crusty pan-fried fish with the fresh explosion of pesto. This meal is very easy to prepare, especially if you keep pesto and candied tomatoes on hand as I do.

4 medium zucchini
Extra-virgin olive oil
4 6-ounce halibut fillets (or other white flaky fish)

Sea salt and freshly ground black pepper
1 recipe Candied Roma Tomatoes (page 204)
1 recipe Parsley Pesto (page 189)

Peel the zucchini ribbons as described on page 209 and set aside uncooked.

Drizzle olive oil over the halibut to coat. Season liberally with salt and pepper. Heat a large sauté pan on medium high. Add about 2 tablespoons olive oil and the halibut fillets to fit comfortably in the pan. Sear for 2 minutes per side, or until just cooked through.

Remove the fish from the pan and set aside to keep warm. Return the pan to medium heat and add the zucchini ribbons. Season with salt and pepper and sauté for about 30 seconds, until just warmed through.

Place the fish on individual dishes along with zucchini ribbons and three Candied Roma Tomatoes per plate. Top the fish with a generous spoonful of Parsley Pesto and serve immediately.

Crispy-Skinned Salmon with Roasted Garlic Aïoli and Warm Radicchio–Shiitake Mushroom Salad

PRO/FATS AND VEGGIES—LEVEL ONE

SERVES 2

As many of you know, I am not known for my love of salmon. In fact, I generally don't eat it. This recipe bears no resemblance to the lousy salmon one gets at banquets! If you can get wild, river-caught salmon from the Copper River or the Yukon River in Alaska, you have really hit the jackpot. If not, fresh from the market will do. Serve this with the radicchio and mushroom salad and for Level Two add French Lentils (page 216). Yum.

Extra-virgin olive oil
2 6-ounce salmon fillets, $1^1/_2$ inches thick, with skin on
Sea salt and freshly ground black pepper
6 shiitake mushrooms, stemmed and julienned

$^1/_2$ head radicchio
1 cup arugula, loosely packed
1 recipe Roasted Garlic Aïoli (page 194)

Preheat the oven to 350 degrees.

Drizzle olive oil on the salmon and season with salt and pepper. Heat a sauté pan on high, then add about 2 tablespoons olive oil. Add the salmon fillets and sear on each side for about 3 minutes. Place onto a serving dish and set aside to keep warm.

Add the shiitake mushrooms to the pan and toss over medium heat until crusty, about 5 minutes. Add the radicchio and arugula and toss quickly for 15 seconds, or until just wilted. Season with salt and pepper.

Place the warm salad beside the salmon, then spoon aïoli over the top of the fish. Serve immediately.

Grilled Scallops Wrapped in Pancetta with Baby Greens

PRO/FATS AND VEGGIES—LEVEL ONE

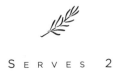

SERVES 2

There's something about the combination of grilled scallops with bacon that just sends me! I make these on the Home Shopping Network with my Somersize Thai Red Curry Sea Salt Rub. So good! Here I've used fresh thyme and served them over greens. A lovely lunch.

4 large scallops
4 slices pancetta (or bacon)
Extra-virgin olive oil
Sea salt and freshly ground black pepper

4 sprigs thyme, leaves only (or 1 teaspoon dried thyme)
1 recipe Baby Greens with Sherry Shallot Vinaigrette (page 180)

Preheat the grill to high.

Wrap the scallops in pancetta and secure with a skewer through the middle. Drizzle with olive oil, then season with salt, pepper, and thyme. Sear on the grill for 3 minutes per side.

Serve immediately over a bed of Baby Greens with Sherry Shallot Vinaigrette.

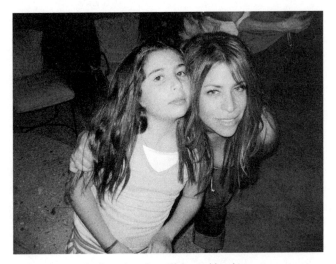

Leslie and my beautiful granddaughter.

Bouillabaisse with Red Pepper Rouille

PRO/FATS AND VEGGIES—LEVEL ONE

SERVES 4

This seafood stew will knock your socks off! Bouillabaisse is a French fish stew that is traditionally served over crusty slices of bread with red pepper rouille. Its Italian counterpart, cioppino, is more tomato based, while this version is more delicate and sophisticated. To keep with tradition, I serve this with Whole-Wheat Crostini with Red Pepper Rouille (page 198) for Level Two. For Level One, I simply drizzle the red pepper rouille right over the dish. For best results, try to get fresh shellfish from a fish market. Ask them to clean the shells for you and to remove the beards from the mussels. Then give another good scrub when you get home to avoid getting sand and grit in the broth. Another good tip: If the mussels are open before they are cooked, tap on the shell. If they close, they are alive. If they stay open, they are dead and should be discarded.

2 tablespoons extra-virgin olive oil
1 onion, thinly sliced
1 head fennel, thinly sliced
2 cloves garlic, smashed
10 to 12 saffron threads
$1^1/_2$ cups white wine
8 cups chicken broth
1 tablespoon sea salt
Freshly ground black pepper

12 clams (preferably Littleneck)
16 mussels
$^1/_2$ pound bay scallops
$^1/_2$ pound rock shrimp (or peeled and deveined shrimp)
8 crab legs (optional)
1 tomato, seeds removed and diced
8 tablespoons butter, cut into 8 pieces
Juice from 1 lemon

Place a large stockpot on medium heat. Add the olive oil, onion, fennel, and garlic. Cook for 10 to 15 minutes, until the vegetables are soft. Add the saffron threads and wine and continue cooking until reduced by half. Add the broth, salt, and a few turns of freshly ground black pepper. Cook slowly over medium heat for another 20 to 30 minutes to let the flavors combine.

Add all the seafood (if the clams are particularly large, add them 3 minutes before the other seafood since they will take longer to open). Add the tomato, cover, and cook for about 5 minutes. Remove the lid and check on the seafood. The shellfish should be opened and the shrimp just cooked through. Discard any unopened shells. Add the butter and swirl to dissolve. Drizzle with lemon juice and serve in large bowls. Garnish with Red Pepper Rouille or with 2 slices of Whole-Wheat Crostini with Red Pepper Rouille for Level Two.

Grilled Tuna with Lemon-Thyme Aïoli

PRO/FATS AND VEGGIES — LEVEL ONE

SERVES 2

This grilled tuna dish is simple and elegant and very easy to prepare. Feel free to substitute any fish you prefer. I like the tuna paired with Lemon-Thyme Aïoli (page 195) because the light, lemony herb sauce cuts the richness of the meaty fish. Delicious!

Extra-virgin olive oil
2 6-ounce tuna steaks, 1$^{1}/_{2}$ inches thick
Sea salt and freshly ground black pepper

Zest from 1 lemon
1 recipe Lemon–Thyme Aïoli
2 sprigs fresh thyme, for garnish

Preheat the grill to high.

Drizzle olive oil on the tuna. Season with salt, pepper, and lemon zest. Grill for 2 minutes per side for medium-rare tuna. If you like it cooked through, keep it on for 3 minutes per side.

Place the fish onto serving plates. Drizzle with Lemon–Thyme Aïoli and garnish with a fresh sprig of thyme. Serve immediately.

Pan-Roasted Sole with Thyme Butter Sauce

PRO/FATS AND VEGGIES—LEVEL ONE

SERVES 2

Petrale sole is one of my favorite types of fish. For those of us living on the West Coast, it's readily available so it's always fresh. The thyme leaves in this butter sauce literally dance in your mouth! Serve this with Grilled Asparagus (page 207) for a lovely pairing.

THYME BUTTER SAUCE

1 shallot, thinly sliced
3 sprigs fresh thyme
5 black peppercorns
1 cup white wine
4 tablespoons ($^1/_2$ stick) unsalted butter
1 tablespoon freshly chopped thyme

SOLE

2 6-ounce pieces petrale sole
Sea salt and freshly ground black pepper
3 tablespoons extra-virgin olive oil

TO MAKE THE SAUCE

In a medium saucepan over medium heat, add all the ingredients except the butter and chopped thyme. Cook until reduced by three fourths. Lower the heat and add the butter. Whisk until melted. Strain through a sieve, then add the chopped thyme.

TO MAKE THE SOLE

Season the fish with salt and pepper.

In a medium sauté pan over high heat, add the oil, then add the fish and cook for 2 to 3 minutes on each side, until golden brown. Remove from the heat and place onto plates. Spoon Thyme Butter Sauce over the top. Serve immediately.

CHAPTER 24

Beef, Pork, and Lamb

Pan-Roasted Rib-Eye Steak with Slow-Roasted Sweet Onion and Sautéed Spinach

PRO/FATS AND VEGGIES—LEVEL ONE

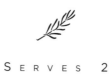

SERVES 2

This is the way I like to cook... with lots of flavor. The slow-roasted sweet onion turns an everyday steak into a gourmet meal. The flavors of the bacon and thyme infuse into the onion to give the entire dish a smoky, wonderful taste. This recipe gives you your entrée and side dish all in one. It is so worth the effort, and your house will smell divine in the process. When I made this for my little granddaughter, she was licking the plate.

1 red onion
1 tablespoon balsamic vinegar
Extra-virgin olive oil
Sea salt and freshly ground black pepper
2 slices bacon
1 bunch fresh thyme (or 3 teaspoons dried)

1 pound rib-eye steak, 2 inches thick (or Spencer or New York strip steak)
2 cloves garlic, minced
12 ounces baby spinach leaves
Juice from 1 lemon

Preheat the oven to 350 degrees.

Peel the red onion and slice it through the middle into thirds. Stack back together and drizzle with the balsamic vinegar, about 1 tablespoon olive oil, salt, and pepper. Wrap the slices of bacon around the onion and tuck one sprig of fresh thyme (or 1 teaspoon dried) under the bacon. Wrap the onion in aluminum foil and place onto a baking sheet. Roast for about 1 hour, or until soft. Unwrap and discard the foil. Remove the bacon, coarsely chop, and

reserve to cook with the spinach. Coarsely chop the onion and set aside.

Preheat the oven to 500 degrees. Drizzle olive oil to coat the steak. Season with salt, pepper, the remaining sprigs of thyme, and 1 clove of the minced garlic. Heat an oven-proof sauté pan on high. Add about 2 tablespoons olive oil. Sear the steak for about $2^1/_2$ minutes on each side. Place the sauté pan into the oven for 2 minutes. Turn the steak over and continue cooking for another 2 minutes. Remove the steak from the pan, being extremely cautious of the hot handle. Pour off any fat and add the chopped roasted onion, warming on medium heat while scraping bits off the bottom of the pan.

Heat a separate sauté pan over medium high. Add 1 tablespoon olive oil, the reserved bacon, and the remaining minced garlic. Sauté for about 2 minutes. Add the spinach leaves and lemon juice and toss until just wilted, about 3 minutes. Slice the steak on the diagonal and divide between two plates. Place sautéed spinach next to each steak. Then spoon onions atop the steak and serve immediately.

Christmas Roast

PRO/FATS—LEVEL ONE

SERVES 6

This is one of my family's favorite meals. It's a Christmas tradition in our house and surprisingly easy to prepare. The house smells divine and reminds my family of all the good times. One of the most important steps in preparation is to sear the roast in a sauté pan first. This seals in the flavor and makes a crispy crust that is delicious. Another important step in making a roast is to let it rest for 20 minutes before slicing. This seals in the juices so they stay in the meat rather than run all over the carving board. These extra steps make the difference between a good roast and an awesome roast. Merry Christmas and Happy Holidays.

2 tablespoons extra-virgin olive oil
1 7- to 8-pound standing rib roast (ask
    your butcher to tie it but leave the
    bone attached)
Sea salt and freshly ground black pepper
1 bunch fresh rosemary, stems attached
1 bunch fresh thyme, stems attached

1 head garlic, full cloves
2 shallots, finely diced
1 cup good red wine (Bordeaux or Merlot)
1 cup veal demi-glace (see Ingredients
    Source Guide, page 298)
$^1/_2$ cup beef broth
2 tablespoons butter

Preheat the oven to 450 degrees.

Preheat a large sauté pan over high. Add the olive oil. Season the meat heavily with salt and pepper, then carefully sear it on all sides until it forms a dark crust (but not burned), about 3 minutes per side. Make sure all sides are evenly browned. (I use tongs to make it easier to handle.)

Remove the meat from the sauté pan and place into a roasting pan bone side down. Using the string as an anchor, stick the stems of rosemary and thyme under the string so they are secure. Attach the cloves of garlic in the same manner. Place the roasting pan into the oven and roast for

30 minutes. Reduce the oven temperature to 350 degrees. Continue cooking for 1 hour more, or until a meat thermometer registers 125 to 130 degrees for medium rare, 140 degrees for medium.

Remove the roast from the pan and let it rest for at least 20 minutes before carving.

Meanwhile, pour the fat out of the roasting pan and place the pan over medium heat. Add the shallots and allow them to caramelize while scraping bits from the bottom of the pan. Add the wine and reduce by half. Add the veal demi-glace and beef broth. Simmer for 2 to 3 minutes. Stir in the butter and season with salt and pepper. Serve with the meat.

Grilled Lamb Chops with Lavender Lamb Jus

PRO/FATS AND VEGGIES—LEVEL ONE

SERVES 2

There is nothing quite as romantic as the fields of lavender in the South of France. Alan and I spent every summer there for eighteen years, and this recipe is one I came up with while living there. The combination of lamb with lavender and rosemary is simply divine. If you can get fresh herbs, that's always best. If not, the dried works well. You might try my Somersize Provence Sea Salt Rub as a quick and easy substitution. It's loaded with these same herbs. The base of this sauce is made with a veal demi-glace, which can be found prepared at a gourmet market. If you can't find it, try beef-flavored Bettter Than Bouillon, which is available at most grocery stores. Serve this with Grilled Fennel and Zucchini (page 213).

$2^1/_2$ tablespoons butter
2 shallots, thinly sliced
1 cup red wine
$^1/_2$ cup veal demi-glace (or $^1/_2$ cup prepared Better Than Bouillon)
$^1/_4$ cup chicken broth

3 sprigs fresh lavender (or 1 teaspoon dried)
3 sprigs fresh rosemary (or 1 teaspoon dried)
Extra-virgin olive oil
Sea salt and freshly ground black pepper
4 T-bone lamb loin chops, 2 inches thick
4 sprigs fresh lavender, for garnish

Place a small saucepan on medium heat. Add $^1/_2$ tablespoon of the butter and the shallots; sauté until the shallots become golden and slightly caramelized, 15 to 20 minutes. Add the red wine to deglaze the pan and reduce it by half. Add the veal demi-glace, chicken broth, 1 of the lavender sprigs, and 1 of the rosemary sprigs. Bring to a boil, then reduce to a simmer until it reduces again by half. Whisk in the remaining 2 tablespoons of butter. Remove the sprigs of herbs. Adjust seasoning with salt and pepper as needed.

Preheat the grill to high.

Drizzle olive oil on the lamb chops. Season liberally with salt and pepper. Remove the stems from the remaining herbs and sprinkle leaves onto the chops. Grill for 4 minutes per side for medium rare.

Place 2 chops onto each plate and generously spoon sauce over the top. Garnish each plate with 2 crisscrossed sprigs of lavender and serve immediately.

Leg of Lamb with Porcini Mushroom Rub

S E R V E S 8 T O 1 0

I love to serve leg of lamb in the spring. It's so easy to make and everyone loves it. In this recipe I use my Somersize Spicy Italian Porcini Mushroom Rub. It makes a wonderful coating. You may also use fresh or dried herbs with salt and pepper. I serve this warm or at room temperature with my Easter brunch that includes Herb and Leek Frittata (page 164), Chilled Asparagus with Lemon Thyme Aïoli (page 208), and Caesar Salad (page 183).

1 7- to 8-pound whole leg of lamb
3 tablespoons olive oil
2 tablespoons Somersize Spicy Italian
   Porcini Mushroom Rub

(or 1 tablespoon dried rosemary and
1 tablespoon dried thyme, with sea salt
and freshly ground black pepper)

Preheat the oven to 350 degrees.

Rub the leg of lamb with the olive oil, then coat all over with the mushroom rub. Place the lamb, fat side up, on a rack in a roasting pan. Set the pan in the oven and roast for 1¼ to 1½ hours. Baste several times during cooking with the accumulated juices. After 1 hour, start testing for doneness with a meat thermometer: 130 degrees for medium rare, 140 degrees for medium.

When the lamb is done, remove from the oven and let rest for at least 10 minutes. Slice on the diagonal and serve warm or at room temperature.

Lamburger with Tomato Chutney and Mint

PRO/FATS AND VEGGIES—LEVEL ONE

SERVES 2

Ground lamb has its own distinct flavor completely different from lamb chops or leg of lamb. Ground lamb cooks quickly, and the combination of lamb and chutney is spectacular. Keep these ingredients on hand at all times and you can whip up this spectacular flavorful meal to impress your family in minutes.

CHUTNEY

2 tablespoons extra-virgin olive oil
1 onion, medium dice
2 tablespoons minced fresh ginger
1 tablespoon rice wine vinegar
1/4 teaspoon SomerSweet
Sea salt and freshly ground black pepper
1/4 cup diced tomatoes (or whole baby cherry tomatoes)
1 tablespoon chopped fresh mint

LAMBURGER

12 ounces ground lamb
2 tablespoons minced onion
Sea salt and freshly ground black pepper
Fresh julienned basil leaves, for garnish

TO MAKE THE CHUTNEY

In a saucepan over medium heat, add the olive oil, onion, and ginger and cook until soft, about 5 minutes. Add the vinegar, SomerSweet, salt, pepper, and tomatoes. Cook slowly, stirring occasionally, until the tomatoes are broken down. Remove from the heat and add the mint. Set aside.

TO MAKE THE LAMBURGER

Heat the grill.

In a mixing bowl, combine the lamb with the minced onion. Season with salt and pepper and form patties.

Place the patties on the hot grill and cook for 4 minutes on each side. Remove the patties from the grill and put onto plates. Spoon chutney onto the top of each burger. Sprinkle with basil and serve immediately.

Braised Veal Stew
with Gremolata

PRO/FATS AND VEGGIES — LEVEL ONE

SERVES 6

This is comfort food gone gourmet! The demi-glace is an intense reduction of veal stock that adds flavor and viscosity to the sauce. You can find it at gourmet markets or check the Ingredients Source Guide (page 298). Serve this stew with Celery Root Puree in *Eat Great, Lose Weight,* page 98. I like to make this in my Somersize Slow Cooker; but if you don't have one, you can cook it in a pot in the oven.

$^1/_4$ cup olive oil

2 pounds veal stew meat (or beef stew meat)

1 veal shank (or beef shank)

1 onion, medium dice

6 stalks celery, medium dice

2 carrots, medium dice (for Level Two)

3 tablespoons tomato paste

$1^1/_2$ cups red wine

2 tablespoons veal demi-glace (or 1 cup prepared beef-flavored Better Than Bouillon)

4 cups chicken broth (or more to cover)

2 sprigs fresh thyme (or 1 teaspoon dried)

4 sprigs fresh flat-leaf parsley (or 2 teaspoons dried)

$^1/_2$ head garlic

1 recipe Gremolata (page 196)

Heat a large sauté pan on high. Add the olive oil, stew meat, and shank. Sauté the meat until browned on the outside, about 5 minutes. Transfer the meat to the porcelain crock of a slow cooker. Return the sauté pan to the heat and add the onion, celery, and carrots (for Level Two). Cook for 3 to 4 minutes, until they become slightly browned. Add the tomato paste and stir into the vegetables for 2 to 3 minutes. Add the red wine, scraping any bits off the bottom of the pan to release the flavor. Cook for about 10 minutes, then pour the entire contents into the slow cooker.

Add the veal demi-glace, chicken broth, thyme, parsley, and garlic (with skin) to the slow cooker. Cover and cook on low for 8 hours. (If you don't have a slow cooker, bring the stew to a simmer in a Dutch oven, then cover and cook in a 375-degree oven for $2^1/_2$ hours.)

Ladle into serving bowls and sprinkle with Gremolata.

Veal Patties with Lemon-Caper Sauce

PRO / FATS — LEVEL ONE

SERVES 4

Here's another great way to make something special from ground meat. In this recipe I use ground veal, but feel free to substitute ground turkey if you prefer. Rather than flour the patty, I use egg as the coating and it creates a delicious crust. As for the sauce . . . lemon, wine, and butter work every time!

2 tablespoons olive oil
1 pound ground veal (or ground dark-
   meat turkey)
Sea salt and freshly ground black pepper
1 cup freshly grated Parmesan cheese
2 eggs, slightly beaten

2 teaspoons capers
1 garlic clove, finely minced
Zest and juice from 1 lemon
$^1/_4$ cup dry white wine
2 tablespoons unsalted butter

Heat a sauté or nonstick pan over high. Add the olive oil.

Form the veal into 4-ounce patties and season with salt and pepper. Dip each patty first into the Parmesan cheese and then into the eggs. Gently place the patties into the sauté pan, being careful not to splash the oil. Cook each side until golden brown, about 3 minutes. Transfer to a warm platter and set aside.

Reduce the heat to medium. In the same sauté pan add the capers, garlic, lemon zest, lemon juice, and wine, carefully scraping any bits from the bottom of the pan. Allow the wine to reduce by half. Add the butter and stir until melted. Pour the sauce over the patties and serve immediately.

Herb-Roasted Loin of Pork with Pan Drippings

PRO/FATS — LEVEL ONE

SERVES 6

One of the things I love about making a roast is that it looks like you spent all day making such an incredible feast. Truly, nothing could be further from the truth. Roast dinners are the easiest. You simply rub the roast with oil, season it, sear it, and roast it for about 15 minutes per pound. Try serving this with Warm Cranberry Relish (page 193). Roast pork can be dry if overcooked. This relish keeps it exciting and moist, plus it's simple to make. The drippings from roasted pork have exceptional flavor, and the addition of veal demi-glace raises the sauce to restaurant quality. Veal demi-glace is available in most gourmet sections of your grocery store. If you can't find it, check out my Ingredients Source Guide (page 298).

1 4-pound loin of pork, ribs attached
Extra-virgin olive oil
Sea salt and freshly ground black pepper
1 bunch fresh sage
1 bunch fresh thyme

1 bunch fresh marjoram
$^{1}/_{2}$ cup red wine
1 cup veal demi-glace (optional)
$^{1}/_{4}$ cup chicken broth
2 tablespoons butter

Preheat the oven to 450 degrees.

Rub the pork loin with olive oil, then season the pork liberally with salt and pepper. In a large sauté pan over high heat, add oil to coat the pan and sear the pork on all sides, 2 to 3 minutes on each side, until golden brown all over.

Remove from the sauté pan and place into a roasting pan bone side down. Place the herbs with their stems all over the roast, tucking between bones and through the skin to hold in place. Place into the oven

and roast for 15 minutes. Lower the heat to 350 degrees and continue roasting for approximately 45 minutes, or until the internal temperature on a meat thermometer reads 160 degrees. Remove from the pan and set aside to rest while preparing the pan drippings.

Place the roasting pan on the stovetop over medium heat. Add the red wine, scraping any bits off the bottom of the pan. Continue cooking until the wine is reduced by half. Add the veal demi-glace and chicken broth and cook until the mixture begins to boil, about 7 to 10 minutes. When the sauce is thickened, turn off the heat and stir in the butter until combined.

Slice the pork roast into single-rib chops and spoon the pan drippings over the top. Serve immediately.

Peppered Pork Chops with Fried Sage Leaves

PRO/FATS — LEVEL ONE

SERVES 4

This recipe brings pork chops to a whole new level. The sage leaves add wonderful flavor and turn an everyday dinner into a gourmet treat. This is a great meal to pull together at the last moment and it can be prepared in about 12 minutes. For Level Two, try these with Smashed Tuscan Potatoes (page 217).

1 tablespoon black peppercorns
Extra-virgin olive oil
4 center-cut pork chops on the bone, about 1 inch thick

Sea salt
1 bunch fresh sage leaves (or 1 teaspoon dried sage)

Place the peppercorns onto a cutting board. Using the bottom of a heavy skillet, press onto the peppercorns until they crack. You do not want any whole peppercorns.

Drizzle olive oil to coat the pork chops, then season with cracked pepper and sea salt. Place a large skillet on medium-high heat. Add 2 tablespoons olive oil and the pork chops. Cook for 3 minutes on each side. Remove from the pan and set aside.

Add another 3 tablespoons olive oil to the pan over medium heat. After about 30 seconds toss in the fresh sage leaves and sauté for 30 seconds. Remove with a slotted spoon and scatter over the pork chops. Season the fried sage leaves with a sprinkle of sea salt.

Chipotle-Glazed Pork with Candied Tomato Salsa

PRO/FATS AND VEGGIES—LEVEL ONE

SERVES 2

My favorite way to serve this pork tenderloin is with three salsas: the Candied Tomato Salsa plus the Mango Salsa and Tomatillo Salsa. The latter two create a Level Two dish. The combination of the slightly spicy pork and the three fabulous salsas is amazing!

1 whole pork tenderloin, $1^1/_2$ to 2 pounds
2 tablespoons adobo sauce from canned
    chipotle peppers
2 tablespoons extra-virgin olive oil, plus
    more for the pan
Sea salt and freshly ground black pepper
1 recipe Candied Tomato Salsa (page 202)

FOR LEVEL TWO

1 recipe Tomatillo Salsa (page 201)
1 recipe Mango Salsa (page 200)

Place the pork in a medium bowl. Mix together the adobo sauce, oil, and salt and pepper; pour over the pork and cover with plastic wrap. Marinate in the refrigerator for at least an hour, or overnight.

Preheat the oven to 450 degrees.

Coat the bottom of a medium ovenproof sauté pan with olive oil. Place the pork in the pan and sear on all sides. Place into oven and bake until cooked through, about 8 minutes. Remove from the oven and allow to rest before slicing.

Serve immediately with the three salsas.

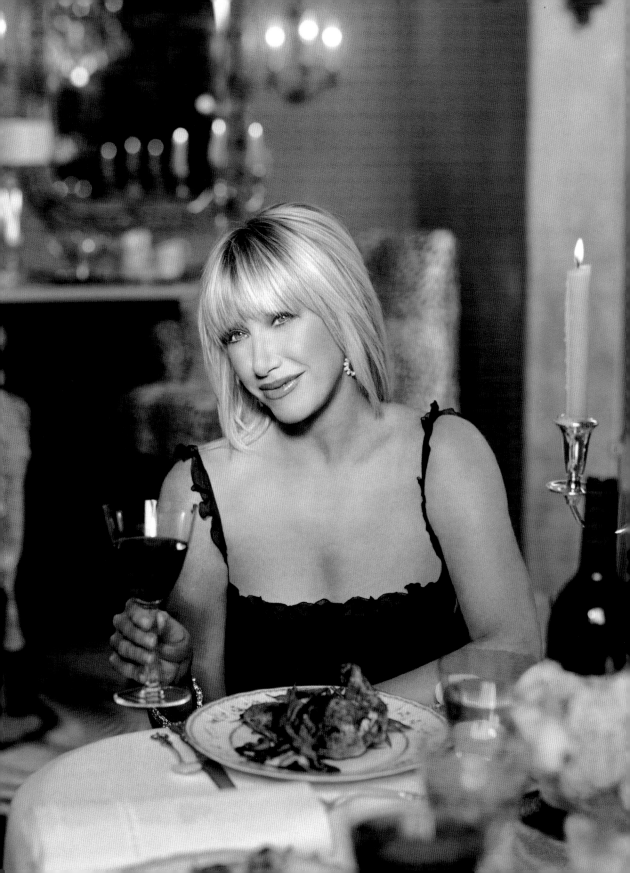

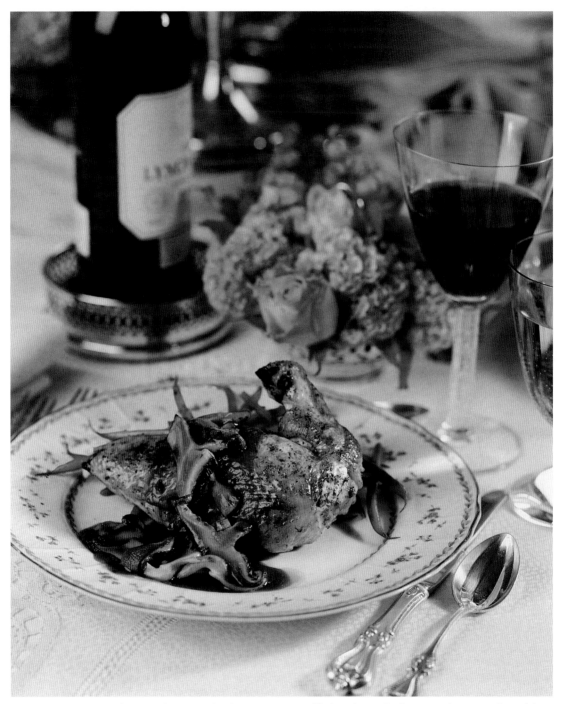

Our New Year's dinner of Roast Chicken Breast Stuffed with Herbed Goat Cheese with Wild Mushroom Sauce.

PRECEDING PAGE: Just another New Year's Eve looking into my husband's eyes.

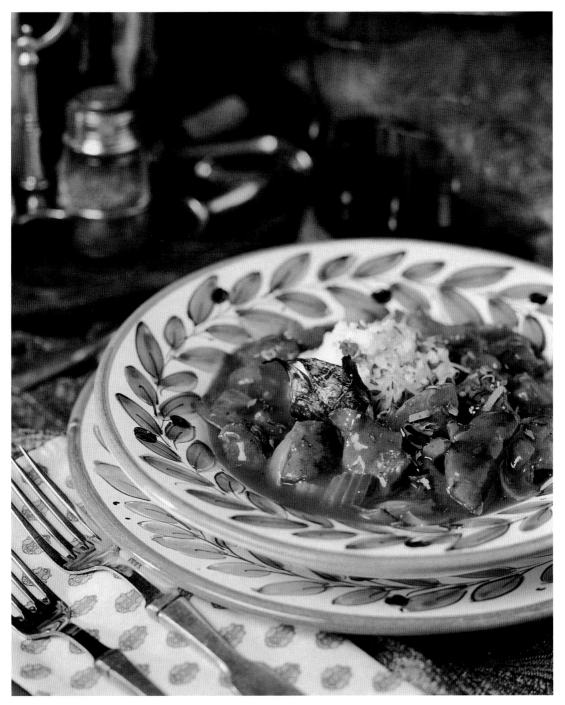

A wonderful winter meal of Braised Veal Stew with Gremolata.

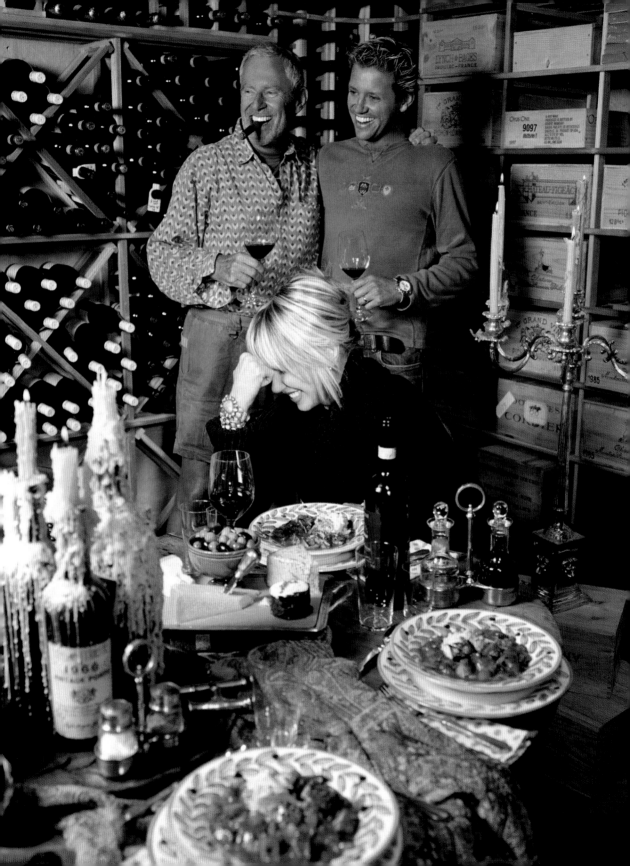

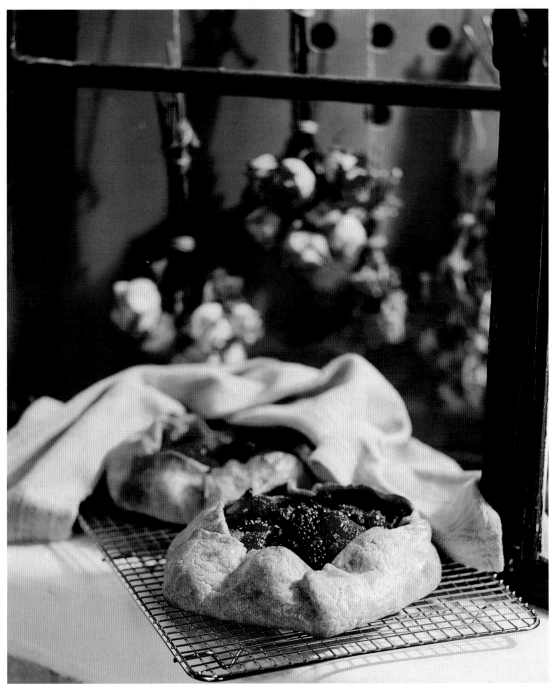

My Wild Berry Crostadas cooling on a rack on the windowsill.

PRECEDING PAGE: My boys, Alan and Bruce, being naughty in the wine cellar while I serve a delicious stew.

A cool and refreshing Tangerine Soufflé with Tangerine Crème Anglaise.

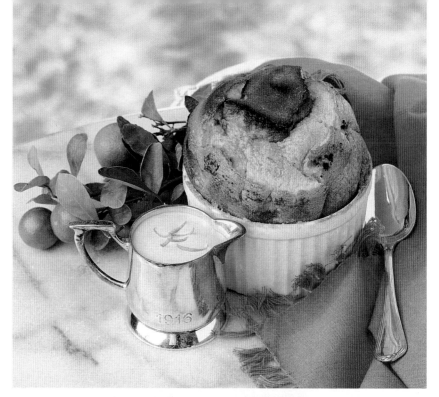

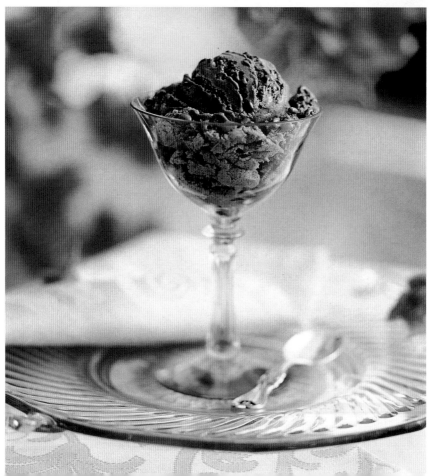

Sometimes the most simple desserts are best— here, a scoop of Chocolate Espresso Gelato.

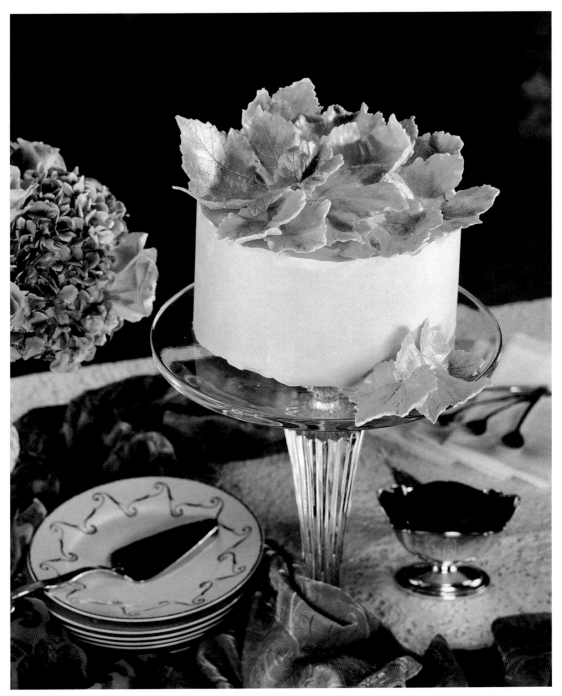

This Gold Leaf Cake has the Midas touch—white chocolate leaves with gold leafing!

FOLLOWING PAGE: Finishing off a fancy dinner party with my Gold Leaf Cake.

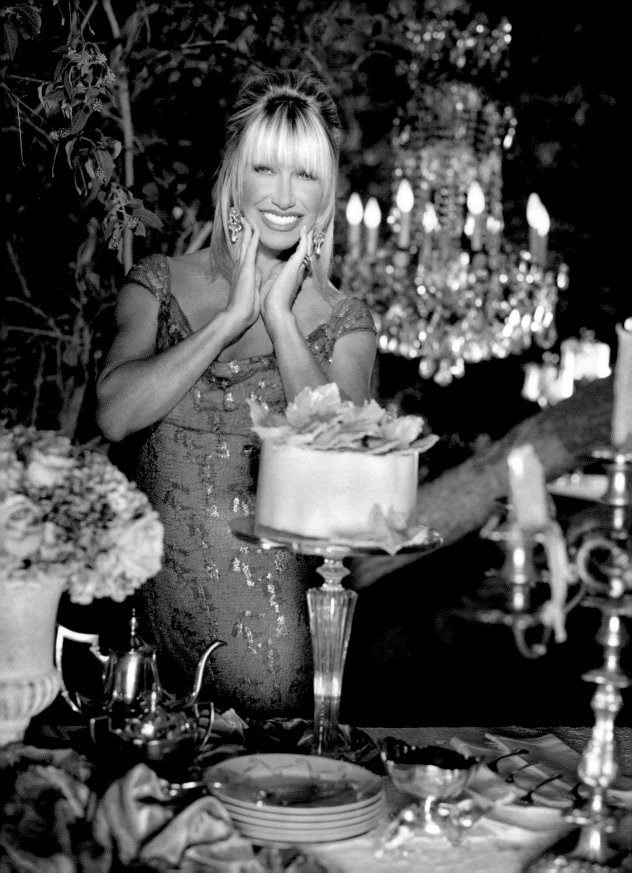

CHAPTER 25

Desserts

Velvet Chocolate Pudding

S E R V E S   6

One of the beautiful aspects of Somersizing is our ability to have sinful rich desserts while we are losing weight. This is one of my favorite recipes, which I have been enjoying since I was a little girl. Of course, when I was a child my mother used real sugar to make this for me. Now we can enjoy this yummy treat without guilt because I have substituted SomerSweet for sugar.

$^1/_2$ vanilla bean, halved lengthwise
$1^1/_2$ cups whole milk
$^1/_2$ cup heavy cream
1 to 2 tablespoons SomerSweet (or more to taste)

$4^1/_2$ ounces SomerSweet baking chocolate (or any dark chocolate), roughly chopped
5 large egg yolks

Put the oven rack in the middle position and preheat the oven to 275 degrees.

With the tip of a paring knife, scrape the seeds from the vanilla bean into a saucepan, then add the pod, the milk, cream, and SomerSweet and bring just to a boil, stirring until the SomerSweet is dissolved.

Add the chocolate and cook over moderately high heat, stirring gently with a whisk, until the chocolate is melted and the mixture just boils. Remove from the heat.

Pour the mixture into a metal bowl. Set the bowl into a larger bowl of ice and cold water and cool to room temperature, stirring occasionally, about 5 minutes.

Whisk in the yolks, then pour the entire mixture through a fine-mesh sieve. Discard the vanilla pod and any other solids.

Divide the mixture among six 4-ounce ramekins. Place the ramekins into a roasting pan. At the oven door, pour water into the roasting pan so that it comes halfway up the sides of the ramekins. Bake until the puddings are just set around the edge but the centers wobble when the ramekins are gently shaken, about 1 hour.

Cool the puddings in the water bath for 1 hour, then remove from the water and chill, uncovered, until cold, at least 1 hour.

Note: The puddings can be refrigerated, if covered with a sheet of plastic wrap after 4 hours, for up to 2 days. Blot very gently with paper towels before serving.

Chocolate Espresso Gelato

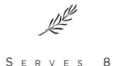

SERVES 8

Use this delectable dessert any way you would use ice cream. It has a strong espresso taste, which is wonderful for coffee lovers. I like to serve this on its own in a lovely martini glass or in my most beautiful dessert dish. It's also great over a chocolate cake.

1 vanilla bean

3 cups heavy cream

2 tablespoons plus $1/2$ teaspoon
  SomerSweet

2 tablespoons ground decaf espresso roast
  coffee beans

6 egg yolks

$2 1/4$ ounces SomerSweet Dark Chocolate
  Baking Bar (or any dark chocolate),
  finely chopped

Slice the vanilla bean lengthwise and scrape the seeds into a medium saucepan. Add the pod as well. Add the cream, SomerSweet, and coffee. Stir over medium heat until bubbles form around the edge. Lower the heat to a simmer.

In a small bowl, whisk the egg yolks until blended. Gradually whisk in $1/2$ cup of the warm cream mixture, whisking constantly. Pour the egg mixture back into the saucepan and return to low heat. Cook until the custard thickens enough to coat the back of a wooden spoon, about 10 minutes. Be careful not to let it boil. Remove from the heat and strain through a fine-mesh sieve. Add the chocolate and whisk until melted. Place the custard into the refrigerator until cool, about an hour.

Freeze in an ice-cream maker according to the manufacturer's instructions.

Tangerine Soufflé

PRO / FATS — ALMOST LEVEL ONE

S ERVES 4

A soufflé with a twist—the sprightly flavor of tangerines!

Unsalted butter for the soufflé dish
$^1/_2$ cup tangerine juice
6 large egg yolks at room temperature
1 tablespoon plus 2 teaspoons SomerSweet

2 teaspoons tangerine zest
$^1/_4$ cup heavy cream
6 large egg whites at room temperature

Preheat oven to 450 degrees and butter a 1-quart soufflé dish.

Pour the tangerine juice into a saucepan over medium-high heat. Let the juice reduce by three-quarters, until it becomes thick and syrupy. Remove from heat and set aside.

Beat the egg yolks and 1 tablespoon of the SomerSweet until light and tripled in volume, about 6 to 8 minutes. Add 2 table-spoons of the reduced tangerine syrup, the tangerine zest, and the heavy cream. Continue to beat for another minute. Set aside.

In another bowl, beat the egg whites until frothy. Add 2 teaspoons of the Somersweet and beat until stiff peaks form. Gently fold the egg whites into the yolk mixture until well incorporated. Transfer to the soufflé dish and bake for 15 to 20 minutes. Serve immediately.

Tangerine Crème Anglaise

PRO/FATS — ALMOST LEVEL ONE

MAKES 2 1/4 CUPS

This delicious custard sauce is divine on nearly any dessert and delicious with the addition of tangerine zest.

6 large egg yolks
1 3/4 teaspoons vanilla extract
1 teaspoon tangerine zest

2 cups heavy cream
2 1/4 teaspoons SomerSweet

Whisk the egg yolks, vanilla, and tangerine zest in a bowl and set aside. Heat the cream in a saucepan over medium heat until hot but not boiling. Remove the cream from the heat and add the Somer-Sweet. Slowly pour the cream over the egg yolk mixture, whisking constantly. Return the mixture to the saucepan over low heat, whisking constantly until the mixture thickens and coats the back of a spoon. Serve warm or cover and refrigerate until ready to use.

Gold Leaf Cake

LEVEL TWO

SERVES 8

This cake is an ode to my love of white chocolate. It's a lot of steps, but it's simply stunning. Your family and friends will think they're enjoying dessert from a bakery in Paris! The gold powder gives this such an elegant look. If you cannot get the gold powder, the cake still looks beautiful without it.

GOLD LEAVES

1 4.9-ounce SomerSweet White Chocolate Baking Bar, finely chopped

24 fresh, stiff leaves, wiped clean with moist paper towels and patted dry

Edible gold powder (available at restaurant and bakery supply stores)

MERINGUE CAKE LAYERS

14 egg whites (about 1^1/$_2$ cups) at room temperature

^{1}/$_2$ cup SomerSweet

2 teaspoons vanilla extract

1 recipe Chocolate Marquise (page 263)

WHITE CHOCOLATE FROSTING

1 4.9-ounce SomerSweet White Chocolate Baking Bar, chopped

16 tablespoons unsalted butter, softened

2 tablespoons SomerSweet

2 teaspoons vanilla extract

4 ounces of cream cheese

WHITE CHOCOLATE RIBBON

2 4.9-ounce SomerSweet White Chocolate Baking Bars, chopped

To make the chocolate leaves

Line a baking sheet with wax paper or foil and set aside. Place the chocolate in a glass bowl and microwave in 30-second intervals at medium power, stirring in between, until the chocolate is melted and smooth.

Hold a leaf veined side up. Using a pastry brush, carefully coat the surface completely with the melted chocolate. Wipe away any chocolate overflow from the edges of the leaf. Place the leaf, chocolate side up, on the prepared baking sheet. Repeat with the remaining leaves. Refrigerate the coated leaves until the chocolate is cold and set, about 10 minutes.

Carefully peel the leaves off the chocolate. Barely dip a small, dry paint brush into the gold powder and brush the powder on the leaves. Return the leaves to the baking sheet and refrigerate them until ready to use.

To make the cake layers

Preheat the oven to 250 degrees. Line two 8-inch springform pans with wax or parchment paper.

Place the egg whites in the clean stainless-steel bowl of an electric mixer. Beat on medium speed until frothy. Add the Somer-Sweet and increase the speed to high. Beat until the egg whites form soft peaks, about 6 minutes. Add the vanilla extract and continue to beat until the egg whites holds stiff peaks.

Spoon the egg whites evenly into prepared pans, being careful not to deflate them. Bake for 1 hour. Remove the cakes from the oven and allow them to cool for 5 minutes. Carefully run a thin-bladed knife around the edge of each cake to loosen it, then remove the outside edge of the springform pans. Run a spatula underneath each cake to loosen it from the wax paper. Set aside until the cakes are at room temperature before assembling.

To make the frosting

Melt the chocolate in a double-boiler over gently simmering water, or in a microwave. Allow the chocolate to cool to room temperature.

In an electric mixer, beat together the butter, SomerSweet, and vanilla until light and fluffy. Gradually add the melted chocolate, beating constantly. Beat in the cream cheese. Beat at high speed until light and fluffy.

To assemble the cake

Place one meringue cake layer on a serving platter. Carefully spread Chocolate Marquise evenly and thickly over the top of the layer. (An easy way to do this is to fill a large pastry bag fitted with a large round tip with marquise, then squeeze out the marquise in a thick, tight spiral, beginning in the center. If any marquise is left over, squeeze it out on top and smooth with a spatula.) Place the remaining cake layer on top of the marquise filling.

Spread White Chocolate Frosting over the entire top and sides of the cake. Don't worry about it being perfect. Nobody is going to see it. Refrigerate the cake for 10 minutes or until the ribbon is ready.

TO MAKE THE WHITE CHOCOLATE RIBBON

Don't make this ahead of time or it will cool down too much and crack. Cover a work surface with a piece of wax paper about 36 inches long. Tape edges down so it won't curl. Measure the height of the frosted cake (it should be about 4 inches) and cut another strip of wax paper 32 × 4 inches wide (or the height of your cake if not 4 inches). It's okay if it's a little taller than your cake. Place this strip of wax paper on top of the larger piece of wax paper.

Place the white chocolate in a glass bowl and microwave in 30-second intervals at medium power, stirring in between, until the chocolate is melted and smooth.

Brush the melted chocolate generously and evenly over the 4"-high strip of wax paper. Let it sit until the chocolate has begun to set but is still malleable enough to bend without breaking, 20 to 30 minutes. Lift the 4"-high strip of wax paper with the chocolate on it. Wrap it carefully around the cake, wax paper side out, pressing gently so that the chocolate sticks to the frosting. Cut off any overlap. Refrigerate the cake until the chocolate ribbon has set completely, about 30 minutes. Carefully peel off the wax paper.

Decorate the top of the cake with the chocolate leaves and serve.

Perfectly Whipped Cream

PRO/FATS — LEVEL ONE

MAKES ABOUT 3 CUPS

2 cups heavy cream
1 teaspoon vanilla extract
2 teaspoons SomerSweet

With an electric mixer, whip the cream until it starts to thicken. Add the vanilla and the SomerSweet. Continue whipping until soft peaks form.

Chocolate Marquise

SERVES 6

Creamy, dreamy, yummy. Look at the ingredients . . . how can this be bad? This dessert is light and makes a beautiful ending to a roast-lamb dinner. It's also a great filling for my Gold Leaf Cake (page 260).

8 ounces SomerSweet Dark Chocolate (or any dark chocolate), chopped
1 cup (2 sticks) unsalted butter

$^1/_4$ cup SomerSweet
6 eggs, separated
2 tablespoons Grand Marnier

Place the chocolate, butter, and 3 tablespoons of the SomerSweet in a metal or glass bowl or the top of a double-boiler and melt over a pot of simmering water, stirring to combine. Set aside.

Place the egg yolks into a bowl and beat on high for 10 minutes, gradually adding the chocolate mixture.

In another bowl, beat the egg whites until stiff. Add the remaining tablespoon of SomerSweet, the egg yolk mixture, and the Grand Marnier. Beat on high for 10 minutes more.

Pour the mixture into buttered dessert dishes and refrigerate for 6 to 8 hours, until set.

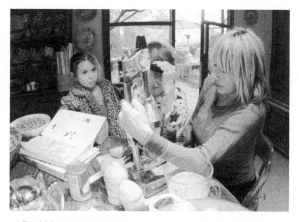

The kids love to help squeeze the lemons, fresh off the tree, for my homemade lemon tarts.

Wild Berry Crostada

LEVEL TWO

SERVES 8

A crostada is a beautiful free-form tart. The filling is placed into the center of the dough, then the dough is wrapped in from the edges. This style of tart is especially helpful when you are working with whole-wheat tart dough, since it's not quite as pliable as dough made with white flour. I also happen to think this shape is rustic and beautiful.

This is not a very sweet tart. Double the SomerSweet if you like things more sweet. You may use any type of fruit as a filling. Peaches, cherries, and apples all work well. I have used a combination of berries because they cause the least imbalance. The citrus zest gives it a brightness that I love.

This recipe makes two small tarts. Each one will serve about four people. If you add a dollop of whipped cream or vanilla ice cream, it creates more of an imbalance, but it sure tastes good!

4 cups mixed berries (blackberries,
   raspberries, blueberries)
1 teaspoon SomerSweet
Zest of 1 lemon

Zest of 1 orange
1 recipe Whole-Wheat Tart Dough
   (page 265)
2 tablespoons unsalted butter

Preheat the oven to 425 degrees.

In a bowl combine the berries, Somer-Sweet, and zests. Gently stir to combine.

Place the two rounds of rolled-out tart dough onto a baking sheet. Spoon half of the berries onto the center of each piece of dough. Bring the edges of the tart dough up around the sides of the fruit to create a crust that encloses the fruit, but leaves the center open. Top each tart with a tablespoon of butter.

Bake for about 20 minutes, until the crust is golden and the center is bubbly. Cool for 15 minutes before cutting.

Whole-Wheat Tart Dough

LEVEL TWO

MAKES TWO 9-INCH TARTS

This is the fabulous dough I use with my Wild Berry Crostada (page 264). Desserts are a treat at any time in your weight-loss program. Because it is such a novelty to indulge in them, I have spent a great deal of time finding sweets that will not cause too much of an insulin spike. That is why whole-wheat pastry dough is so important to your program. The glycemic index for whole-wheat flour is much lower than that for white flour, and the fiber is good for you. Over the years I have found that I prefer the yummy, nutty texture of whole-wheat flour. Make this in advance and keep it in your freezer; then you will have it ready any time you are in the mood to make a fruit tart or pie. Use King Arthur white whole-wheat flour for best results.

$2^1/_2$ cups white whole-wheat flour or
    whole-wheat pastry flour, plus more
    for rolling
1 teaspoon SomerSweet

2 teaspoons salt
1 cup (2 sticks) unsalted butter, chilled
$^1/_4$ cup ice water
1 teaspoon vanilla extract

In a food processor combine the flour, SomerSweet, and salt and pulse to blend. Add the butter to form crumbs. Sprinkle in the ice water and vanilla just until the dough forms a ball.

Remove the dough from the processor; divide in half and pat into two 1-inch-thick disks. Cover with plastic wrap and refrigerate for at least 45 minutes. (The dough may also be frozen at this point and thawed for later use. Wrap each disk individually in plastic if you freeze them.)

Preheat the oven to 425 degrees.

Remove the dough from the refrigerator.

Place the dough between two pieces of parchment paper, adding flour as necessary to avoid sticking. Roll the dough into a large round shape, about $^1/_4$ inch thick.

For tarts that call for prebaked shells, preheat the oven to 425 degrees. Gently lay the dough over a rolling pin and very slowly flip it over into a well-greased tart pan. Press the dough into the pan gently and trim the edges to $^1/_4$ inch. Bake for about 10 minutes or until golden brown. For pies or crostadas, bake as specified in the recipe.

Warm Chocolate Soufflé Cakes

LEVEL TWO

SERVES 4

Every Christmas my mother always made her famous steamed puddings. It's one of those great taste memories from my childhood. The textures were exciting, the insides dense, firm, and moist. This recipe reminds me of that steamed treat. Even though this cake is baked in the oven and not steamed in water, the result is very similar: rich, warm, and satisfying. Serve it swimming in cherry compote with fresh whipped cream. This dessert is made without any flour, so it keeps you on your program, creating only a slight imbalance because of the carbohydrate inherent in chocolate. This is one of Alan's favorites.

4 ounces semisweet chocolate
6 tablespoons ($^3/_4$ stick) unsalted butter,
   plus 1 tablespoon for greasing the molds
3 tablespoons SomerSweet

$1^3/_4$ tablespoons cornstarch
2 eggs
2 egg yolks

In a medium saucepan, melt the chocolate and 6 tablespoons of the butter over low heat. Set aside.

In a medium bowl, combine the SomerSweet and cornstarch.

In a separate bowl, whisk the eggs and yolks.

Add the chocolate mixture to the SomerSweet mixture. Add the eggs, stirring until smooth. Refrigerate overnight.

Preheat the oven to 400 degrees.

Grease four 6- to 8-ounce cake molds with butter, then scoop mixture into the molds, filling them two-thirds full. Bake for 20 minutes on the top rack in the oven, until set. They should spring lightly to the touch.

Serve warm.

Strawberry Rhubarb Cobbler

LEVEL TWO

SERVES 8

Use your best-looking baking dish for this cobbler so you are able to take it right from the oven to your dinner table. Strawberries and rhubarb together bring out the best in each other. The sourness of the rhubarb and the sweetness of the berries, served warm with light, flaky pastry cutouts, make a fantastic combination.

FRUIT FILLING

4 cups strawberries, quartered

4 cups rhubarb, cut into 1-inch pieces

1 teaspoon vanilla extract

2 tablespoons plus 1 teaspoon SomerSweet

2 tablespoons orange juice

2 tablespoons cornstarch

1 recipe Perfectly Whipped Cream (page 262) or vanilla ice cream

TOPPING

$1^1/_3$ cups white whole-wheat flour, (or whole-wheat pastry flour) plus more as needed

1 teaspoon SomerSweet

$1^1/_4$ teaspoons baking powder

1 teaspoon baking soda

$^1/_4$ teaspoon salt

4 tablespoons ($^1/_2$ stick) cold unsalted butter, cut up

$^1/_2$ cup buttermilk

TO MAKE THE FILLING

In a large bowl, combine the strawberries, rhubarb, vanilla, SomerSweet, orange juice, and cornstarch. Mix well and set aside.

Preheat the oven to 350 degrees.

TO MAKE THE TOPPING

In a stand mixer fitted with a paddle (or in a bowl), combine the flour, SomerSweet, baking powder, baking soda, and salt. Add the butter and mix until coarse (or cut the butter into the dry ingredients with a pastry cutter or two knives). Add the buttermilk and, using a fork, mix until a dough forms. Turn onto a work surface and knead gently, but do not overwork. Roll the dough out until it is $^1/_2$ inch thick, adding flour as needed. Using a cookie cutter, cut out biscuits and place on a cookie sheet while setting up the dish.

Place the fruit filling into an ovenproof 9 × 13 inch baking dish and top with the biscuits. Bake for 30 to 40 minutes until the fruit is bubbling and the biscuits are golden brown. Serve hot, topped with Perfectly Whipped Cream or vanilla ice cream.

Tropical Fruit Soup with Coconut Sorbet

SERVES 2

I love fruit soups, especially when made with tropical fruit. I first had this at a fabulous restaurant in Kauai. The balmy breezes and the cold mango soup with coconut ice cream made from frozen coconut milk left me swooning. Light, creamy, and delicious, it's one of my favorite desserts.

COCONUT SORBET

1 can unsweetened coconut milk
4 teaspoons SomerSweet
2 teaspoons vanilla extract

FRUIT SOUP

1 whole mango, peeled, fruit carved away
    from the seed and diced
1 whole papaya, peeled, seeded, and diced
3 teaspoons SomerSweet
1 teaspoon vanilla extract

2 tablespoons toasted, shredded
    unsweetened coconut, for garnish

TO MAKE THE SORBET

Mix the ingredients together and freeze in an ice-cream maker according to the manufacturer's directions.

TO MAKE THE SOUP

Put half of the diced mango and papaya into a blender. Add $1/2$ cup water, the SomerSweet, and the vanilla. Purée until smooth. Adjust the SomerSweet if you want it sweeter. Place a ladleful of the soup into a bowl. Add the reserved diced fruit and a scoop of sorbet, and garnish with coconut. Serve cold immediately.

Bittersweet Chocolate Citrus Tart

LEVEL TWO

SERVES 6 TO 8

This is awesome. Yes, it's Level Two, but the crust is made with whole wheat and there is no refined sugar. By melting the butter for the crust it comes out sweet and crumbly, like a graham-cracker crust. I made this for my family recently and all I heard was oohs and aahs. Try this one. It's delicious.

FOR CRUST

$^1/_2$ cup (1 stick) unsalted butter, melted
2 tablespoons SomerSweet
$^3/_4$ teaspoon vanilla extract
1 teaspoon salt
1 cup whole-wheat pastry flour

FOR FILLING

8 ounces SomerSweet Dark Chocolate
    Baking Bar (or other dark chocolate),
    finely chopped
5 tablespoons unsalted butter, cut up
Zest of 1 tangerine
Zest of 1 ruby red grapefruit
1 egg yolk
$^1/_4$ cup boiling water

TO MAKE THE CRUST

Preheat the oven to 350 degrees.

In a medium bowl, combine all the ingredients except the flour. Slowly add the flour and stir until just blended. Press the dough into the bottom and sides of an 8-inch tart pan and chill for 30 minutes. Remove from the refrigerator and bake until deep golden brown, about 25 minutes. Cool in the pan on a rack.

TO MAKE THE FILLING

In a stainless-steel bowl, combine the chocolate, butter, and zests. Melt over a pan of simmering water.

In a separate bowl, whisk the egg yolk slowly with the boiling water. Cook over a pan of simmering water, stirring constantly, until the temperature reaches 160 degrees, about 3 minutes. Strain into the chocolate mixture and mix until smooth. Pour into the crust and refrigerate until ready to serve, at least 30 minutes.

CHAPTER 26

Convenience Cooking

When I first started the Somersize program, my intent was simply to teach you how to eat real food that would help you to lose weight. Then the letters came pouring in and although people were getting great results, they wanted an easier and more convenient way to Somersize—and they missed their sweets. I went on a hunt and after more than two years of work I developed

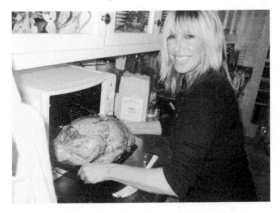

I roast my second turkey in my Somersize Convection oven. Handy!

SomerSweet. Yeah! Now we finally had a way to eat sweets while we were Somersizing. After SomerSweet, I naturally started making chocolate truffles. How wonderful to have no refined sugar and still enjoy our beloved chocolate.

Well, we've come a long way since the first can of SomerSweet and the first box of SomerSweet Chocolate Truffles. Now we have a huge line of products. It started with all sweets: Somersize Crème Brûlée—delicious and instant! Somersize Chocolate Mousse—divine and instant! Somersize Hot Cocoa—sinful and instant! My Somersizers gobbled up these delicious foods and the demands for more kept pouring in. Now I have a full line of chocolates as well as kitchen helpers to make your favorite meals.

My pantry is filled with Somersize products and I use them every day. I never thought I would use packaged products. I have always been a person who buys and cooks with fresh food. However, my products are so delicious and I am so busy—they solve a big problem for me. I don't have a whole lot of time to cook. I love to, but I was finding that Alan and I would go out to eat more and more because I didn't have the time or energy to prepare something at home. That's when I started working on foods and appliances for what I call Convenience Cooking.

SOMERSIZE STOCK-UP!

Let me start by saying that you do not need ANY Somersize products or appliances to stay on the program. You can purchase everything you need from a regular grocery store. However, if the idea of Convenience Cooking interests you, here's a way to feed yourself and your family incredible meals in minutes while you still stay on your Somersize program. All you need to have at home are meat, chicken, seafood, and fresh vegetables and you can have an amazing meal. The time-consuming part of cooking is the chopping and sautéing to make a sauce. Now the sauces and seasonings are all done for you! This is goof-proof gourmet.

Here are just a few samples of the types of meals you can make with my Somersize products.

SOMERSIZE GRILL WITH SOMERSIZE MARINADES AND CONDIMENTS

Throw a few burgers on the grill (and you can even melt cheese on them since my grill opens up flat), then serve them in lettuce cups with sliced tomato, red onion, pickles, Somersize Ketchup, or Somersize Secret Sauce. Yum! My grill has removable trays that pop out and go right into the dishwasher for easy cleanup. No more stinky grills hanging out on the counter waiting to cool.

Or quickly marinate some chicken breasts in my Ginger Teriyaki Marinade or try lamb chops in my Balsamic Thyme Marinade or a fillet of fish in my Lemon Pepper Rosemary Marinade. All of them are perfectly balanced with just the right amount of seasoning. I can't tell you how easy it is to open a jar and throw some food on the grill. In less than ten minutes you can have dinner on the table—and you are Somersizing—and it tastes great!

SOMERSIZE SLOW COOKER WITH SEA SALT RUBS AND SIMMER SAUCES

I love my slow cooker! In the morning I take out a chuck roast and put it into my slow cooker. I add a few pearl onions, a few pieces of chopped celery, and half a jar of Somersize Traditional Burgundy Simmer Sauce. Then I leave for the day and when I come home the aroma of a home-cooked roast wafts through the air. The meat shreds into luscious pieces with a big spoonful of delicious sauce. You can't believe how good this is!

On another day I wake up in the morning and throw a whole chicken into my slow cooker with half a jar of Somersize Garden Vegetable Simmer Sauce. If I feel like it, I add a few cut red bell peppers and some zucchini and maybe a sliced onion. When I arrive home at the end of the day I have fabulous chicken cacciatore!

Or how about a couple of pounds of cubed pork with half a jar of Somersize Chili Verde Sauce? At the end of the day you have the most delicious pork chili verde! Try cut-up chicken legs with Somersize Thai Red Curry Simmer Sauce and you have an exotic meal that will knock your socks off. Or one of my favorites, a few pounds of beef stew meat with Somersize Chili Colorado Sauce and you have chili that could win the contest at your state fair. Awesome!

The best part about it is that with a slow cooker there is no stirring, no basting—you just put it on low and walk away for eight hours and dinner's ready! Plus, with my Somersize Slow Cooker you have two insert dishes so that you can cook two items at the same time. Or you can make one side spicy and one side mild. I tell you, this appliance has transformed my kitchen.

As for my Somersize Sea Salt Rubs, these are my favorite product of all. These rubs are a perfect blend of high-quality sea salt with chunky dried herbs to create tastes from around the globe. I use the Tuscan Sea Salt Rub several times a week. It's perfect for roast chicken. Olive oil, Tuscan Sea Salt Rub, and a chicken; that's all you need for a perfect dinner. Same with the Provence Sea Salt Rub—the lavender and thyme are fabulous on steak, poultry, seafood, and vegetables. The Cajun is brilliant on shrimp or fried fish. And don't forget the Southwest for the best-tasting ribs you can imagine! Especially with my Somersize BBQ Sauce! Oh, my.

SOMERSIZE FAST & EASY COOKER

This amazing appliance is the opposite of the slow cooker—it's the Fast & Easy Cooker. This is very different from your mother's pressure cooker. It has several safety features so that you can never end up with pea soup on the ceiling. What is remarkable about this product is that even if you forgot to take something out of the freezer to thaw, you can still have dinner on the table in thirty minutes! No lie. Take a whole frozen chicken and place it into my cooker. Add water about halfway up the side and a palmful of Provence Sea Salt Rub. Put the pot on the stove with the pressure lid and bring to a boil. The pressure lid brings the temperature inside 40 degrees beyond boiling point so that your food cooks 70 percent faster. That means in about thirty minutes you will have a beautifully cooked chicken that pulls apart with a gorgeous broth that tastes like you cooked it all night. The remarkable thing about pressure cooking is how the flavors infuse into the food. Unbelievable flavor!

SOMERSIZE SU-CHEF

One of my most exciting products is my Somersize Su-Chef. It's your biggest helper in the kitchen. It's a hand immersion blender on steroids. You can purée soups right in the pot. You can blend salad dressing with ease. And, with all the extra attachments you can also whisk egg whites, whip cream, froth milk, and blend milkshakes. But my favorite part of all is the Fancy Food Cutter. This attachment grates cheese and chocolate and also makes beautiful julienne and ribbon slices. It even makes zucchini noodles! Then I take a jar of my Somersize Pasta Sauce and have zucchini spaghetti with meatballs and sauce! Or I make wide ribbon noodles and make zucchini alfredo—divine. Believe me, you won't miss the pasta.

And That's Not All!

I also have a Smoothie Maker that is perfect with my Somersize Protein Shakes or my fruit smoothie mixes made from fruits that are picked and canned in the rain forests of Colombia. And I have an awesome Somersize Ice Cream Maker with very easy ice cream mixes and even dessert sauces with no refined sugars! Imagine, ice cream with Somersize Triple Hot Fudge Sauce and Hot Caramel Sauce—and you're still losing weight. I have a Somersize Electronic Hand Mixer for all your baking needs and even SomerSweet Chocolate Baking Bars.

Try my Somersize Deep-Fryer and my Bake 'n Fry Mix—it's breading made with no bread. You can actually have deep-fried foods with a crunchy, crispy coating. Unbelievable!

I could go on and on and on. I know it sounds like I am shamelessly selling, but I tell you because these appliances and mixes are such problem-solvers for me. I'm busy and I still want to eat home-cooked foods. Now I can, and the best part is that I can't beat the flavor. I now have hundreds of products and they are truly amazing. They are all available at SuzanneSomers.com and I invite you to check them out.

I have included some recipes here that take advantage of some of my products and mixes. Enjoy!

Somersize Chicken Cacciatore

PRO/FATS AND VEGGIES — LEVEL ONE

SERVES 4 TO 6

Chicken Cacciatore is so easy and so delicious. In this method you just dump everything into your Somersize Slow Cooker and 8 hours later you have a wonderful dinner. I have added some vegetables here, but you can just make this with the chicken and the sauce if you don't have the 5 minutes to prep the vegetables.

2 pounds cut-up chicken pieces
$^{1}/_{2}$ jar Somersize Garden Vegetable
 Simmer Sauce
1 zucchini, cut into $^{1}/_{4}$-inch slices

1 red bell pepper, seeded and sliced into
 wide strips
1 onion, thinly sliced

Place all the ingredients into the porcelain pot of a Somersize Slow Cooker. Cover with the lid and set to Low for 8 hours.

Chicken Parmigiana

PRO / FATS AND VEGGIES — LEVEL ONE

SERVES 4

With a jar of my Somersize Marinara Sauce and a Somersize Fast and Easy Cooker, you can have dinner in about 10 minutes! If you like a little spice, try my Somersize Arrabiata Sauce. You can even start with frozen chicken breasts and still have dinner in just minutes. Talk about a problem solver!

2 tablespoons unsalted butter
4 boneless, skinless chicken breasts
1 25-ounce jar Somersize Marinara Sauce
6 ounces mushrooms, sliced

1 tablespoon Italian seasoning
Sea salt and freshly ground black pepper
$1^1/_2$ cups grated mozzarella cheese

Pour 2 cups water into an 8-quart pressure pot. Grease the bottom of the large separator pot with the butter.

Lay the chicken breasts in a single layer on the bottom of the large separator pot. Pour the marinara sauce over the chicken breasts. Scatter the sliced mushrooms over the chicken breasts. Sprinkle with Italian seasoning, salt, and pepper.

Divide the grated cheese and spread evenly on top of each chicken breast. Cover with the separator lid, then place the separator pot with the rack into the water in the pressure pot. Lock the pressure lid into place. Bring to high pressure (regulator setting number 2) over high heat. When the pressure builds, the pressure indicator will pop up. When you hear the hissing of releasing steam, set the timer for 10 minutes.

After 10 minutes, release the steam and open the lid. Remove the separator pot and serve the chicken immediately.

Somersize Tex-Mex Chicken Drumettes and Meatballs

PRO/FATS AND VEGGIES—LEVEL ONE

MAKES ABOUT 12 DRUMETTES
AND 18 MEATBALLS

Chicken drumettes are the tiny piece from the wing bone. They make the yummiest appetizers, especially when you cook them with my Somersize Tex-Mex Simmer Sauce. They are perfect side by side in my Slow Cooker with the double-dish inserts—drumettes on one side and Tex-Mex Meatballs on the other. These are great to serve to sports fans watching a game. They stay nice and warm until everyone is ready to eat. Serve the wings with my Somersize Ranch Dressing!

$1^1/_2$ pounds chicken drumettes
1 jar Somersize Tex-Mex Simmer Sauce

$1^1/_2$ pounds ground beef (or turkey)

Place the chicken drumettes into one of the double dishes of the Somersize Slow Cooker. Pour half a jar of Somersize Tex-Mex Simmer Sauce over the chicken. Form small 1-inch meatballs out of the meat and place into the other double-dish insert. Pour the remaining sauce over the meatballs. Cover with the lid and set to Low for 8 hours.

Maple Vanilla Rotisserie Duck

PRO/FATS—LEVEL ONE

SERVES 2 TO 4

I may be famous as Chrissy Snow to the public, but in my family I am famous for my Maple Vanilla Duck. I used to make it with maple syrup, rosemary, and vanilla. Now it's easier than ever because I bottled my recipe in Somersize Maple Vanilla Grilling and Basting Sauce. You can add an extra layer of flavor with the Somersize Provence Sea Salt Rub, if you like. I cook it on the rotisserie in my Somersize Convection Oven. It makes a delicious, sweet, crispy duck that will have you licking your fingers! And it has no refined sugars!

$^1/_2$ cup extra-virgin olive oil
1 cup Somersize Maple Vanilla Grilling
   and Basting Sauce

1 tablespoon Somersize Provence Sea Salt
   Rub
1 5-pound duck

Combine the olive oil, Somersize Maple Vanilla Grilling and Basting Sauce, and Somersize Provence Sea Salt Rub in a sealable plastic bag. Tie the wings of the duck to the body and tie the drumsticks together with kitchen twine. Add the duck to the bag and let it marinate in the refrigerator for at least 4 hours, turning the bag over after 2 hours to marinate both sides.

Remove the rack and bake pan from the Somersize Convection Oven. Preheat the oven to 350 degrees for 10 minutes.

Remove the duck from the marinade. Reserve the marinade. Secure the duck onto the rotisserie rod using the rotisserie forks. Tighten the screws to secure the forks on the rotisserie rod. Insert the pointed end of the rotisserie rod into the hole on the right side of the oven wall. Place the squared end into the harness on the left side of the oven wall. Insert the oven rack and bake pan in the lowest oven position under the duck.

Set the Somersize Convection Oven and Rotisserie to 350 degrees. Set the function to Rotisserie. Set the timer to 120 minutes. Use the reserved marinade to baste the duck 3 or 4 times during the cooking process.

For conventional baking, roast the duck on a rack at 350 degrees, basting frequently, for about $1^1/_2$ hours.

When the duck is almost finished roasting, pour the leftover marinade into a saucepan. Bring to a boil over medium-high heat and let reduce by half. Use the warm sauce as a dipping sauce for the crispy duck.

Somersize Thai Red Curry Shrimp

PRO/FATS AND VEGGIES—LEVEL ONE

SERVES 4

These spicy shrimp are awesome and they take only minutes to prepare. For an extra layer of exotic flavor, add $1/4$ cup of unsweetened coconut milk. This makes it Level Two, but it's so delicious. This tastes great over zucchini noodles.

Olive oil
2 zucchini, cut into long, thin ribbons
   (see page 209)
Sea salt

$1^1/_2$ pounds peeled, deveined shrimp
$^1/_2$ jar Somersize Thai Red Curry
   Simmer Sauce

Place 1 teaspoon of olive oil into a sauté pan on high heat. Add the zucchini noodles to the pan until just warmed through, about 30 seconds. Season with sea salt. Divide noodles among 4 plates.

Add about 1 tablespoon olive oil to the sauté pan over medium-high heat. Add the shrimp and sauté until cooked through, about 4 minutes. Add the Somersize Thai Red Curry Simmer Sauce and continue cooking until the sauce is hot and slightly reduced.

Pour the shrimp and sauce over the zucchini noodles and serve immediately.

Somersize Beef Bourguignonne

PRO/FATS AND VEGGIES—LEVEL ONE

SERVES 6

The combination of my Slow Cooker with Somersize Simmer Sauces is fabulous! This is a knockout meal. You won't believe that you can prepare it in minutes. It's like having Mom in the kitchen! Great with mashed celery root.

1 3-pound chuck roast
4 stalks celery, coarsely chopped
2 cups pearl onions, peeled

$^{1}/_{2}$ jar Somersize Traditional Burgundy
    Simmer Sauce

Place the chuck roast into the porcelain pot of a Somersize Slow Cooker. Add the celery, onions, and Somersize Traditional Burgundy Simmer Sauce. Cover with the lid and set to Low for 8 hours.

Somersize Chili Colorado

PRO/FATS AND VEGGIES—LEVEL ONE

SERVES 6 TO 8

Chili Colorado is one of my favorite things to order at Mexican restaurants. It's a red sauce that is not too spicy. I top mine with Cheddar cheese, sour cream, and scallions for a zippy dinner.

2 pounds beef stew meat
$1/2$ jar Somersize Chili Colorado
    Simmer Sauce
1 cup grated Cheddar cheese

Sour cream
1 bunch scallions, chopped

Place the beef stew meat and Somersize Chili Colorado Simmer Sauce into the porcelain pot of a Somersize Slow Cooker. Cover with the lid and set to Low for 8 hours.

Spoon the chili into serving bowls and garnish with Cheddar cheese, sour cream, and scallions.

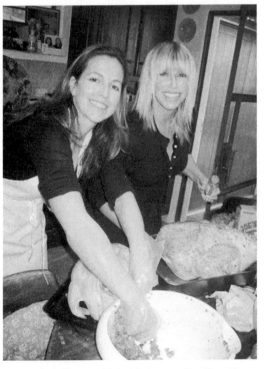

Caroline is stuffing one bird while I season the other. We are a great team for holiday meals.

Somersize Slow Cooker Lasagna

PRO/FATS AND VEGGIES—LEVEL ONE

SERVES 10

1^1/$_2$ pounds ground beef
1 32-ounce jar Somersize Roasted Garlic
   & Mushroom Sauce
1 32-ounce container whole-milk
   ricotta cheese

5 ounces shredded Parmesan cheese
^{1}/$_2$ cup Somersize Basil Pesto
8 Somersize Egg Crepes (see recipe right)
2 cups shredded mozzarella cheese

Brown the ground beef in a large skillet, then add a jar of Somersize Roasted Garlic & Mushroom Sauce. Heat thoroughly.

In a separate bowl, combine the ricotta, Parmesan, and pesto until well blended.

Coat the bottom of the porcelain pot of a Somersize Slow Cooker with 2 ladles of meat sauce. Cover with a layer of 2 egg crepes. Next, spread half of the ricotta cheese mixture over the crepe layer and top with two more crepes. Pour two more ladles of meat sauce over the crepes and cover with half of the shredded mozzarella. Continue layering with two crepes on top of the mozzarella. Spread the remaining ricotta cheese mixture evenly over the crepes. Place two crepes on top. Cover with the remaining meat sauce and top with the rest of the mozzarella.

Set the Slow Cooker to High for 2 hours or Low for 4 hours.

Somersize Egg Crepes

PRO / FATS — LEVEL ONE

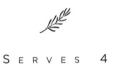

SERVES 4

These egg crepes are so versatile! You've seen them in many of my books. Try them to make lasagna with no pasta!

6 eggs
Sea salt and freshly ground black pepper
Butter

In a mixing bowl, lightly beat the eggs. Season with salt and pepper. Heat a crepe or omelette pan over medium to medium-high heat and lightly coat the bottom and sides of the pan with butter.

Using a ladle, put enough egg into the pan to make a thin coating. When it sets, lift up with a spatula, being careful not to tear the crepe, and turn. Cook for 1 more minute and then slide the crepe out of the pan and onto a dish. Continue making egg crepes in this way until you have used all the batter. Stack the crepes as you would pancakes.

Somersize Pork Chili Verde

PRO/FATS AND VEGGIES — LEVEL ONE

SERVES 6 TO 8

I have eaten Pork Chili Verde too many times to count at my favorite little restaurant in Santa Fe. The sauce is perfectly seasoned—not too spicy, with just enough oomph! Top with sour cream. Use an inexpensive cut of meat for best results. The slow cooker will break down the tendons and leave you with the most tender pork.

2 pounds pork shoulder or butt, cut into chunks
$^1/_2$ jar Somersize Chili Verde Simmer Sauce

Sour cream, for garnish
1 bunch scallions, chopped, for garnish

Place the pork and Somersize Chili Verde Simmer Sauce into the porcelain pot of a Somersize Slow Cooker. Cover with the lid and set to Low for 8 hours.

Spoon the chili into serving bowls and garnish with sour cream and scallions.

Super-Easy Mint Chocolate Cheesecake

ALMOST LEVEL ONE

SERVES 8

1 Chocolate Cookie Crust (page 286)
4 8-ounce packages cream cheese, softened
1 package Somersize Mint Ice Cream Mix
4 eggs
$^1/_2$ cup sour cream

1 Somersize Dark Chocolate Baking Bar, broken into 1-inch chunks
3 tablespoons Somersize Mint Chocolate Hot Fudge Sauce

Preheat the oven to 350 degrees. Prepare the crust in a 9-inch springform pan according to the recipe and bake it for 10 minutes. Set it aside to cool.

In a large mixing bowl, combine the cream cheese with the packet of mint ice cream mix. Blend well. Add the eggs one at a time and continue blending. Gradually add the sour cream and continue mixing until well blended. Add the dark chocolate chunks to the mixture.

Pour the cheesecake mixture into the prepared pie crust. Reduce the oven temperature to 325 degrees and bake for 45 minutes. Turn the heat off in the oven and let the cheesecake stand in the oven for an hour longer.

Remove the cheesecake from the oven and cover with the mint fudge sauce. Refrigerate for at least 30 minutes before serving.

Chocolate Cookie Crust

ALMOST LEVEL ONE

MAKES 1 PIE CRUST

4 tablespoons ($^1/_2$ stick) ice-cold butter
1 box Somersize Flourless Chocolate
   Brownie Mix

Preheat the oven to 350 degrees. Grease a 9-inch springform or pie pan.

Cut the cold butter into small cubes. The butter must be very cold; place the cubes in the freezer for 10 minutes if not thoroughly chilled. Place the Brownie Mix and butter into the bowl of a food processor or blender with a blade attachment. Process for 10 to 15 seconds, or until the mixture has a smooth, powdered consistency. Pour the mixture into the springform pan and smooth into an even layer without pressing into the pan (to avoid having the crust stick to the pan).

Bake for 10 minutes. Let cool and use with any pie recipe.

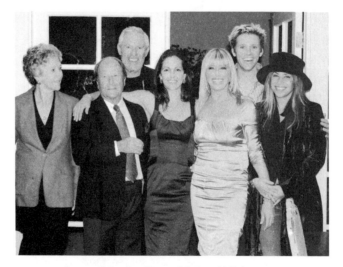

Bruce and Caroline threw a fabulous birthday party.

REFERENCE GUIDE

Here is a complete list of all the foods available in each of the categories:

PRO/FATS

CHEESE
American
asiago
Babybel
bel paese
blue
Bonbel
Brie
buffalo mozzarella
Camembert
Cheddar
Colby
cream cheese
farmer
feta
fontina
goat
Gouda

Gruyère
Havarti
hoop
Jarlsberg
Limburger
mascarpone
Monterey Jack
mozzarella
Muenster
Parmesan
pecorino
provolone
queso blanco
ricotta
Romano
Roquefort
string
Swiss

OTHER DAIRY PRODUCTS
butter
cream
eggs
margarine
mayonnaise
sour cream
whey protein

FISH
anchovy
bass
bluefish
bonito
burbot
carp
catfish

cod
eel
flatfish
flounder
gefilte fish
grouper
haddock
halibut
herring
mackerel
mahi-mahi
monkfish
ocean perch
orange roughy
pollack
pompano
red snapper
sablefish

salmon
sardine
sea bass
shark
smelt
snapper
sole
sturgeon
swordfish
tripe
trout
tuna
turbot
whitefish
wolf fish
yellowtail

MEAT
bacon
Canadian bacon
beef
bologna
bratwurst
capocollo
cold cuts
frog's legs
ham
hot dogs
lamb
pastrami
pepperoni
pork
prosciutto
rabbit
salami
sausage
veal
venison

OILS
canola oil
chili oil
olive oil
peanut oil
safflower oil
sesame oil
vegetable oil

POULTRY
capon
chicken
Cornish game hen
duck
goose
guinea hen
pheasant
quail
squab
turkey

SEAFOOD
abalone
caviar
clams
crab
crayfish
lobster
mussels
octopus
oysters
scallops
shrimp
squid

CARBOS

BEANS
adzuki beans
Anasazi beans
black beans
black-eyed peas
cannellini beans
fava beans
garbanzo beans
great northern beans
green peas
kidney beans
lentils
lima beans
mung beans
navy beans
pinto beans
red beans
split peas
white beans

BREADS, BAGELS, CRACKERS, HOT CEREALS, COLD CEREALS, OR PASTA MADE FROM WHOLE GRAINS
amaranth
barley
bran
brown rice
buckwheat
kamut
millet
oat
pumpernickel
rye
spelt
wheat

NONFAT DAIRY PRODUCTS
nonfat cottage cheese
nonfat milk
nonfat rice milk
nonfat ricotta cheese
nonfat sour cream
nonfat soy milk
nonfat yogurt

RICE
brown rice
brown rice cakes
wild rice

VEGGIES

alfalfa sprouts
artichoke
arugula
asparagus
bamboo shoots
basil
bean sprouts
beet greens
bok choy
broccoli
Brussels sprouts
cabbage
cauliflower
celery
chervil
chicory greens
chives
cilantro
clover sprouts
collard greens
crookneck squash

cucumber
daikon
dandelion greens
dill weed
eggplant
endive
escarole
fennel
garlic
ginger
green beans
horseradish
jícama
kale
kohlrabi
leeks
lettuce
   Boston or bibb
   frisée
   iceberg
   limestone

red oak
romaine
mushrooms
mustard greens
okra
onion
parsley
peppers
   bell peppers
   cherry peppers
   chili peppers
   pepperoncini
   piccalilli
pickles (except sweet)
purslane
radicchio
radish
rhubarb
rosemary
sage
salsify

sauerkraut
scallions
shallots
snow peas
spinach
sugar snap peas
Swiss chard
tarragon
thyme
tomatillo
tomato
tomato (green)
turnip
turnip greens
water chestnut
watercress
wax beans
yard-long beans
yellow beans
zucchini

FRUIT

apples
apricots
Asian pear
berries
   blackberry
   blueberry
   boysenberry
   cranberry
   currant
   elderberry
   gooseberry
   mulberry
   ollalaberry
   raspberry

strawberry
cherimoya
cherry
crabapple
fig
grapefruit
grapes
guava
kiwi
kumquat
lemon
lime
loquat
lychee

mandarin oranges
mangoes
melons
   cantaloupe
   casaba
   Crenshaw
   honeydew
   orange flesh
   Sharlyn
   watermelon
nectarines
oranges
papaya
passion fruit

peaches
pears
persimmon
pineapple
plums
pomegranate
prickly pear
pommelo
quince
star fruit
tamarind
tangerine

YOUR ONE-PAGE
REFERENCE GUIDE

For the first few days or weeks on the program, you might want to make a copy of this page and slip it into your purse or wallet. Somersizing will soon become second nature to you, but this summary will help remind you of the plan until you no longer need this for reference.

1. Eliminate all Funky Foods.
2. Eat Fruits alone, on an empty stomach.
3. Eat Proteins/Fats with Veggies.
4. Eat Carbos with Veggies and no fat.
5. Keep Proteins/Fats separate from Carbos.
6. Wait three hours between meals if switching from a Proteins/Fats meal to a Carbos meal, or vice versa.
7. Do not skip meals. Eat three meals a day, and eat until you feel satisfied and comfortably full.

PROTEINS AND FATS

Butter	Mayonnaise
Cheese	Meat
Cream	Oil
Eggs	Poultry
Fish	Sour cream

VEGGIES

Asparagus	Green beans
Broccoli	Lettuce
Cauliflower	Mushrooms
Celery	Spinach
Cucumber	Tomato
Eggplant	Zucchini

CARBOS

Beans	Whole-grain
Nonfat milk	breads, cereals,
products	pastas
Nonfat soy milk	

FRUITS

Apples	Oranges
Berries	Papaya
Grapes	Peaches
Mangoes	Pears
Melons	Plums
Nectarines	

ELIMINATE FUNKY FOODS

SUGAR

Beets	Maple syrup
Carrots	Molasses
Corn syrup	Sugar
Honey	

STARCHES

Bananas	Potatoes
Corn	Sweet potatoes
Pasta made from	White flour
semolina or	White rice
white flour	Winter squashes
Popcorn	(acorn, butternut)

COMBO PROTEINS/FATS AND CARBOS

Avocados	Nuts
Buttermilk	Olives
Coconuts	Tofu
Liver	
Low-fat or	
whole milk	

CAFFEINE AND ALCOHOL

Alcoholic beverages
Caffeinated coffees, teas, and sodas
Cocoa (including unsweetened cocoa)

Resources: Doctors and Compounding Pharmacies

NATURAL HORMONE REPLACEMENT
THERAPY

DAVID R. ALLEN, M.D.
2211 Corinth Avenue, Suite 204
Santa Monica, CA 90064
(310) 966-9194

AMERICAN ACADEMY OF ANTI-AGING
   MEDICINE
1510 West Montana Street
Chicago, IL 60614
(773) 528-4333
www.worldhealth.net

Contact the academy to learn more about natural hormone replacement therapy. It is the leading organization of its kind, dedicated to the advancement of all therapeutic approaches that play a role in antiaging medicine, including natural bioidentical HRT.

AMERICAN COLLEGE FOR ADVANCEMENT IN
   MEDICINE (ACAM)
23121 Verdugo Drive, Suite 204
Laguna Hills, CA 92653

(800) 532-3688
www.acam.org
ACAM is dedicated to establishing certification and standards of practice or preventive medicine and the ACAM protocol.

JENNIFER BERMAN, M.D.
Female Sexual Medicine Center at UCLA
924 Westwood Boulevard, Suite 515
Los Angeles, CA 90024
(310) 794-3030
(866) 439-2835
www.urology.medsch.ucla.edu/fsmc-
   jberman.html

LAURA BERMAN, PH.D.
Berman Center
211 East Ontario Street
Chicago, IL 60611
(800) 709-4709
www.bermancenter.com

NETWORK FOR EXCELLENCE IN WOMEN'S
   SEXUAL HEALTH
www.newshe.com

Newshe is the official Web site of Drs. Laura and Jennifer Berman.

JOE FILBECK, M.D.
The Palm LaJolla Medical Spa
4510 Executive Drive, Suite 125
San Diego, CA 92121
(858) 457-5700
www.palmlajolla.com
Dr. Filbeck specializes in quality of life and antiaging medicine.

MICHAEL GALITZER, M.D.
12381 Wilshire Boulevard, Suite 102
Los Angeles, CA 90025
(310) 820-6042
www.ahealth.com

THE CENTER FOR ANTIAGING MEDICINE
1270 Coast Village Circle, Suite 2
Montecito, CA 93108
(805) 969-7322
mikegal@att.net
Dr. Galitzer specializes in antiaging and natural bioidentical hormone replacement therapy.

AMERICAN HEALTH INSTITUTE
12381 Wilshire Boulevard
Los Angeles, CA 90025
(800) 392-2623
www.ahealth.com
Cofounded by Dr. Michael Galitzer, the institute is a pioneering research organization in the field of longevity medicine and the use of natural hormone replacement therapy.

ROBERT GREENE, M.D.
1255 East Street, Suite 201
Redding, CA 96001
(530) 244-9052
www.specialtycare4women.com
Dr. Greene specializes in natural bioidentical hormone replacement therapy.

PRUDENCE HALL, M.D.
1148 4th Street
Santa Monica, CA 90403
(310) 458-7979
(800) 442-4517
www.thehallcenter.com

DR. DANIELA PAUNESKY
3400 Old Milton Parkway
Bldg. C, Suite 380
Alpharetta, GA 30005
(770) 777-7707 Phone
(770) 777-7789 Fax
www.atlantaantiaging.com

UZZI REISS, M.D.
414 North Camden Drive, Suite 750
Beverly Hills, CA 90210
(310) 247-1300
www.uzzireissmd.com
Dr. Reiss, an ob/gyn, specializes in natural bioidentical hormone replacement therapy.

DR. DIANA SCHWARZBEIN
5901 Encina Road, Suite A
Goleta, CA 93117
(805) 681-0003
www.drhormone.com
Dr. Schwarzbein is an endocrinologist who specializes in menopause and a pioneer in natural bioidentical hormone replacement therapy.

EUGENE SHIPPEN, M.D.
9 East Lancaster Avenue
Shillington, PA 19607
(610) 777-7896
Dr. Shippen specializes in male menopause (andropause).

DR. LARRY WEBSTER
719 Green Valley Road, Suite 101
Greensboro, NC 27406
(866) 266-8869
www.webster.com

WWW.SUZANNESOMERS.COM
My Web site has a link to information on bioidentical hormone replacement, including a reprint of the Women's Health Initiative Study.

WEB SITES FOR SEXUAL AIDS

www.goodvibes.com
www.grandopening.com

TESTING HORMONE LEVELS

AERON LIFECYCLES
1933 Davis Street, Suite 310
San Leandro, CA 94577
(800) 631-7900
www.aeron.com

SABRE SCIENCES, INC.
910 Hampshire Road, Suite P
Westlake Village, CA 91361
(888) 490-7300
www.sabresciences.com

COMPOUNDING PHARMACIES

APOTHÉCURE, INC.
4001 McEwen Road, Suite 100
Dallas, TX 75244
(972) 960-6601
(800) 969-6601
www.apothecure.com

THE COMPOUNDING PHARMACY OF BEVERLY HILLS
9629 West Olympic Boulevard
Beverly Hills, CA 90212
(310) 284-8675
(888) 799-0212
www.compounding-expert.com

HEALTH PHARMACIES
2809 Fish Hatchery Road, Suite 103
Madison, WI 51713
(800) 373-6704

INTERNATIONAL ACADEMY OF COMPOUNDING PHARMACISTS
P.O. Box 1365
Sugar Land, TX 77487
(800) 927-4227
www.iacprx.org
You may call them or go to their Web site and enter your zip code for a referral to the closest compounding pharmacy in your area.

KRONOS PHARMACY
3675 South Rainbow Boulevard
Las Vegas, NV 89103
(800) 723-7455

SOLUTIONS PHARMACY
4632 Highway 58 North
Chattanooga, TN 37416
(423) 894-3222
(800) 523-1486
www.solutions-pharmacy.com/index2.ivnu

STEVEN'S PHARMACY
1525 Mesa Verde Drive East
Costa Mesa, CA 92626
(800) 352-DRUG
www.stevensrx.com

TOWN CENTER DRUGS AND COMPOUNDING PHARMACY
72840 Highway 111
Westfield Shopping Town
Palm Desert, CA 92260
(760) 341-3984
(877) 340-5922

WOMEN'S INTERNATIONAL PHARMACY
12012 North 111th Avenue
Youngtown, AZ 85363

INGREDIENTS SOURCE GUIDE

Some of the ingredients I call for in the recipe section may be new to you or hard to find in certain areas. I try to give you alternatives, when possible, but I hope you will try to get some of these ingredients so that you can experience these recipes at their finest. I love experimenting with new flavors. Here are some descriptions of ingredients and sources of where you can find them.

All Somersize products are available at SuzanneSomers.com.

For other hard-to-find ingredients try Surfas Restaurant Supply and Gourmet Foods in Culver City, California (310-559-4770) or order online at surfasonline.com.

Achiote (ground annatto seed) This slightly musky seed of the annatto tree is available whole or ground in East Indian, Spanish, and Latin American markets. In its paste form, annatto is used to color butter, margarine, cheese, and smoked fish.

Adobo Sauce This dark, red paste is made of ground chiles, herbs, and vinegar. It's used as a marinade, as well as a serving sauce. Chipotle chiles are often packed in adobo sauce. I have used adobo sauce only from a can of chipotle chiles, which are available at most grocery stores.

Arugula (also called Italian cress, rocket, roquette, rugula, and rucola) This bitterish, aromatic salad green has a peppery, mustardy flavor. Some find it too strong, although it has long been a favorite of Italians. Available at most supermarkets or fine grocery stores. If you can't find it you may substitute dandelion greens or the much milder spinach.

Baby Black Lentils (Beluga lentils) These tiny lentils hold their shape beautifully. They do not turn mushy when you cook them so they are perfect for salads or for warm dishes. Available at surfasonline.com.

Better Than Bouillon Just like the brand name says, it's better than bouillon. I still prefer demi-glace, when it's available, but this is a less expensive option that is easy to find at most grocery stores. It comes in a paste and needs to be made into broth to use as a substitution for the recipes in which demi-glace appears.

Black Kale Kale is a member of the cabbage family. It has an extremely high vitamin content and a mild cabbagelike flavor. Although it comes in many colors, the black version has a very interesting earthy flavor, like a hearty spinach. Many people prefer to remove the center stalk, since it can be quite tough. Available at specialty produce or farmers' markets. Of course, you may substitute more common colors such as deep green tinged with blue or purple.

Cannellini Beans are white Italian kidney beans available in dry and canned form. I prefer them dry. Available at Italian markets, gourmet grocery stores, or surfasonline.com.

Chicken Demi-Glace This rich sauce is made with chicken bones and Madeira or sherry and is then reduced until it is a thick glaze that coats the back of a spoon. It is used as the base for many sauces in fine restaurants. It can take all day to make or you can purchase it at gourmet markets. I prefer the Vatel brand. Available at surfasonline.com.

Chile de Arbol (red chile) These are the tiny dried red chiles from Mexico. Available at most grocery stores or specialty produce markets.

Chipotle This hot, smoky chile is actually a dried, smoked jalapeño. It has a wrinkly, dark brown skin and a smoky, sweet, almost chocolate flavor. Chipotles can be found dried, pick-led, and canned in adobo sauce (page 294). They are available at most grocery stores.

Crème Frâiche is a thickened mature cream with a tangy, velvety texture. In France, the cream used to make crème frâiche is unpasteurized and contains the bacteria necessary to thicken it naturally. In America, where all commercial cream is pasteurized, the fermenting agents necessary for crème frâiche can be obtained by adding buttermilk or sour cream. You can find American crème frâiche at gourmet markets or you can make your own. Combine 1 cup heavy cream with 2 table-spoons buttermilk in a glass container. Cover and let stand at room temperature (about 70 degrees) for 8 to 24 hours or until very thick. Stir well and refrigerate for up to 10 days. The small amount of buttermilk creates a very slight imbalance, making your homemade crème frâiche Almost Level One.

Extra-Virgin Olive Oil The cold-pressed result of the first pressing of the olives, it is only 1 percent acid. It's considered the finest and fruitiest of the olive oils and therefore is the most expensive. It can range from golden color to deep green. In general, the deeper the green color, the more intense the olive flavor. Available at Italian markets and fine grocery stores.

Farro This Italian grain is nutty and delicious. I first discovered it in Italy as an addition to their soups. It's also made into pasta. A wonderful whole grain to add to your repertoire. Available at gourmet Italian markets and surfasonline.com.

Farro Pasta A wonderful whole-grain alternative to regular whole-wheat pasta. Available at gourmet Italian markets and surfasonline.com.

Fontina Cheese This Italian cheese is made from cow's milk. It is semifirm with a dark golden brown rind with a pale yellow interior dotted with tiny holes. It melts easily and smoothly. Available in gourmet markets. If you can't find it you may substitute a very mild Swiss cheese.

Forbidden Rice This black rice is used in Asian cooking. It's nutty and interesting and holds its shape and texture after cooking. Available at surfasonline.com.

French de Puy Lentils These tiny French brown lentils are delicious. They are available at gourmet markets and surfasonline.com.

Fresno Chile This short, cone-shaped chile is as hot as the better-known jalapeño. It ranges in color from light green to bright red when fully ripe.

Frisée A member of the chicory family, frisée has delicate slender, curly leaves that range in color from yellow-white to yellow-green. This feathery vegetable has a mildly bitter flavor and is often used in the salad mix mesclun. You may substitute butter lettuce or escarole if you can't find frisée.

Honey Crisp Apples These delicious apples are available for only two months of the year—October and November. They are sweet and crisp and a bit tart. A delightful apple. If you cannot find them, substitute Gala or Fuji.

Lemongrass (also called citronella root or sereh) This is a very important flavor in Thai and Vietnamese cooking. This herb has long, thin, light green leaves and a woody scallionlike base. It has a sour-lemon flavor and fragrance.

Available in Asian markets, produce markets, and some supermarkets. Store in tightly wrapped plastic in the refrigerator for two weeks. Use to flavor tea, sauces, soups, and curry dishes. Discard lemongrass before serving.

Littleneck Clams (littlenecks) These small hard-shelled clams have a shell diameter of less than 2 inches. They are sweet and delicious. Available at specialty seafood markets.

Mascarpone Cheese This double to triple cream cheese is made from cow's milk. It's a soft cheese that ranges in texture from clotted cream to that of room-temperature butter. It is mostly known as the cheese used in the Italian dessert tiramisu. It is available at Italian specialty shops or gourmet markets. If you can't find it, you may substitute cream cheese.

Pancetta This Italian bacon is cured with salt and spices but not smoked. Full of flavor and slightly salty, it comes in a roll and is then sliced to your liking. I prefer it thinly sliced. Available at Italian markets and in the deli department of fine grocery stores. If you cannot find pancetta, you may substitute prosciutto or regular bacon.

Prosciutto Literally, this term is Italian for "ham" but it differs greatly from the traditional ham we are accustomed to in America. Prosciutto is a ham that has been seasoned, salt-cured, and air-dried. It is not smoked. I prefer it sliced very thinly. Look for it in the deli section of Italian specialty markets or gourmet grocery stores.

Quinoa The Incas called this "the mother grain." This grain contains more protein than any other grain. It is considered a complete protein because it contains all eight essential amino acids. It also has a lower glycemic index than most other grains. Available at natural food stores and some supermarkets.

Radicchio This red-leafed Italian chicory is most often used as a salad green. It has burgundy leaves with white ribs. Radicchio di Verona grows in small, loose heads similar to butter lettuce. Radicchio de Treviso is narrow and pointed and forms tighter, more tapered heads. This salad green is slightly bitter. It is also delicious sautéed, grilled, or baked. Available at most supermarkets or fine grocery stores.

Red Jalapeño This is simply a ripe jalapeño chile. It ranges from hot to very hot and is about 2 inches long and $^3/_4$ inch to 1 inch in diameter.

Red Rice This delicious rice has the nutty shell, as does brown rice. It is often used in French or Himalayan cuisine. Available at gourmet markets and surfasonline.com.

Rhubarb This thick, celery-shaped stalk of the buckwheat family can reach up to 2 feet long. Some varieties are available year round, but most peak from April to June. Because of the intense tartness, rhubarb is usually combined with a considerable amount of sugar or sweetener. It makes delicious jams, sauces, desserts, and most commonly pie. Traditionally, it is combined with strawberries.

Rice Wine Vinegar There are Japanese and Chinese versions of this slightly mild vinegar, made from fermented rice. Comes in white (the most common type, which is clear or amber), red, and black. The Japanese variety is used in sushi rice and sunomono (vinegared sal-

ads). Can be found in Asian markets and some supermarkets.

Rock Shrimp These small, compact shrimp have a wonderful lobster taste and texture. Available at seafood stores. If you can't find them, you may substitute small prawns.

Saffron This is the world's most expensive spice. It comes from the small purple crocus and each flower provides only three stigmas, which must be carefully hand-picked, then dried. One ounce of saffron consists of 14,000 of these tiny stigmas! Fortunately, a little goes a long way.

Shiitake Mushrooms This exotic mushroom was originally grown in Japan and Korea. It's now being cultivated in the United States. The cap of the shiitake mushroom is dark brown and averages 3 to 6 inches across. The stems are extremely tough and should be removed. Rather than discard them, I add them to stocks and sauces as flavoring. Both fresh and dried shiitakes are available almost year-round in many supermarkets. They are quite expensive. You may substitute regular button mushrooms if you cannot find them or if they are too expensive.

Soba Noodles These Japanese noodles are made from buckwheat and wheat flour. They are available at Asian markets, fine grocery stores, and surfasonline.com.

Tomatillo (also called jamberry) This small Mexican green tomato is covered with a thin parchmentlike covering. They are used when they are bright green and quite firm. The flavor includes hints of lemon, apples, and herbs. They are available sporadically year round in specialty grocery stores, Latin American markets, and some supermarkets. Remove husk and wash off sticky coating before using. Store in a paper bag in the refrigerator for up to a month.

Veal Demi-Glace This rich sauce is made with veal bones, wine, Madeira or sherry, and is then reduced until it is a thick glaze that coats the back of a spoon. It is used as the base for many sauces in fine restaurants. It can take all day to make or you can purchase it at gourmet markets. I prefer the Vatel brand. Available at surfasonline.com.

White Whole-Wheat Flour Don't confuse white whole-wheat flour with white flour—they are not the same. Most flour is made from red wheat. Whole-wheat flour is the whole grain of red wheat. White whole-wheat flour is made from the hard white kernel of wheat. The white whole-wheat version tastes and blends more like white flour than regular whole-wheat flour. King Arthur makes an excellent white whole-wheat flour. It is available at many grocery stores and at KingArthurFlour.com.

Yukon Gold Potatoes These potatoes have a skin and flesh that range from buttery yellow to golden. They have a moist, succulent texture and are great roasted, boiled, or mashed. Available at some grocery stores.

ACCESSORIES GUIDE

For everyone who is as interested in what we serve our food on as in how it's prepared, I have included a list of the fabulous accessories that you see throughout the book.

FIRST PHOTO INSERT

Suzanne at table and three tomato soups: Yellow-footed bowl by Primitive Artisan available at *Corners of the World,* 1 Malaga Cove Plaza, Palos Verdes Estates, California 90274. 310-791-7322.

Celedone "Batter Bowl" by Primitive Artisan available at *Corners of the World,* 1 Malaga Cove Plaza, Palos Verdes Estates, California 90274. 310-791-7322.

French white ceramic covered soup tureen available at *Maison Midi,* 148 South La Brea Avenue, Los Angeles, California 90036. 323-935-3157.

Antique clay terra-cotta pots, antique wood tray with handle, and tall tin flower buckets available at *Bountiful,* 1335 Abbott Kinney Boulevard, Venice, California 90291. 310-450-3620.

Tomato plants from *Country Fresh Herbs,* 18211 Emelita Street, Tarzana, California 91356. 818-345-8810.

Crab Bisque: "Belvedere" dinner plate and rimmed soup bowl in terra-cotta available at *Williams-Sonoma,* 142 South Lake Avenue, Pasadena, California 91101. 626-795-5045. For the store nearest you, call 800-391-1262 or visit www.williams-sonoma.com.

Fork and napkin from Suzanne's private collection.

Bruschetta Artichokes: All from Suzanne's private collection.

Omelette: Ruffled-edge sage dinner plate made exclusively for *Sur La Table,* 161 West Colorado Boulevard, Pasadena, California 91105. 626-744-9987. For the store nearest you, call 800-243-0852 or visit www.surlatable.com.

Hand-forged silver fork, "Starlit" by Allan

Adler, available at *Allan Adler,* 1626 Ohms Way, Costa Mesa, California 92627. 949-722-8484; www.allanadler.com.

New Mexican Huevos: Plate by Aletha Soele. Available at *New Stone Age,* 8407 W. 3rd Street, Los Angeles, California 90048. 323-658-5969.

Poolside lunch and Grilled Scallops: White wood riser antique, antique glass pitcher available at *Bountiful,* 1335 Abbott Kinney Boulevard, Venice, California 90291. 310-450-3620.

Hand-painted green ceramic dishes with violets from the Suzanne Somers Collection. www.suzannesomers.com.

Thai Beef and Cucumber Salad: "Apple Green Love" plate and "Marshmallow Dinner Love" plate both available at *Geary's Beverly Hills,* 351 North Beverly Drive, Beverly Hills, California 90210. 310-273-4741 or 800-793-6670; www.gearys.com.

"Triad" sterling silver fork by Christofle. For the store nearest you, call 877-PAVILLON or visit www.christofle.com.

Grains: "Vegetable Jacquard" linens by April Cornell available at *Cornell Trading Company,* 340 East Colorado Boulevard, Pasadena, California 91101. For the store nearest you, call 802-879-5100 or visit www.aprilcornell.com.

All else from Suzanne's private collection.

SECOND PHOTO INSERT

Cobbler: Ruffled baker by Vietri available at *Buyers Service Ltd.,* 379 South Robertson Boulevard, Beverly Hills, California 90211. 310-273-8526 or 800-551-8710; www.buyersservice.com.

Pan-Roasted Halibut: "Queen Anne" dinner plate available at *Williams-Sonoma,* 142 South Lake Avenue, Pasadena, California 91101. For the store nearest you, call 800-391-1262 or visit www.williams-sonoma.com.

"Perles" crystal goblet by Lalique. For the store nearest you, call 310-271-7892 or visit www.lalique.com.

"Aria" sterling silver fork by Christofle. For the store nearest you, call 877-PAVILLON or visit www.christofle.com.

Antique ceramic pitcher circa 1930 from *Bountiful,* 1335 Abbott Kinney Boulevard, Venice, California 90291. 310-450-3620.

All linens from Suzanne's private collection.

Crispy-Skinned Salmon: "Vintage Port" dinner plate in off-white by Casafina available at *Table Top Elegance,* 73470 El Paseo, Palm Desert, California 92260. 760-674-9234.

Silver-plate salt cellar by Erquis available at *Geary's of Beverly Hills,* 351 North Beverly Drive, Beverly Hills, California 90210. 310-273-4741 or 800-793-6670; www.gearys.com.

"Marly" sterling silver fork and knife by Christofle. For the store nearest you, call 877-PAVILLON or visit www.christofle.com.

All linens from Suzanne's private collection.

Grilled Lamb Chops: "Romantic Blue" dinner plate by April Cornell available at *Cornell Trading Company,* 340 East Colorado Boulevard, Pasadena, California 91101. For the store nearest you, call 802-879-5100 or visit www.aprilcornell.com.

"Bugatu Diamante-Chartreuse" fork and knife by Vietri available at *Room with a View,* 1600 Montana Avenue, Santa Monica, California 90403. 310-998-5858 or 800-410-9175; www.roomview.com.

"Song Jacquard Breakfast" tablecloth in periwinkle by April Cornell available at *Cornell Trading Company,* 340 East Colorado Boulevard, Pasadena, California 91101. For the store nearest you, call 802-879-5100 or visit www.aprilcornell.com.

"Essential" napkin in light periwinkle by April Cornell available at *Cornell Trading Company,* 340 East Colorado Boulevard, Pasadena, California 91101. For the store nearest you, call 802-879-5100 or visit www.aprilcornell.com.

Fresh lavender grown and loved by *Country Fresh Herbs,* 18211 Emelita Street, Tarzana, California 91356. 818-345-8810.

Bouillabaisse/Patio lunch: Bowls imported from Italy by *Intrada.* For the store nearest you call 800-752-7576.

Hand-pounded, imported copper stockpot available at *Williams-Sonoma,* 142 South Lake Avenue, Pasadena, California 91101. For the store nearest you, call 800-391-1262 or visit www.williams-sonoma.com.

Herb and flower arrangement by *Country Fresh Herbs,* 18211 Emelita Street, Tarzana, California 91356 (818) 345-8810.

Peppered Pork Chops: Reactive-glaze dinner plate from the *Ambiance Collection.* For the store nearest you, call Gus Dallas at 888-857-4894.

"Talisman" sterling silver fork and knife by Christofle. For the store nearest you, call 877-PAVILLON or www.christofle.com.

Gold jacquard napkin by April Cornell available at *Cornell Trading Company,* 340 East Colorado Boulevard, Pasadena, California 91101. For the store nearest you, call 802-879-5100 or visit www.aprilcornell.com.

Pan-Roasted Rib-Eye: Two-handled, imported pewter platter by Arte Italica available at *Neiman Marcus.* For the store nearest you,

call 800-937-9146 or visit www.neimanmarcus.com.

All other pieces from Suzanne's private collection.

Chicken Lemon Piccata: "Lilac Sorbette" dinner plate by Vietri available at *Room with a View,* 1600 Montana Avenue, Santa Monica, California 90403. 310-998-5858 or 800-410-9175; www.roomview.com.

"Argos" crystal goblet by Lalique. For the store nearest you, call 310-271-7892 or visit www.lalique.com.

"Empire" sterling silver fork by Erquis available at *Room with a View,* 1600 Montana Avenue, Santa Monica, California 90403. 310-998-5858 or 800-410-9175; www.roomview.com.

In bed with pudding: "Martini Verre" martini glass/compote by Baccarat available at *Geary's Beverly Hills,* 351 North Beverly Drive, Beverly Hills, California 90210. 310-273-4741 or 800-793-6670; www.gearys.com.

THIRD PHOTO INSERT

New Year's dinner/Chicken and Goat Cheese: Silver candelabra and "Artos Vert" dinner plates by Bernardand available at *Geary's Beverly Hills,* 351 North Beverly Drive, Beverly Hills, California 90210. 310-273-4741 or 800-793-6670; www.gearys.com.

Braised Veal Stew: Pewter-and-glass salt and pepper set by Arte Italica available at *Neiman Marcus.* For the store nearest you, call 800-937-9146 or visit www.neimanmarcus.com.

All else from Suzanne's private collection.

Wine cellar: Wood and pewter cheese board,

pewter-and-glass salt and pepper set, pewter corkscrew, pewter-and-glass oil and vinegar set, and pewter stew ladle by Arte Italica available at *Neiman Marcus.* For the store nearest you, call 800-937-9146 or visit www.neimanmarcus.com.

Wild Berry Crostada: Cooling rack available at *Sur La Table,* 161 West Colorado Boulevard, Pasadena, California 91105. 626-744-9987. For the store nearest you, call 800-243-0852 or visit www.surlatable.com.

Imported French towels available at *Maison Midi,* 148 South La Brea Avenue, Los Angeles, California 90036. 323-935-3157.

Tangerine Soufflé: White soufflé cups available at *Williams-Sonoma,* 142 South Lake Avenue, Pasadena, California 91101. For the store nearest you, call 800-391-1262 or visit www.williams-sonoma.com.

"Essential" napkin in coral by April Cornell available at *Cornell Trading Company,* 340 East

Colorado Boulevard, Pasadena, California 91101. For the store nearest you, call 802-879-5100 or visit www.aprilcornell.com.

Chocolate Espresso Gelato: All from Suzanne's private collection.

Gold Leaf Cake: Cake server available at *Cornell Trading Company,* 340 East Colorado Boulevard, Pasadena, California 91101. For the store nearest you, call 802-879-5100 or visit www.aprilcornell.com.

"Foller" dessert plates by Lacroix available from *Christofle.* For the store nearest you, call 877-PAVILLON or visit www.christofle.com.

White antique urn with flowers available at *Bountiful,* 1335 Abbott Kinney Boulevard, Venice, California 90291. 310-450-3620.

Domed-glass footed cake plate by Vagabond available at *The Art of Living,* 1933 South Broadway, Los Angeles, California 90007. 213-744-1330.

BIBLIOGRAPHY

American Academy of Pediatrics, "Prevention of Pediatric Overweight and Obesity," *Pediatrics,* 112, no. 2 (August 2003): pp. 424–30, http://aappolicy.aappublications.Org/cgi/content/full/pediatrics;112/2/424

Anderson, K. M., W. P. Castelli, and D. Levy, "Cholesterol and Mortality: 30 Years of Follow-up from the Framingham Study," *Journal of the American Medical Association* 257 (1987): pp. 2176–80.

Aude, Y. W., A. S. Agatson, F. Lopez-Jimenez, E. H. Lieberman, M. Almon, M. Hansen, G. Rojas, G. A. Lamas, C. H. Hennekens, "The National Cholesterol Education Program Diet vs a Diet Lower in Carbohydrates and Higher in Protein and Monounsaturated Fat," *Archives of Internal Medicine,* 164 (2004): pp. 2141–46.

Bailes, J. R., M. T. Strow, J. Werthammer, et al., "Effect of Low-Carbohydrate, Unlimited Calorie Diet on the Treatment of Childhood Obesity: A Prospective Controlled Study," *Metabolic Syndrome and Related Disorders,* 1, no. 3 (2003): pp. 221–25.

Brehm, B. J., R. J. Seeley, S. R. Daniels, et al., "A Randomized Trial Comparing a Very Low Carbohydrate Diet and a Calorie-Restricted Low Fat Diet on Body Weight and Cardiovascular Risk Factors in Healthy Women," *The Journal of Clinical Endocrinology and Metabolism,* 88, no. 4 (2003): pp. 1617–23.

Center for Disease Control and Prevention, "Heart Disease & Stroke," Leading Causes of Death: Heart Disease & Stroke, http://www.cdc.gov/washington/overview/heartstk.htm; "Obesity," Genomics and Disease Prevention, Public Health Perspectives, http://www.cdc.gov/genomics/oldWeb01_16_04/info/perspectives/files/obesomim.htm; "Obesity and Genetics: A Public Health Perspective" (February 2002), http://www/cdc.gov/genomics/oldWeb01_16_04/info/perspectives/obesity.htm.

Dansinger, M. L., J. L. Gleason, J. L. Griffith, et al., "One Year Effectiveness of the Atkins, Ornish, Weight Watchers, and Zone Diets in Decreasing Body Weight and Heart Disease Risk," presented at the American Heart

Association Scientific Sessions, November 12, 2003 in Orlando, Florida.

DeFronzo, R. A., "Insulin Secretion, Insulin Resistance, and Obesity." *Int J Obes* 6, Suppl. 1 (1982): 73–82.

DeFronzo, R. A., and E. Ferrannini, "Insulin Resistance: A Multifaceted Syndrome Responsible for NIDDM, Obesity, Hypertension, Dyslipemia, and Atherosclerotic Cardiovascular Disease," *Diabetes Care* 14, no. 3 (March 1991): p. 173.

Dotinga, Randy, "As Weight Goes Up, Life Span Goes Down," *HealthDayNews,* ABCNEWS.com.

"Evidence Proves Sugar-Sweetened Beverages Contributing to Obesity in Children," *Nutrition Research Newsletter,* March 2001. FINDarticles.com 11 Dec. 2001. http://www.findarticles.com/cf_0/M0887/3_20/72606626.

Fackelmann, K., "Hidden" Hazards: Do High Blood Insulin Levels Foretell Heart Disease?" *Science News* 136 (September 16, 1989): p. 184.

"Fatter Parents, Fatter Kids: Childhood Obesity Is a Hefty Problem," *CNN In-Depth Health,* September 8, 1998, http://www.cnn.com/HEALTH/9809/08/child.obesity/.

Foster, Gary D., Holly R. Wyatt, James O. Hill, et al., "A Randomized Trial of a Low-Carbohydrate Diet for Obesity," *The New England Journal of Medicine,* 348, no. 21 (2003): pp. 2082–90.

Fouad, Tamer, M.D., "Obesity Approaching Tobacco as Top Preventable Cause of Death," April 5, 2004, www.thedoctorslounge.net/medlounge/articles/obesity_death.

Gannon, M. C., F. Q. Nuttall, "Effect of a High-Protein, Low-Carbohydrate Diet on Blood Glucose Control in People with Type 2 Diabetes," *Diabetes,* 53, no. 9 (2004): pp. 2375–82.

Gillman, M. W., L. A. Cupples, B. E. Millen, R. C. Ellison and P. A. Wolf, "Inverse Association of Dietary Fat with Development of Ischemic Stroke in Men," *Journal of the American Medical Association,* 278, no. 24 (December 24, 1997).

Greene, P. J., J. Devecis, W. C. Willett, "Effects of Low-Fat vs Ultra-Low-Carbohydrate Weight-Loss Diets: A 12-Week Pilot Feeding Study," abstract presented at Nutrition Week 2004, February 9–12, 2004, in Las Vegas, Nevada.

Harvard School of Public Health, "Carbohydrates" http://www.hsph.harvard.edu/nutrition-source/carbohydrates.html; "Fiber" http://www.hsph.harvard.edu/nutritionsource/fiber.html; "Fruits & Vegetables" http://www.hsph.harvard.edu/nutritionsource/fruits.html.

Hays, J. H., A. DiSabatino, R. T. Gorman, et al., "Effect of a High Saturated Fat and No-Starch Diet on Serum Lipid Subfractions in Patients with Documented Atherosclerotic Cardiovascular Disease," *Mayo Clinic Proceedings,* 78, no. 11 (2003), pp. 1331–36.

Jackson, S. J., and K. W. Singletary, "Sulforaphane Inhibits Human MCF-7 Mammary Cancer Cell Mitotic Progression and Tubulin Polymerization," *Journal of Nutrition* 134, no. 9 (September 2004), pp. 2229–36.

Jamieson, Bob, "Big Business—Products for the Obese Can Be Added Cost for Some, Business Opportunity for Others," ABCNEWS.com.

Jenkins, J. A., et al., "Starchy Foods and Glycemic Index," *Diabetes Care* 11, no. 2 (February 1998): 149.

Ludwig, David S., Karen E. Peterson, and Steven L. Gortmaker, "Relation Between Consumption of Sugar-Sweetened Drinks and Childhood Obesity: A Prospective, Observational Analysis," *The Lancet,* 357 (February 17, 2001).

Meckling, K. A., C. O'Sullivan, D. Saari, "Comparison of a Low-Fat Diet to a Low-Carbohydrate Diet on Weight Loss, Body Composition, and Risk Factors for Diabetes and Cardiovascular Disease in Free-Living, Overweight Men and Women," *Journal of Clinical Endocrinology and Metabolism,* 89, no. 6 (2004): pp. 2717–23.

MSNBC.com, "Doctors Seek Ban on Soda in School," http://msnbc.msn.com/id/3879023.

National Center for Chronic Disease Prevention and Health Promotion, "Improving Nutrition and Increasing Physical Activity," *Chronic Disease Prevention,* http://www.cdc.gov/nccdphp/Bb_nutrition.

National Center for Chronic Disease Prevention and Health Promotion, "1991–2001 Prevalence of Obesity Among U.S. Adults by State," *Overweight and Obesity—Obesity Trends, Nutrition & Physical Activity,* http://www.cdc.gov/nccdphp/dnpa/Obesity/trend/prev_reg.htm.

National Center for Chronic Disease Prevention and Health Promotion, "Overweight and Obesity—Defining Overweight and Obesity," *Nutrition & Physical Activity* http://www.cdc.gov/nccdpdphp/Dnpa/obesity/defining.htm.

National Center for Chronic Disease Prevention and Health Promotion, "Overweight and Obesity—Economic Consequences," *Nutrition & Physical Activity,* http://www.cdc.gov/nccdphp/Dnpa/obesity/economic_consequences.htm.

National Center for Chronic Disease Prevention and Health Promotion, "Overweight and Obesity—Health Consequences," *Nutrition and Physical Activity* http://www.cdc.gov/nccdphp/Dnpa/obesity/consequences.htm.

National Center for Chronic Disease Prevention and Health Promotion, "2001 Obesity and Diabetes Prevalence Among U.S. Adults, by Selected Characteristics," *Nutrition & Physical Activity, Overweight and Obesity—Obesity Trends,* http://www.cdc.gov/nccdphp/dnpa/obesity/trend/obesity_diabetes_characteristics.htm.

National Geographic, "The Heavy Cost of Fat—Why Are We So Fat?" August 2004.

Nickols-Richardson, S. M., J. J. Volpe, R. E. Coleman, M. D., "Premenopausal Women Following a Low-Carbohydrate/High-Protein Diet Experience Greater Weight Loss and Less Hunger Compared to a High-Carbohydrate/Low-Fat Diet," Abstract Presented at FASEB Meeting on Experimental Biology: Translating the Genome, April 17–21, 2004, in Washington, D.C.

"Polymorphism of the UCP2 Promoter Region and Obesity," *Human Genome Epidemiology Network,* e-journal club, Office of Genomics and Disease Prevention, Center for Disease Control, http://www.cdc.gov/genomics/oldWeb01_16_04/hugenet/ejournal/UCP2.htm.

Rao, A.V., S. Agarwal, "Role of Antioxidant Lycopene in Cancer and Heart Disease" *Journal of the American College of Nutrition,* no. 5 (October 19, 2000): pp. 563–69.

Reaven, G. M., C. B. Hollenbeck, and Y-DI Chen, "Relationship Between Glucose Tolerance, Insulin Secretion, and Insulin Action in Non-Obese Individuals with Varying Degrees of Glucose Tolerance," *Diabetologia* 32 (1989): pp. 52–55.

Samaha, F. F., N. Iqbal, P. Seshadri, et al., "A Low-Carbohydrate as Compared with a Low-Fat Diet in Severe Obesity," *The New England Journal of Medicine,* 348, no. 21 (2003): pp. 2074–81

Seshadri, P., N. Iqbal, L. Stern, M. Williams, K. L. Chicano, D. A. Daily, J. McGrory, E. J. Gracely, D. J. Rader, F. F. Samaha. "A Randomized Study Comparing the Effects of a Low-Carbohydrate Diet and a Conventional Diet on Lipoprotein Subfractions and C-Reactive Protein Levels in Patients with Severe Obesity," *American Journal of Medicine,* 117, no. 5 (2004): pp. 398–405.

Sondike, S. B., N. M. Copperman, M. S. Jacobson, "Low Carbohydrate Dieting Increases Weight Loss but not Cardiovascular Risk in Obese Adolescents: A Randomized Controlled Trial," *Journal of Adolescent Health,* 26 (2000): p. 91.

Stern, L., N. Iqbal, P. Seshadri, et al., "The Effects of Low-Carbohydrate Versus Conventional Weight Loss Diets in Severely Obese Adults: One-Year Follow-up of a Randomized Trial," *Annals of Internal Medicine,* 140 no. 10 (2004): p. 778–85.

Taubes, Gary, "What If It's All Been a Big Fat Lie?" *New York Times Magazine,* July 7, 2002, http://www.nytimes.com/2002/07/07/Mag azine/07FAT.html?ex=1027151477&ei=1&e n=bb41d22c6b88108.

"Overcoming Obesity in America," *Time,* June 7, 2004.

Volek, J. S., M. J. Sharman, A. L. Gómez, "Comparison of a Very Low-Carbohydrate and Low-Fat Diet on Fasting Lipids, LDL Subclasses, Insulin Resistance, and Postprandial Lipemic Responses in Overweight Women," *Journal of the American College of Nutrition,* 23, no. 2 (2004): pp. 177–84.

Volek, J. S., M. J. Sharman, and A. L. Gómez, et al., "An Isoenergetic Very Low Carbohydrate Diet Improves Serum HDL Cholesterol and Triacylglycerol Concentrations, the Total Cholesterol to HDL Cholesterol Ratio and Postprandial Lipemic Responses Compared with a Low Fat Diet in Normal Weight, Normolipidemic Women," *The Journal of Nutrition,* 133, no. 9 (2003): pp. 2756–61.

Volek, J. S., M. J. Sharman, D. M. Love, et al., "Body Composition and Hormonal Responses to a Carbohydrate Restricted Diet," *Metabolism,* 51, no. 7 (2002): pp. 864–70.

Volek J. S., Ph.D., R.D., and Eric C. Westman, M.D., M.H.S., "Very-Low-Carbohydrate Weight-Loss Diets Revisited," *Cleveland Journal of Medicine,* 69, no. 11 (November 2002).

Yancy, W. S., Jr., M. K. Olsen, J. R. Guyton, et al., "A Low-Carbohydrate, Ketogenic Diet Versus a Low-Fat Diet to Treat Obesity and Hyperlipidemia," *Annals of Internal Medicine,* 140, no. 10 (2004): pp. 769–77.

Young R. Lisa, Ph.D., R.D., and Marion Nestle, Ph.D., M.P.H., "The Contribution of Expanding Portion Sizes to the U.S. Obesity Epidemic," *American Journal of Public Health* 92, no. 2 (February 2002).

RECOMMENDED READING ABOUT
HORMONES AND HEALTH

These books have assisted me in my journey to understand the importance of hormones and our health.

Berman, Jennifer, M.D., and Laura Berman, Ph.D. *For Women Only: A Revolutionary Guide to Overcoming Sexual Dysfunction and Reclaiming Your Sex Life.* New York: Holt, 2001.

Colgan, Michael. *Hormonal Health.* Vancouver, B.C.: Apple Publishing, 1996.

Collins, Joseph, N.D. *What's Your Menopause Type?* Roseville, Calif.: Prima Health, 2000.

Gershon, Michael D., M.D. *The Second Brain.* New York: HarperCollins, 1998.

Hanley, Jesse Lynn, M.D., and Nancy Deville. *Tired of Being Tired.* New York: Putnam, 2001.

Lee, John R., M.D., with Jesse Hanley, M.D., and Virginia Hopkins. *What Your Doctor May Not Tell You About Premenopause.* New York: Warner Books, 1999.

Lee, John R., M.D., with Virginia Hopkins. *What Your Doctor May Not Tell You About Menopause.* New York: Warner Books, 1996.

Nelson, Miriam E., Ph.D., with Sarah Wernick, Ph.D. *Strong Women, Strong Bones.* New York: Perigee, 2000.

Regelson, William, M.D., and Carol Colman. *The Super-Hormone Promise: Nature's Antidote to Aging.* New York: Simon & Schuster, 1996.

Reiss, Uzzi, M.D., with Martin Zucker. *Natural Hormone Balance for Women.* New York: Pocket Books Health, 2001.

Sapolsky, Robert M. *The Trouble with Testosterone.* New York: Scribner, 1997.

Schwarzbein, Diana, M.D., with Marilyn Brown. *The Schwarzbein Principle II.* Health Communications, 2002.

Schwarzbein, Diana, M.D., and Nancy Deville. *The Schwarzbein Principle.* Health Communications, 1999.

Shippen, Eugene, M.D., and William Fryer. *The Testosterone Syndrome.* New York: M. Evans, 1998.

INDEX

Ischemic stroke, 82
Itching, 2

J

Journal of the American College of Nutrition, 68, 69, 83
Journal of the American Medical Association, 49

K

Kale
  Black Kale (Cavello Nero), 210
  health benefits from, 83
  Tuscan White Bean Soup, 171
Kennedy, John F., 37

L

Lamb
  Chops, Grilled, with Lavender Lamb Jus, 247
  Lamburger with Tomato Chutney and Mint, 249
  Leg of, with Porcini Mushroom Rub, 248
Lasagna, Somersize Slow Cooker, 282
Leaky gut, 38
Leek and Herb Frittata, 164
Lemon-Caper Sauce, Veal Patties with, 251
Lemon Piccata, Chicken Patty, 230
Lemon-Thyme Aïoli, 195
Lentil, Baby Black, Salad, 185
Lentils, French, 216
Leptin, 140
Level One, 108–26
  Almost Level One, 124–26
  breakfasts, 114–16
  cheating in, 121–22
  desserts in, 132
  forbidden foods in, 57, 66, 108–11
  general guidelines for, 119–20
  goal of, 7, 63, 108, 124–25
  lunch and dinner, 117–19
  menus, 158–60
  moving back to, 129, 133

portion sizes in, 130, 133, 138–39
  sample week on, 122–24
Level Two, 127–35
  breakfasts, 133–35
  carbohydrates in, 2, 76–77, 78, 128–29
  cheating in, 129, 137–38
  cravings in, 132–33, 141
  desserts in, 132
  fruits in, 131
  Funky Foods in, 131–32
  general guidelines for, 129–31
  goal of, 7, 63, 127
  lunch and dinner, 133–35
  portion sizes in, 130, 133, 141–42
  sample week on, 133–35
  slipups in, 132–33
  sugars in, 131
  when to move to, 127
Licorice, 40
Linguine, Whole-Wheat, with Candied Roma Tomatoes, 221
Liver disease, 47
Low-carb programs, 5, 67–68, 79
Low-density lipoproteins (LDLs), 68, 70
Low-fat diets, 68–69
Low-fat/high-carb programs, 56
Lunch and dinner
  Level One, 117–19
  Level Two, 133–35
Lycopene, 80–82

M

Macular degeneration, 82
Mango(s)
  Mango Salsa, 200
  Tropical Fruit Soup with Coconut Sorbet, 268
Maple Vanilla Rotisserie Duck, 278
Margarine, 70
Meals, skipping, 34–35
Meat. *See also* Beef; Lamb; Pork; Veal
  approved list of, 288

Meatballs and Chicken Drumettes, Somersize Tex-Mex, 277
Men
  decreased sex drive in, 38
  high cortisol in, 38
  hormonal loss in, 2, 4, 16, 26, 38
  hormone replacement for, 26
Menopause
  hormone loss during, 1–2, 14–15
  in men (andropause), 4, 26
  symptoms of, 2–3, 12
  "toughing it out," 17–18, 24
Menstrual cramps, 71
Menstruation, 23–24
Metabolism, 55–56, 62, 140, 146
Mint Chocolate Cheesecake, Super-Easy, 285
Monounsaturated fats, 70
Mood swings, 2
Mushroom(s)
  Porcini, Rub, Leg of Lamb with, 248
  Shiitake, -Radicchio Salad, Warm, Crispy-Skinned Salmon with Roasted Garlic Aïoli and, 238
  Wild, Fontina, Pancetta and Sage, Omelette with, 162
  Wild, Sauce, 197
Mustard Vinaigrette, Champagne, 190

N

National Geographic magazine, 47
New England Journal of Medicine, 68
"Night-eating syndrome," 2
Noodles, Soba, 225
Norepinephrine, 40

O

Oat bran, 81
Obesity, 45–52
  causes of, 49–52, 65

Trans fats, 70–71, 79–80
Trazadone, 33
Triglycerides, 38, 68
Tuna, Grilled, with Lemon-Thyme Aïoli, 241
Turkey Breast, Roast, Stuffed with Prosciutto, Fontina Cheese, and Sage, 234
Tuscan White Bean Soup, 171

U

Ulcers, 38
Undereating, 34–35, 138–39
Unsaturated fats, 70
USDA Food Pyramid, 51

V

Vaginal dryness, 3
Varicose veins, 47
Veal, Braised, Stew with Gremolata, 250
Veal Patties with Lemon-Caper Sauce, 251
Vegetables. *See also specific vegetables*
    approved list of, 289
    combining with other foods, 66, 112–13
    daily requirements, 82
    growing your own, 82–84
    health benefits from, 79–82
    Root, Caramelized, 212
Vegetarians, 65, 76
Veggies food group, 112–13, 289
Vinaigrette, Champagne Mustard, 190
Vitamin A, 83, 112
Vitamin B_5, 40
Vitamin B_6, 80
Vitamin C, 40, 80, 83
Vitamin D, 112
Vitamin E, 112
Vitamin K, 112

W

Water, 120–21, 144
Webster, Larry, 292
Weepiness, 16
Weight gain
    antidepressants and, 31
    causes of, 49
    hormonal imbalance and, 6, 7, 18–19, 20
    insulin resistance and, 55–62
    stress and, 20
    synthetic HRT and, 18–19, 23
Weight loss
    helpful hints for, 143–45
    in Level One, 7, 63, 108, 124–25
    plateaus in, 5–6, 136–43
    roadblocks to, 140
    Schwarzbein's strategy for, 77
Weight training, 146
Wheat bran, 81
Whipped Cream, Perfectly, 262
Whole grains. *See* Grains, whole
Whole-Wheat Crostini with Red Pepper Rouille, 198
Whole-Wheat Linguine with Candied Roma Tomatoes, 221
Whole-Wheat Tart Dough, 265
Willett, Walter C., 68–69
Wine, 110, 111
Women's Health Initiative, 15, 16
Women's Health Study, 80

Z

Zucchini
    Grilled Fennel and, 213
    Red Rice, 226
    Ribbons, 209
    Ribbons, Candied Roma Tomatoes, and Parsley Pesto, Pan-Roasted Halibut with, 237
    Somersize Chicken Cacciatore, 275
    Somersize Thai Red Curry Shrimp, 279

ABOUT THE AUTHOR

SUZANNE SOMERS is the author of thirteen books, including the *New York Times* bestsellers *Keeping Secrets; Eat Great, Lose Weight; Get Skinny on Fabulous Food*; *Eat, Cheat, and Melt the Fat Away;* and *Fast and Easy.* The former star of the hit television programs *Three's Company* and *Step by Step,* Suzanne is one of the most respected and trusted brand names in the world, representing cosmetics and skincare products, apparel, jewelry, a computerized facial fitness system, fitness products, and a dessert line called SomerSweet.

C O N V E R S I O N   C H A R T
EQUIVALENT IMPERIAL AND METRIC MEASUREMENTS

American cooks use standard containers, the 8-ounce cup and a tablespoon that takes exactly 16 level fillings to fill that cup level. Measuring by cup makes it very difficult to give weight equivalents, as a cup of densely packed butter will weigh considerably more than a cup of flour. The easiest way therefore to deal with cup measurements in recipes is to take the amount by volume rather than by weight. Thus the equation reads:

$$1 \; cup = 240 \; ml = 8 \; fl. \; oz. \quad 1/2 \; cup = 120 \; ml = 4 \; fl. \; oz.$$

It is possible to buy a set of American cup measures in major stores around the world.

In the States, butter is often measured in sticks. One stick is the equivalent of 8 tablespoons. One tablespoon of butter is therefore the equivalent to ½ ounce/15 grams.

SOLID MEASURES

U.S. and Imperial Measures		Metric Measures	
Ounces	Pounds	Grams	Kilos
1		28	
2		56	
3½		100	
4	¼	112	
5		140	
6		168	
8	½	225	
9		250	¼
12	¾	340	
16	1	450	
18		500	½
20	1¼	560	
24	1½	675	
27		750	¾
28	1¾	780	
32	2	900	
36	2¼	1000	1
40	2½	1100	
48	3	1350	
54		1500	1½
64	4	1800	
72	4½	2000	2
80	5	2250	2¼
90		2500	2½
100	6	2800	2¾

LIQUID MEASURES

Fluid Ounces	U.S.	Imperial	Milliliters
	1 teaspoon	1 teaspoon	5
¼	2 teaspoons	1 dessertspoon	10
½	1 tablespoon	1 tablespoon	14
1	2 tablespoons	2 tablespoons	28
2	¼ cup	4 tablespoons	56
4	½ cup		120
5		¼ pint or 1 gill	140
6	¾ cup		170
8	1 cup		240
9			250
10	1¼ cups	½ pint	280
12	1½ cups		340
15		¾ pint	420
16	2 cups		450
18	2¼ cups		500
20	2½ cups	1 pint	560
24	3 cups		675
25		1¼ pints	700
27	3½ cups		750
30	3¾ cups	1½ pints	840
32	4 cups or 1 quart		900
35		1¾ pints	980
36	4½ cups		1000
40	5 cups	2 pints or 1 quart	1120
48	6 cups		1350
50		2½ pints	1400
60	7½ cups	3 pints	1680
64	8 cups or 2 quarts		1800
72	9 cups		2000

OVEN TEMPERATURE EQUIVALENTS

Fahrenheit	Celsius	Gas Mark	Description
225	110	¼	Cool
250	130	½	
275	140	1	Very Slow
300	150	2	
325	170	3	Slow
350	180	4	Moderate
375	190	5	
400	200	6	Moderately Hot
425	220	7	Fairly Hot
450	230	8	Hot
475	240	9	Very Hot
500	250	10	Extremely Hot

EQUIVALENTS FOR INGREDIENTS

all-purpose flour—plain flour
arugula—rocket
confectioners' sugar—icing sugar
cornstarch—cornflour
eggplant—aubergine
granulated sugar—castor sugar
half and half—12% fat milk
lima beans—broad beans
scallion—spring onion
shortening—white fat
squash—courgettes or marrow
unbleached flour—strong, white flour
vanilla bean—vanilla pod
zest—rind
zucchini—courgettes